THE PRACTICE
OF
HYPNOTHERAPY

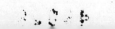

MEDICAL HYPNOSIS

By

LEWIS R. WOLBERG, M.D.

Assistant Clinical Professor of Psychiatry, New York Medical College

Volume II

THE PRACTICE OF HYPNOTHERAPY

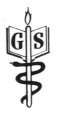

GRUNE & STRATTON

NEW YORK

First printing, April 1948
Second printing, December 1949
Third printing, October 1951
Fourth printing, January 1955
Fifth printing, August 1956
Sixth printing, January 1958
Seventh printing, February 1959
Eighth printing, April 1960
Ninth printing, May 1965
Tenth printing, September 1971

GRUNE & STRATTON, INC.
111 Fifth Avenue, New York, New York 10003

Library of Congress Catalog Card Number   48-2929
International Standard Book Number   0-8089-0537-6

Printed in the United States of America (E-B)

CONTENTS

v

PREFACE

THE PRACTICE of hypnotherapy is dependent upon the use of the coordinated skills of hypnotic induction and psychotherapy. In Volume One the principles of hypnotic induction, as well as general applications of psychotherapy, were discussed in detail. The present volume describes the joint technics of hypnosis and psychotherapy by presentation of actual case material through complete transcription of a number of treatment sessions. In addition to several briefer examples, three complete psychosomatic cases are included, illustrative of the three main divisions of therapy presented in this volume. The first case is that of a patient with enuresis who was treated by means of symptom removal through prestige suggestion. The second case is one of premature ejaculation, treated by hypnosis with psychobiologic therapy. The third patient complained of severe, persistent headaches and was treated by re-education through hypnoanalysis.

The use of complete case records makes it possible for the reader to follow the therapeutic process, the transference manifestations, the evidence of resistance, as well as the specific technics as they were applied in each particular case.

The conclusions which have been presented in each of the three types of therapy—symptom removal, psychobiologic therapy and psychoanalytic therapy—are based on clinical experience with a fairly wide variety of cases. As more experience is gained in the different treatment methods, however, a modification and revision of these conclusions will undoubtedly be required.

Acknowledgment is made to the Editor of *The American Journal of Psychotherapy* for permission to reprint material from an article written by myself and published in the Journal under the title "Hypnosis and Psychoanalysis."

LEWIS R. WOLBERG, M.D.

New York City
January, 1948

Part One

HYPNOSIS IN SYMPTOM REMOVAL

SYMPTOM removal by hypnotic command is the oldest of hypnotherapeutic technics. It is still employed extensively throughout the world, particularly in Europe. Reported results vary from unbounded enthusiasm to discreditment of the method as an irrational form of psychotherapy. On the whole it is the least successful of all hypnotic procedures.

Because it deals with effects rather than with causes, the method has many limitations. Judiciously employed, nevertheless, symptom removal can serve a valuable purpose in carefully selected cases.

Results are best where the symptom has a minimal defensive purpose, and where the need for symptom-free functioning constitutes a powerful incentive. Psychosomatic symptoms, alcoholic addiction, and certain habit disturbances, such as nail-biting, insomnia, excessive eating, inordinate smoking and drinking, are often remarkably susceptible to symptom removal, since they are so incapacitating to the person and have no great protective values.

Results are also most pronounced where the patient has no other motivation for therapy than to abandon his symptoms or bring them under control, and where he refuses to explore the genesis of his neurosis or to inquire into deviations in interpersonal relationships.

The removal of a symptom can have an important effect on the total personality functioning. An individual handicapped by a disturbing symptom often loses self respect.

He withdraws from people and gets more and more involved within himself. The symptom becomes a chief preoccupation around which he organizes his insecurity and his inferiority feelings. The removal of a symptom for this reason can alter his whole pattern of adjustment. A man addicted to alcohol, for instance, may suffer more from the social consequences of drinking than from the physical effects of alcohol. Removing his desire for alcohol by hypnotic command may start a process of personality rehabilitation. An individual with a hysterical tic may isolate himself because of embarrassment caused by his symptom. Eliminating his tic can have an important influence on his social adjustment. A patient with a paralytic limb may be restored to economic usefulness and benefit immeasurably from this restoration.

In spite of its limitations and disadvantages, there are instances when symptom removal has to be resorted to as an expedient measure. A symptom may be so disabling, may cause such great suffering, that all psychotherapeutic efforts will be blocked until the person obtains some relief. There are patients, as has been indicated, whose motivations for therapy are so inadequate, whose ego strength is so minimal, that psychotherapeutic methods aimed at increasing self growth are destined to failure. The most that can be expected at the start is that the patient will respond to palliative or supportive procedures.

Such therapies need not block preparation for a deeper form of treatment. In the course of symptom removal, efforts may be made to demonstrate to the patient the meaning of his symptoms. He may be shown how his distorted character patterns contribute to fears of the world and to difficulties with others. In this way he may develop the motivation to explore the sources of his difficulty.

TECHNICS IN SYMPTOM REMOVAL

ONCE SYMPTOM removal has been decided upon, it is necessary to determine whether to attempt the removal at one session, or whether to extend therapy over a period of several weeks. The severity of the symptom, its duration, the nature of the patient's personality, and his aptitude for hypnosis have to be considered. The approach is an individual one, and suggestions must be so framed that they will conform with the patient's personality, the type of symptom, and its symbolic significance. It is essential to adapt one's language to the patient's intelligence and to his education. Many failures in symptom removal are due to the fact that the patient does not clearly comprehend what the hypnotist is trying to convey to him.

If removal of the symptom at one session is decided upon, sufficient time must be set aside to devote oneself exclusively to the problem. As many as two to three hours may be necessary. At first the patient is encouraged to discuss his history and his symptom in order to determine his reaction to his illness, as well as to gain clues to his attitudes, motivations and character strivings. It is essential to get the patient to verbalize how uncomfortable he is with his symptom, and to get him to see that his life is hampered by his illness. Once the physician is convinced that the patient has an intense incentive to relinquish his symptom, he may tell him that if he has a strong enough desire to overcome his ailment, he will want to cooperate and do what is necessary to get well.

An optimistic attitude on the part of the physician is important because many patients are terrified by their illness and have convinced themselves of the impossibility of cure. Where the patient has a psychosomatic or hysterical disorder, and where a thorough physical examination has not been made, it may be necessary to perform a physical or neurologic examination to rule out possibilities of organic disease. If

3

the examination is negative, the patient is informed in simple language that many emotional problems may express themselves in terms of physical symptoms.

A cure should not be promised, and the physician must insist that relief will depend upon how well the person cooperates. However, an attempt must be made to inculcate in the patient's mind a firm conviction that he will get well. He may be told that hypnosis has helped other people recover and can help him, too, if he will let it. Symptom removal will not succeed in a medium of discouragement or where there is a conviction of ultimate failure.

The patient may then be informed that it is necessary to determine how he will respond to suggestions. He is instructed that he need not try to concentrate too hard on what is said, because even though his attention wanders, suggestions will get to his subconscious mind and he will find himself reacting to them. If he has the desire to rid himself of his symptom, he will have the desire to relax and to follow suggestions. No indication is given the patient at this time that hypnosis will be used to remove his symptom, since the latter may have unconscious values for him, and he may show resistance if he feels he will be deprived of it immediately.

Hypnosis is then induced, and confidence in his ability to follow suggestions is built up by conducting the patient through light, medium and, finally, deep trance states. In the event the patient has a symptom which consists of loss of a physical function, it may be expedient to suggest that he is unable to use the part. This is done in order to associate malfunction with the hypnotist's command instead of with a personal inadequacy.

The next phase in treatment is to get the patient, if he so desires, to discuss under hypnosis his immediate life situation and his reaction to his illness. A persuasive talk may be given to the patient, avoiding for the time being reference to his symptom.

SYMPTOM REMOVAL WITH A STRONG AUTHORITARIAN APPROACH

A STRONGLY directive approach, in which the patient participates minimally, is indicated in certain emotional problems. Persons who express a desire to have their will power reinforced in order to control excessive drinking, eating and smoking, or to alter uncomfortable habit patterns, are often susceptible to this technic. The method is particularly suited to extremely ill and very dependent people.

The following patient illustrates the use of symptom removal with a strongly authoritarian approach. In this case symptom removal based on prestige suggestion was decided on because of the age of the patient, the severity of his symptom, and the lack of any motivation other than a desire to have his insomnia removed. As will be seen from the following transcribed record of the interview, his insomnia was the product of a severe neurosis, exaserbated temporarily by an intercurrent somatic illness in the form of a heart ailment. Treatment was oriented around removing insomnia by authoritative command. The patient was responsive to these suggestions, and on the evening following the trance slept well for the first time since his insomnia developed.

Pt. What, what moved me to come to see you, doctor, was that I thought that hypnoanalysis would really do something for me because I'm sort of too old and too worn down to go through a long psychoanalysis now. It never had occurred to me before that I needed it.

Dr. Yes, how old are you?

Pt. I'm fifty-four.

Dr. And your marital status?

5

Pt. Yes, I've been married and divorced and married again. My daughter is the daughter of the first marriage.

Dr. How long have you been married? Present marriage.

Pt. Fifteen years.

Dr. Are you living with your wife?

Pt. Yes.

Dr. I see, and no children by the second wife?

Pt. No, none.

Dr. And how old is your daughter?

Pt. She is twenty-two going on twenty-three.

Dr. And your occupation?

Pt. I'm an artist, a painter.

Dr. And your chief complaint is insomnia?

Pt. Right now, yes. Of course I had a heart attack a while ago and there were severe pains in both arms, across the neck. I was hospitalized and kept under chloral and stuff.

Dr. Yes.

Pt. And I seemed to come out of it fairly well, and I stayed there for nearly a month, not quite; then I went down to my sister-in-law's in Canada and I began to develop insomnia. Not paroxysmic at first, but the onset of the paroxysmic insomnia now is about three weeks. During those three weeks I have slept maybe from five to fifteen minutes a night. The night before last I slept for three hours. I thought it was broken, but this last night I didn't sleep for a minute.

Dr. The insomnia occurred how many weeks ago?

Pt. About three weeks ago, the paroxysmic onset about three weeks ago. But almost immediately, when I came out of the hospital, I began having, you know, two or three hours a night.

Dr. Now, when the insomnia occurs do you have any thoughts that come to your mind at that time? Do you feel merely helpless in your inability to sleep, or is your mind pre-occupied with thoughts?

Pt. It's something, it's not, it's preoccupied with certain things, but I've come to feel that there are other things connected with it. The one thing is that I've had conferences with a psychiatrist and he says there are two or three things. One is that, of course, this heart attack was a great shock to me, this latest one, and he thinks that it has something, it has to do with a subconscious death fear, that the idea, the subconscious equating of sleep with death, you see. That's one thing. The other is that I figured out by myself certain guilt feelings. I have a terrible, a terribly bad family history. You see, my father and mother separated before I ever knew my father, when I was less than two. Ah, my mother married immediately again, and she divorced that man and remarried my father when I was about five. They never got along; they quarreled and fought all the time. And I took my mother's part, and the result was that I had the most, the utmost contempt for my father. I wouldn't say hatred; I don't know whether it was hatred, but it was contempt anyway. And there was a situation of terrible insecurity, emotional insecurity and economic insecurity too. My parents were poor people. Then when I was, ah, ten years old, my father and mother separated for good and I was sent out to live with relatives. As I look back upon it now, I realize certain things. For instance, I remember when I went to live with those relatives. I was between nine and ten years old, and I developed a habit of wetting the bed, and I don't remember that I ever wet the bed before, but that went on for a couple of years, and, of course, I would get the most frightful scolding. I'd feel awfully degraded and inferior about it, but as I understand it now, it was really a reaction to the insecurity.

Dr. Yes.

Pt. Then, then, you see, I never—then I stayed with

relatives until I was about thirteen years old. Then my mother married another man, and that to me, that was a terrible shock to me in the adolescent period. My mother came to me and told me about this thing. Because I had developed the usual boy's middle class American's attitude towards sex, I thought it was just horrible, you know. And then I didn't realize the sort of incestuous jealousy I had towards this man. The result was that it made in the end, a complete break between my mother and myself. I never saw her again, until she died, from the time I was about fourteen on.

Dr. Where did you go at fourteen?

Pt. I went up north to stay with some relatives, and worked for about a year, and then I came back. When I came back I wanted to see my mother. I was then fifteen. She had married this man and they had gone away to live, far away from where I was. It was not possible for me to see her because it was the economic situation. I had to look after myself. I had to earn my own living, you know. I earned my own living from the time I was about fourteen years old until the present time. I educated myself and never had any help.

Dr. What sort of a person was your mother? Her personality, I mean.

Pt. Why, I think she was a very sweet and emotional person. Ah, I had a great affection for her as a child, and I had terrible, I have had terrible guilt feelings about the whole situation as I look back upon it. And, of course, I waked up in the night many times and saw how tragic it was, how too bad it was that my mother and I had to go through that. And it was probably the accidents of life because I was so busy trying to make my own way, trying to educate myself, trying to find a place for myself in the world that it just never came about.

Dr. And what sort of a person was your father?

Pt. Well, I never knew him very well, because I never knew him in my childhood; but, as I say, I took my mother's part and I developed a kind of contempt for him, but as I think about it later I say to myself, "Well, in many ways he was rather a sensitive man." I don't know just what there was about it.

Dr. Because of the time element I am going to ask you just a few questions.

Pt. Yes.

Dr. You feel depressed?

Pt. Yes, I do.

Dr. How about anxiety?

Pt. Oh, I'm sure I'm filled with it. I don't know, I mean I—ah—ah.

Dr. Do you get any heart palpitations?

Pt. Well, there's—I always have since I've had this heart attack some of the days. I get along, but now last night and today I've very strong heart consciousness, and a little pain shooting through there. It's not too much like an attack, but soreness.

Dr. Any phobias of any kind?

Pt. I don't know of any specific phobias.

Dr. Any headaches or dizziness?

Pt. Very severe headaches. All my life very severe headaches, but one time there, in 1942, where I had this severe attack of dizziness, and it was diagnosed as a condition of the heart. I've never had an occurrence of that.

Dr. What about sexual problems of any kind?

Pt. Well, they're not very severe, except I have, since I had this, well, these operations, I, I've had more or less not a very strong libido.

Dr. Now, can you tell me about your dreams? Do you dream?

Pt. Yes, I dream all the time.

Dr. Can you tell me the last dream that you remember?

Pt. The last dream I remember was last night. I came in a room and there were two men. It seemed to me one of the men was fighting against me. He was going to do something, planning against me. And I went over to where he was and took hold of him and threw him on the floor though I was afraid he'd beat me, because he was younger and stronger than I. But he lay there, and I said, "For God's sake, why do we have to go on like this? Why can't we straighten this thing out?" And that's a dream I often have, but there are guilt dreams too. For instance, there's a dream that I've committed a crime. I've killed somebody, and that I'm free and try to get away. And then a desperate dream that says, "Well, after all you're guilty, I mean you can never run away from yourself." Also of having nothing on but a suit of underwear, and having to cross the street, or go through a long hotel corridor, and trying to run up to the room, and trying to get away so people won't see me. That's a very frequent kind of dream.

Dr. What about nightmares, do you have any nightmares?

Pt. Very seldom, but I have had them, I mean they have to do with this capture and this pursuit about being guilty.

Dr. Apparently there are many, many things about which you have a tremendous amount of guilt.

Pt. Yes, yes.

Dr. The reason I've gone into this detail is to get an idea of what we have to deal with. So that suggestions can be given you which will prove more effective.

Pt. I'm very glad you did. Well, I wish you could do that for me. I mean I wish you could put me into a trance and make me sleep, and then we could go on with the thing because I'm so, I'll tell you truly, doctor, I, myself, I'm so desperate about this insomnia. It makes me feel so bad. And this heart thing. And at the same time, I'm very susceptible to cold, and I catch cold at the slightest provocation.

I'm just afraid that, ah, you know I'm, ah, I'm filled with phobias about that.

Dr. Well, supposing we see what sort of a hypnotic subject you'd be. Do you want to put your glasses down?

Pt. Yes.

Dr. Have you ever been hypnotized before?

Pt. No, but I, when I was a boy, one of the reasons I came to see you about was this: When I was a boy, I was interested in hypnosis, and read up on it, and I tried to hypnotize another boy. I was about fifteen years old. He was about two years older than I. I put him to sleep, but I couldn't get him to do anything. Whether I put him to sleep, or he put himself to sleep, I don't know. He was in such a deep sleep that I could hardly get him awake, and it frightened me so I never did it again.

Dr. I see. Well now, hypnosis, as you know, is merely a state of suggestibility.

Pt. Yes.

Dr. And some subjects get the idea they are required to sleep deeply and actually go to sleep. This is rare, of course.

Pt. Yes.

Dr. Be assured that a person always wakes up from a trance.

Pt. Yes.

Dr. Now, just to give you an example of what hypnosis feels like, I'm going to ask you to clasp your hands together, this way, and to close your eyes for a moment. Visualize a vise, one of those heavy, metal vises with the great big jaws that clamp together with a screw. I want you to visualize that vise, and, as I count from one to five, imagine that your hands are just like the jaws of that vise. I'll count slowly from one to five. When I reach the count of five, your hands will be so firmly clasped together that it will be difficult or impossible to open them up. One, tight, bring them together very tight. Two, visualize that vise, the jaws of the vise. Three, tighter and tighter. Four, extremely tight, very tight. Five, so tight that they're cemented together, and even though you try to separate them, the harder you try to separate them, the more firmly cemented they become. Even though you try with all your might to pull them apart, your hands are so clasped together that it's difficult or impossible to open them up, until I give you the command to do so. Now, very slowly open your hands and separate them. Slowly they come apart; slowly they open up, slowly, just like that. Good, now you'll be able to pull them apart.

Now I want you to bring your hands down on your thighs. Watch your hands. Keep gazing at your hands, and at your fingers. Gaze at them. I want you to begin experiencing whatever feelings there may be in your hands. Perhaps it will be the feeling of texture. Feel a roughness of the trousers as your hand presses down on the trousers. It may be the feeling of the weight of your hand against your thigh. It may be the warmth of the palm of your hand against your thigh. Whatever feelings there are, I want you to experience them.

I want you to keep gazing at the fingers. Keep watching them. And you'll notice pretty soon that one of the fingers will move. You don't know which one it will be, but one of the fingers will jerk a little, or move in one direction or in the other. It may be the right hand or the left hand. Keep watching the right hand and you'll begin to notice, now, that the fingers move ever so little. There, the little finger moves. And now the space between the fingers will increase. The fingers will separate as you keep gazing at them. The spaces get wider. They separate. Just like that.

Then very slowly the hand becomes light, very light. It becomes so light that it feels as if it's a feather. The fingers now will begin rising. The hand will slowly lift and rise straight up in the air, higher and higher; it will rise towards your face, and as it rises you will become tired and relaxed, even drowsy. But your hand must not touch your face until you're very deeply drowsy.

Now you notice that both hands are rising. The hands rise and you get drowsier and drowsier and drowsier, very tired and drowsy. The hands are moving up, up, up; higher, lifting, lifting, and as they lift, you'll get drowsier and drowsier and drowsier. When the hands touch the face, your eyes will close, and you will feel yourself becoming very drowsy, extremely drowsy, and tired. Your whole body begins to feel heavy, except the arms. Heavier and heavier. As the arms lift, the elbows will be supported by the arms of the chair, and you will lean your head against the palm of your hand. Your eyes are getting heavy, just like lead. They're getting heavier and heavier and heavier. You're getting so tired and so drowsy, that you're going to go into a restful, relaxed, comfortable state. The hands are moving up, up, up, and pretty soon the palm of the hand will touch your face, and when the hand touches your face, just let yourself go. Your eyes are getting heavy, like lead, getting heavier and heavier; very heavy and tired, so tired that they're glued together. They stay glued together, and they're going to stay glued together until I give you the command to wake up. The hands are moving up, straight up. The hands are moving towards the face, and then the palm of your hand will be against your cheek. Lean over and relax. Let yourself go. You are very tired, very sleepy, extremely tired and sleepy and drowsy, very drowsy. You're getting drowsier and drowsier and drowsier. Lean back in the chair, just like that.

I'm going to bring your left hand down now. I'm going to move this hand down just like this. I'm going to stroke this hand, and as I stroke it you begin to notice that a feeling of stiffness comes to the shoulder right down to the finger tips. The hand begins to feel stiff, and firm. Stiffer, and stiffer, and stiffer, so stiff and rigid and firm that it feels as if it's made out of lead.   So firm and stiff that it remains out-stretched.

I'm going to count from one to five, and at the count of five you'll notice that the hand is so stiff and rigid that even though you try to bring it up, it will remain exactly as it is. The harder you try the more stiff and rigid it will become. One, heavy and stiff.   Two, heavier and heavier.   Three, heavier and stiffer.   Four, five, now it's rigid, and when you try to bring it up, it will remain exactly as it is.   The harder you try the more rigid it becomes, until I stroke it again; and only upon my stroking it will it start coming down.   Now, as I stroke it, it will begin to come down, slowly down, straight down, right down to your thigh.   And your breath-ing becomes deep, very deep.   It gets deeper and deeper and deeper, and you're going to go into a very deep, restful, re-laxed state.   And you're going to be able to feel yourself capable more and more of relaxing.

I'm going to stroke your left hand now, and as I stroke your hand you'll notice that the heaviness leaves this hand, and that it's possible for the hand to rise up ever so little when I give you the command.

I'm going to ask you to visualize yourself in a theater, about to observe a play.   The curtain is drawn.   As soon as you visualize yourself in the theater looking at the curtain, indicate that by your hand rising up about an inch.   Visual-ize yourself in a theater looking at the curtain.   As soon as you visualize yourself, your hand will rise.   Good.

Now, as you sit there, you will notice that the curtain draws apart, and you begin to see action on the stage.   As soon as you see action going on on the stage, any action, your hand again will rise up to indicate that you've seen something on the stage.   Now the hand comes up and I bring it down.

Now you are deeply relaxed, your breathing gets deep and automatic, you feel yourself relaxing more and more all over.

You get more restful, more drowsy. Visualize yourself on a mountain top in Maine. You are tired and want to go to sleep. As soon as you see yourself on the mountain top, your hand will rise. Good. You are on a mountain top and want to lie down because you are sleepy. You lie down in the soft grass. Watch the deep blue sky above, all blue, except for one or two billowy clouds. You breathe deeply, and as you look around you notice that you are surrounded by trees, tall fir trees. The scent of pine comes to your nostrils. As soon as you visualize this and smell the pine, indicate it by your hand rising. Good. Now you begin to notice, as you gaze into the distance, many lakes, the surface as smooth as glass. That is how your mind will be, calm, unruffled, and you start going to sleep. As soon as you feel yourself sleeping, indicate it by your hand rising. Good.

Listen carefully to me. You will overcome your insomnia. You will have normal sleep habits. No matter what worries and cares you have, no matter what causes you to be awake at night. From today on you will be able to sleep. You must sleep.

At night you will go to bed at your regular time. You must establish a routine. Go to bed at a set time, and then, as you lie in bed, I want you to visualize yourself on a mountain top in Maine. I want you to have a picture of a blue sky overhead, deep blue sky. You will feel yourself lying on the mountain top in soft, soft grass, warm and pleasant. And you will see the blue sky overhead, blue, deep blue. There will be a few billowy clouds floating by overhead, and you will notice that surrounding you on all sides there are trees, tall trees, fir, spruce, pine. And your nostrils will fill up with the scent of pine. And you become filled with a sense of peace, serenity, a feeling of being at utter peace with yourself and the world.

And as you lie there, I'm going to suggest to you that when you go to bed at nighttime, your eyes will get heavy, you'll breathe deeply and visualize the sky, the trees, the lakes. You will feel at peace with yourself. When you fall asleep, there will be no disturbing dreams. You will sleep, just sleep, sleep very deeply. You'll sleep deeper, and deeper, and deeper, very deep. And as you sleep you may possibly dream, but the dreams must be of a pleasant type. Perhaps you will dream of being on a mountain top looking at the sky, and the trees surrounding you, and off into the distance the lakes. Visualize those lakes, many of them, the surface as smooth as glass, and your mind must become just as serene, just as calm, just as peaceful as the surface of the lake. Not a ripple, just calm, very serene, sleep, sleep, sleep. And if any disturbing thoughts come to you, think of the calm surface, the even, unruffled surface of the water, and your emotions will calm down.

Your sleep will get deeper and deeper and deeper as you visualize that scene in Maine. And your eyes will remain firmly closed, and you relax your muscles; slowly your muscles will relax all over. Your head, your forehead will loosen up. Your face muscles will loosen. The muscles in your neck, your shoulders, will relax. Your arms and legs will feel heavy, just like lead. Your breathing will become deeper and automatic. And then you'll sleep. You'll go into a deep sleep. If you have dreams, they must be pleasant dreams. Disturbing dreams, if they come up, will be crowded out. You must sleep, you must sleep. Your sleep will get deeper and deeper and deeper. And then, when you awaken in the morning, you will be refreshed; you will be refreshed. You must sleep.

I'm going to ask you now to sleep here. In a few moments I'm going to wake you up. When you awaken, you're going to notice something extremely interesting. When you look at me, your eyes will blink; they will blink spasmodically, and the harder you try to control the blinking, the more spastic they will be. It will be impossible to look at me without blinking. And then I will tell you to close your eyes again and I'll say: "The blinking will stop." After this you'll be able to look at me without blinking.

In a moment I'm going to wake you up. You will follow the suggestions that I gave you. Remember, you will be able to sleep; you will go to bed at nighttime and you will sleep. You may not remember everything I say to you here, or you may remember all. Nevertheless, you will still follow the suggestions that I've given you.

Now when you awaken, you will notice that you feel relaxed. You will look at me and your eyes will become spastic. They'll blink; and then I'll tell you to close your eyes again, and I'll say to you at that time: "Your eyes will stop blinking." Then you will be able to look at me without blinking.

I'm going to count from one to five. When I reach the count of five, awaken. One—two—three—four—five. Your eyes start blinking. They blink, blink. Now close them. You will be able to open them when I count five, and your eyes will be steady, they will not blink. One, two, this time awaken fully, three, four, five. Slowly open your eyes, good, steady, fine.

Pt. I, I, doctor, I heard everything you said. I don't know how well I followed you. I tried to, I was, I was trying not to resist. I don't know just how much I was asleep. I want to cooperate, but there may be unconscious resistance.

Dr. It does not matter. When you go to bed at nighttime, you will be able to visualize the scenes that I've mentioned; and you'll notice that in spite of any resistance, it will be possible to relax yourself.

SYMPTOM REMOVAL WITH
ACTIVE PARTICIPATION OF
THE PATIENT

IN OTHER patients active participation is encouraged. A reasonable explanation is given the patient for suggestions that are advanced. In some instances he may even be encouraged to veto suggestions, if he does not wish to follow them or if he believes them to be against his best interests. Active participation is utilized in patients with relatively good ego strength who shy away from too authoritarian a relationship.

Symptom removal by suggestion is far more effective where it is demonstrated to the patient that he has not lost control over his functions, and hence is not the helpless victim of symptoms which cannot be altered or removed. This is achieved by showing the patient, while he is in a trance, that it is possible to create on command such symptoms as paralysis, spasticity and anesthesia. Once the patient responds to these suggestions, he is informed about the important influence that the mind has over the body.

Then a symptom identical with the patient's chief complaint is produced in some other part of the body. Should the patient respond successfully, a partial removal of his own symptom is attempted. For instance, if he has a paralyzed arm, he is told that his fingers will move ever so little. Then paralysis of the other arm, which has been artificially produced, is increased in intensity, while a strong suggestion is made that the patient will find that function is restored to his ailing part. In the case of a paralyzed arm, it is suggested that his hand will move, then his arm, and, finally, that the paralysis will disappear altogether.

The fact that symptoms can be produced and removed so

readily on suggestion may influence the patient to accept the
fact that he is not powerless, that he can exercise control over
his body and his functions.   This self mastery may be enhanced by combining a persuasive, re-educative, and reconditioning approach, and, at a later date, by teaching the
patient the technic of self hypnosis.

In order to protect the patient, should his symptom have
a defensive function, he may be left with some residual symptom which is less disabling than the original symptom, but
which, it is hoped, will absorb its dynamic significance.   For
instance, in the case of a paralyzed arm, paralysis of the little
finger may be induced, and a suggestion may be given the
patient that the finger paralysis will have the same meaning
for him as the arm paralysis, and that the finger paralysis
will remain until he understands fully the reasons for the
original paralysis and no longer needs it.   In the event of an
extensive anesthesia, anesthesia of a limited area may be
suggested as a substitute.

Posthypnotic suggestions are next given the patient to the
effect that his restored functions will continue in the waking
state, except for the induced residual symptom.   An activity
may then be suggested which brings into use the ailing part;
and the patient **may** then be awakened in the midst of this
action.

Subsequent visits repeat these suggestions, and, if desired,
the patient is taught the technic of self hypnosis so that suggestive influences may continue through his own efforts.
Psychobiologic technics may also be instituted to effect a
more constructive change in the personality, or, if the patient
has the motivation and ego strength, an analytic approach
may be employed.

This method may be illustrated by the case of a thirty
year old man who had developed a spastic paralysis of his
left leg with a peculiar gait that interfered with ambulation.
Function was restored in one session.   The patient had no

desire to inquire more deeply into his problems, and was satisfied with mere symptom removal.   It was impossible, in the one session, to gain understanding of the dynamic significance of his symptom.   In this case I was able to demonstrate to the patient quite conclusively that his paralysis could be shifted from his leg into his arm.   He was then able to walk, but his arm was paralyzed.   Then the arm paralysis was shifted to his shoulder.   He was quite amazed by what was happening.   On command he found that he could do the same thing by giving himself suggestions.   This undoubtedly gave him the feeling that since he had the power within himself to shift the paralysis from one part of his body to another, he was not so helpless as he had imagined.   The fact that he could, through his own volition, remove the paralysis gave him a feeling of self confidence and self mastery.   Because it was impossible, on the basis of his lack of motivation, to find out what the paralysis meant to him, there was substituted another symptom that was less incapacitating than his leg paralysis.   One of his toes was paralyzed in the hope that this would have the same symbolic significance as the leg paralysis.   The toe paralysis did not incapacitate him, and he was able to get a job and to work effectively.   When seen briefly several months later, he still had a paralyzed toe about which he complained bitterly.   However, he seemed to have adopted the philosophy that he was really quite brave to be able to face life with a paralyzed toe.   A transcription of the induction of hypnosis follows.

Dr.   Have you ever seen anybody hypnotized?
Pt.   No, I haven't.
Dr.   Well, what ideas come to you when you think about hypnosis?
Pt.   Well, I saw it once on the stage.
Dr.   What happened there?
Pt.   He just did anything the man asked him to do.

Dr. In hypnosis a person is capable of doing many things. Are you capable of walking without a cane?

Pt. It's very hard now.

Dr. It is hard. Do you want to try it for me? (*Patient attempts to stand up, but his leg will not support him. Supported by his cane, he hobbles around the room.*) Are you able to walk around outdoors?

Pt. No, because I can't get my leg to bend.

Dr. You can't lift your leg?

Pt. No, I just don't have confidence and I will fall over.

Dr. Well, I am going to give you an idea of what hypnosis is. Hypnosis is the ability to follow suggestions. I don't want you to try too hard; I want you to have things come just as they will. For instance, put your elbows on the chair—just like this, and clasp your hands together. I want you to close your eyes for a moment and visualize in your mind one of those heavy metal vises. You've seen these heavy metal vises that screw together and bring the jaws together? Well, visualize one of those vises in your mind. And imagine that your hands are just like the jaws of that vise.

I'm going to count from one to five, and at the count of five your hands will be firmly glued together, just like the jaws of a vise. I'm going to count from one to five, and at the count of five, it will be difficult or impossible to separate your hands no matter how hard you try. One, heavy; two, tight; three, you bring them tighter and tighter together just like the jaws of that vise; four, very tight; five, so tight that they're glued together, and even though you try with all your might to separate them, the harder you try, the more firmly clasped together they are. And they're going to stay clasped together until I give you the command to separate them. Now, slowly you will be able to separate them. Open your hands now. Good, just like that.

Now I want you to bring your hands down on your thighs.

And I want you to watch your hands, particularly the right hand. I want you to watch everything your hands do, no matter what they do. Perhaps you'll become aware of sensations in your hands, or you may become aware of the heaviness of your hand as it presses down on your thigh. Perhaps you'll become aware of feelings of pressure in your hand, or a feeling of tenderness or lightness. Whatever feelings you may have, I want you to concentrate your attention on your hands and notice them. Notice everything your hands do.

Now you'll begin to become aware, more and more, of little movements in your hand. You don't know which one of the fingers is going to move first, whether it will be the first finger, or the middle finger, or the thumb, or the ring finger; but one of the fingers is going to move and jerk just a little bit. You don't know which one of the fingers will move. It remains still and quiet, just as it is now. Fairly soon it will begin to wiggle and move. It will begin to move and to wiggle. You don't know exactly when. Perhaps it will be the thumb that will jerk a little, or the ring finger. Just keep watching and gazing at your hand. I want you to become aware of everything your hand does, no matter what it is. Just keep watching and gazing and wondering which finger will move first. Perhaps the fingers will spread apart so that the spaces between the fingers will become wider. Or the finger may move up and down a little bit. There, the little finger just moved. Just watch your hand and you'll become aware of a movement or jerking or separation of the fingers. There, the index finger moved.

Now you're going to notice an interesting thing. The fingers will get light, and will start lifting and rising straight up in the air. The hand will get light, and the hand will move up, slowly, up, up, the hand will get lighter and lighter. It's moving up now and it will begin to rise and lift straight up in the air, right up towards your face. It will begin to lift higher and higher, and as it does your eyes will get heavy, very heavy, and you'll get sleepier and sleepier. But your hand must not and will not touch your face, until you're asleep.

Your eyes are getting heavy now. It's difficult, very difficult to keep them open. And your hand continues slowly to lift, as your eyes get heavier and heavier, and you get sleepier and sleepier and sleepier. You're going to get so tired and sleepy in a moment, your eyes will close, and you'll go to sleep. Your eyes are getting heavy, just like lead; they're becoming very heavy. They blink. Soon they'll burn; they'll feel like lead. It's harder and harder to keep them open. And as the hand slowly continues to lift and rise towards your face, your eyes will get heavier and heavier. You'll get sleepier and sleepier and sleepier. Your eyes are blinking, more and more. They're getting harder and harder to keep open. Slowly your hand continues to rise and lift straight up towards your face, and as it does you get sleepier and sleepier and sleepier.

Soon your hand will touch your face; you'll lean the palm of your hand against your cheek, and you'll go to sleep, deeply asleep, very deeply asleep. Your eyes have closed. Now they're blinking, they're closing, they're closing. Your hand is moving towards your head; it will touch your face, and as soon as it touches your face, you'll sink into a deep sleep. Rest the head on the palm of your hand, and just go to sleep now, go to sleep. It touches your face. Rest your face in the palm of your hand and just go to sleep. Now rest, and when I talk to you next, you will be more deeply asleep. (*Pause*)

You are deeper asleep and will get drowsier and drowsier. Your breathing will get deep and automatic, and you're going to stay asleep until I give you the command to wake up. In a moment I'm going to stroke your arm, and you'll notice an extremely interesting thing. As I stroke it, the arm is going to get heavier and heavier. It will get stiffer and stiffer. I'm going to raise your hand up this way. I'm going to stroke it, and as I do, it will become stiff, very stiff and heavy. I'm going to count from one to five. As I reach the count of five, the arm will have stiffened up, the muscles will have it extended, and it will have become rigid and firm and stiff. One, heavy and stiff; two, heavier and heavier. Three, stiff and heavy and rigid and firm. Four, it is outstretched, just like that. Five, it becomes stiffer and stiffer, and you'll notice that even though you try to move it up in the air, it will not move. The harder you try to move it, the heavier it will feel. And even though you struggle to move it, it will remain exactly as it is, until I stroke it backwards, and only then will it be possible for you to feel it come down. (*Pause*) Do you notice that?

Pt. Yes. (*Pause*)

Dr. Now as I stroke it, it comes down again; just like this, and you'll go into a deeper and deeper and more restful sleep. Your eyelids now have become heavy, very heavy. They become so heavy, so firmly fixed together that they feel like lead. And they're going to get heavier and heavier and heavier, so that they'll feel like lead. They'll get so heavy that it will be impossible for them to open. They're getting heavier and heavier and heavier. And now, even though you try to open them with all your might, they're going to remain closed, fixed together, until I give you the command to open them. They'll remain closed, and you go into a deeper, much deeper, more restful sleep. And as you sit there, your sleep will get deeper, much deeper, and you will begin to feel yourself getting more tired.

Now, in a moment, you're going to find that the arm I had stroked is going to get paralyzed just like your leg. It will be impossible for you to move this arm no matter how hard you try. I'm going to count from one to five, and you'll find that your arm is paralyzed, that you cannot move that arm, no matter how hard you try. As you sit there, it will become

more and more paralyzed.   One, two, three, four, five.   The
arm has become paralyzed now, and even though you try to
move it, it remains exactly as it is.   (*Patient struggles to move
his arm unsuccessfully.*)   You will notice now that the
paralysis extends to your shoulder.   Try to move your
shoulder, and it is impossible to move it.   (*Patient tries to
move his shoulder and finally gives up trying.*)

Now, as you sit there, I'm going to stroke this paralyzed
leg.   As I stroke it, I'm going to make it possible for you to
move your foot easily.   Like this, just like that.   As I
stroke it, I'm going to count from one to five, and your leg
will move a little more easily.   One, two, three, four, five.
Now you'll be able to move your knee, just like that; good.
A little better now, a little better.   Just like that; good.

I want you to sit there and I want you to count from one
to five, and to give yourself the suggestion that as you do so,
your entire body will get rigid and paralyzed.   You're going
to notice that as you count, your whole body will become
rigid and fixed and paralyzed.   You will not be able to move
your legs.   You will not be able to move your arms.   You
will not be able to move your body.   As a matter of fact you
will not be able to come out of your chair, no matter how
hard you try.

Pt.   One, two, three, four, five.   (*Struggles to get out of
chair without success.*)

Dr.   Now you notice the body has become paralyzed and
it is impossible, no matter how hard you try, to get out of
that chair, until you decide you want to.   Count again from
one to five.   When you do, you will be able to move.   Try
it and see if it works.   (*Patient counts to himself, and at the
count of five, he removes the paralysis.*)

Now as you sit there, I want you to feel yourself getting
more tired and drowsy than before.   Even though you sit
there and feel yourself getting sleepier and sleepier and sleepier, you can talk to me.   You'll be able to talk to me just

like a person talks in his sleep. As you sit there, I'm going to ask you to visualize yourself with me walking along a street. As soon as you see both of us walking together, indicate it by this hand rising up. (*Hand rises and comes down.*) Just like that.

Now visualize both of us walking together down the street. We walk into a churchyard, and you look up and notice that the church steeple is in front of you. You see a bell. The bell is moving. The bell is moving and it makes a sound. As soon as you see the bell move and you hear the bell clanging, indicate it by your hand moving up, about an inch. Your hand moves up, good.

As you sit there, we're going, you and I, to go back in your life to where you're little, where you're about thirteen years of age. Perhaps it will be at your birthday, or it will be some other time. You visualize yourself exactly as you were then. As a matter of fact, you feel that you are thirteen. And when I talk to you next, after I count five, you will be thirteen years of age; everything will be exactly as it was at thirteen. One, you're getting little, your arms are getting little, your legs are getting little, you're getting little, smaller and smaller. You're shrinking all over. Two, you're getting very small now. Three, you're getting smaller and smaller, and in a moment you'll be thirteen years of age. Four, you're getting smaller and smaller. Five, you're thirteen years of age; you're exactly thirteen, and when I talk to you next, you'll be exactly thirteen years of age. As soon as you feel yourself to be thirteen years of age, indicate it by your hand rising up about an inch. (*Hand rises.*) How old are you?

Pt. Thirteen.

Dr. Thirteen, good; now bring your hand down, just like that. I want you to stand up and walk with me to the door. (*Patient rises and walks to the door with me without any sign of paralysis.*) Sit down and when I talk to you next, you will be an adult again. (*Pause*) Now, as you sit there, I'm going to give you a suggestion that it will be possible for you to move out of the chair. It will be possible for you to abandon the paralysis of your leg. I'm going to paralyze this toe instead. It will not move. I'm going to stroke the shoe, and even though you stand up, the toe is going to be paralyzed. It is going to be impossible for you to move this toe. This toe, no matter how hard you try, will be paralyzed. No matter how hard you try to move it, it will remain fixed, but you will be able to walk without a cane. You'll be able to stand up and walk along with me. Walk along with me, just the way you walked with me in that vision of yours. (*Patient walks easily with me.*) Now turn around and come back yourself. Good. When you awaken, your toe will continue to be paralyzed, but you will walk well. You will walk better and better. Move your leg, and as I count from one to five, you will move your leg and awaken with your leg moving. One, two, three, four, five. (*Patient moves his leg, opens his eyes and observes his leg moving. He quickly stands up and is able to walk on his leg though he favors it somewhat.*) You will gradually be able to feel more and more confidence in your ability to walk better. Be sure to get in touch with me when you return.

Pt.   I will.

Dr.   Good-by.

Pt.   Good-by.

Results will be most permanent where the patient gains some understanding of the dynamic significance of his symptoms. Under hypnosis, after arm rigidity, paralysis and anesthesia have been induced, the patient may be told that it is possible for thoughts and ideas to produce spasticity, paralysis, anesthesia and other symptoms, in the same way that the physician's suggestions created the present hypnotic effects. He is told that every person has mental conflicts which may act in the same way. For instance, a man may be fearful that he might hurt someone, and his mind will give his body the suggestion that his arm must become weak or paralyzed to prevent this. The most interesting thing is that the person does not know what is going on. The idea that he may even think of hurting anyone is so repulsive that he does not let himself believe it is true. He will be aware only of the result, that is the weakened or paralyzed arm, which may be very uncomfortable or disabling.

The patient can then be told that there may be other reasons why symptoms develop. As a matter of fact his own symptom may be the result of certain suggestions that he gives himself unconsciously, due to conflicts of which he may not be entirely aware. He must now realize from what has happened in hypnosis that his condition is not permanent, that it can be altered. Becoming aware of the factors behind his symptoms will enable him to achieve, in addition to a removal of his symptoms, a real constructive change in his personality. Perhaps he may not see the need for inquiring into the nature of his problem at present, but if, at some future date, he has this desire, the physician will help him to gain a broader understanding.

In many cases such instructions serve to motivate the patient toward an analytic approach, and the patient may actually request further help. Where this happens, the physician may continue therapy in the event he is analytically trained, or if not, he may refer the patient to a psychoanalyst.

A legitimate question is: What effect does the authoritarian, directive relationship—which produces success in symptom removal by prestige suggestion—have on the future ability of the physician to establish the more nondirective relationship necessary in an analytic procedure? When the patient achieves that development where he wants to make his own decisions and to take responsibility for his own growth, he will be able to work with the same therapist, but

in the framework of a different type of relationship.   Experience in psychoanalysis teaches us that it is possible to treat a
sick patient along directive authoritarian lines at first, and
to get him, in the course of therapy, to see the need for a
more cooperative, less authoritarian, relationship.   At the
start of therapy the patient may have been unable to work
analytically, but with preparation he is strengthened to a
point where he can take advantage of the analytic method.
What is necessary, when the patient returns following symptom removal, is to redefine the therapeutic situation for him,
to show him that the deeper personality problems he wants
corrected cannot be approached by the same method of
prestige suggestion, but require a different type of treatment.

TECHNICAL AIDS IN SYMPTOM REMOVAL

ALTHOUGH removal of the patient's symptom at one sitting may be possible and desirable in certain hysterical and psychosomatic conditions, it is usually best to extend therapy over a longer period. Suggestions are carried out very much better where the patient is convinced that hypnosis can have a potent influence on his functions. It may therefore be advisable to delay giving therapeutic suggestions until he achieves as deep a trance as possible, and until he gains confidence in his ability to experience the phenomena suggested to him. The employment of therapeutic suggestions at a time when the patient is skeptical about his ability to comply, and before he has gained sufficient confidence in himself and in the physician, may end in failure and add discouragement and panic to the patient's difficulties.

A deep trance seems to increase therapeutic effectiveness in most patients. Where the person can achieve a deep trance, and where dramatic phenomena can be produced, he will then be able to respond best to therapeutic suggestions. Where only a light trance is possible, the patient may not be able to get to a point where he becomes convinced of his own capacity to control his symptoms.

There are exceptions to this rule of trance depth, and sometimes, even in a light trance, one can remove certain symptoms. In several instances, patients, who were unable to be hypnotized because they were motivated against entering a trance state, were asked simply to close their eyes and ordered in a very authoritarian way to relinquish their symptoms. To my amazement and theirs, their symptoms disappeared. Although the person was motivated against entering a trance state, he was still responsive to suggestion on a waking level. Possibly there was fear of being hypnotized at the same time that there was need to respond to authoritative suggestion. Where the patient cannot be hypnotized, and where symptom removal is the only therapy he can utilize at the time, he may be requested to close his eyes, and suggestions may then be given him as if he were in a light trance.

Patients who have no posthypnotic amnesia react almost universally with the statement that they have not been hypnotized. They may feel, accordingly, that they cannot be helped by the physician's suggestions. Since posthypnotic amnesia may not be possible, it is important to get the patient to understand that amnesia is not essential for success, that suggestions act on the subconscious mind even though a person is aware of what is going on at the time, and that amnesia may even be a detriment. A state of repose and drowsiness alone makes it possible for suggestions to penetrate into deep portions of the mind in spite of existing resistances. The patient may be informed that suggestion does not work immediately in all cases, but that repeated suggestions will be successful.

All suggestions must be as specific as possible and should be repeated several times. The physician should build, as completely as possible, a picture of what he wants the patient to feel or to do. For instance, if the patient is an insomniac, and it is desired to create sleepiness, he should not be told simply that he will fall asleep when he goes to bed at nighttime. Rather, it should be suggested that at a definite hour he will begin to feel drowsy. He will then undress and get into bed. As soon as his head touches the pillow, his eyes will begin to get heavy, and after that he will feel heavy and drowsy all over. A sleepy sensation will sweep over him which will result in his falling asleep. If the sleep is deep as it should be, there will be no disturbing dreams. Furthermore, he will arise at a definite hour in the morning feeling fully refreshed.

If a patient complains of a distressing pain in his leg, he may be instructed that his leg will begin to feel lighter and less tender. It will grow less and less sensitive, but he will continue to feel sensations of touch and temperature. The pain, however, will lessen, and his leg will become much more nimble. He will be able to step out more freely, and, if he happens to strike into things, he will not wince, since he will not feel pain that intensely.

If it is desired to overcome a mild depression, a situation may be described in which a happy chain of events occurs. It is then suggested that the patient participate in this feeling of happiness, as if he, himself, had become a part of it.

Where the patient participates in the therapeutic plan, he should not be ordered to yield his symptoms. Suggestions may be framed so that they will work sometime in the near future, instead of immediately. Rather than demanding that a patient's headache disappear, he may be told: "As you relax, you will discover that the causes of your headache no longer operate to upset you. You will not worry so much or be so tense. You will find that your headache will grow less and less painful and that it will soon disappear." Sometimes, especially in psychosomatic symptoms, symptom removal is not attempted during hypnosis, but posthypnotic suggestions are given the patient, so that the symptom may disappear while he is awake. Erickson[1] has reported a splendid example of this.

The lighter the trance, the less emphatic should be the suggestions. In extremely light hypnotic states, the patient may be instructed that he need not concentrate too closely on the suggestions of the physician, but rather should fixate his attention on a restful train of thought. This technic is based on the idea that the patient's resistances can be circumvented in this way. A logical explanation may be presented of why suggestions will work, along lines of suggestion that the unconscious mind is capable of absorbing and utilizing even though the conscious mind may resist them.

If the patient is in a medium or deep trance, suggestions should be framed in as simple a manner as possible. The patient, especially when he is in a deep trance, should repeat what is expected of him. Otherwise he may be so lethargic that he may not understand clearly the nature of the commands. If he is a somnambule, he may be instructed to carry out instructions even though he does not remember that they were formulated by the physician. It is also a good idea in somnambulistic patients to give them a posthypnotic suggestion that they will be unresponsive to hypnotic induction by any person except the physician. This will prevent the patient from being victimized by an amateur hypnotist who may very well undo therapeutic benefits.

If facts important in the understanding of the patient's condition are uncovered in hypnosis, these may or may not be brought to the patient's attention, depending upon their significance and upon the ability of the patient to tolerate the implications. It is best to make interpretations as superficial as possible, utilizing knowledge one has gained in working with the patient to guide him into activities of a creative nature which do not stir up too much conflict.

Whether to terminate hypnosis abruptly or to have the patient sleep for a few minutes before interruption is another practical point. There is some evidence that a short period of sleep followed by gradual awakening is advantageous. The patient is simply instructed that he will continue to sleep for a designated number of minutes following which he will be awakened. The period of sleep may range from two to fifteen minutes. Where the patient is able to dream on suggestion, this period may be advantageously utilized to induce dreams either of a spontaneous sort or of a nature relevant to the particular trends elicited during the trance.

There is no set rule as to how much time to devote to

hypnosis during each session. Except for the initial induction period, the trance need not exceed one-half hour.
Ample time should be allowed to take up with the patient
his problems both before and after hypnosis. His reaction
to the trance may also be discussed.

The question of the permanency of therapeutic changes
produced by posthypnotic commands is an important one.
Are the suggestions subject to the same laws of forgetting
as learning in the waking state? There is considerable
variation in the length of time that a posthypnotic suggestion
will last without reinforcement. In my experience the
most important factor is the dynamic significance to the
patient of his symptom, and the relative strength of the
motivation to comply with the suggestions of the physician
as compared to the security motivations he gratifies in ex-
ploiting his illness. Whereas innocuous posthypnotic suggestions may continue in force for a considerable period
after hypnosis, those that tend to rob the individual of his
usual defenses may readily be neutralized.

Hypnotic suggestions for symptom removal will usually
need reinforcement. There are various ways by which
reinforcement of posthypnotic suggestions may be secured.
Visits to the physician at monthly intervals, or more frequently if necessary, may provide an opportunity, not only
for reinforcement, but also for gaging the general adjustment of the patient. They will also permit desensitization,
re-education and a modified analytic exploration of conflicts.

Where such visits are not practical, the patient may be
taught the technic of self hypnosis in order to reinforce
suggestions through his own efforts. The ease with which
phonographic recordings may be made these days makes it
possible, in suitable cases, to provide the patient with a
recording of therapeutic suggestions which can provide the
necessary reinforcement.

The giving of medications often helps reinforce suggestions especially where symptoms are somatic or visceral in nature. There are many patients who pattern their lives so much around logic that they cannot permit a circumstance to enter it for which there is the slightest irrational basis. Posthypnotic suggestions smack too much of magic, and the patient may subject his impulses toward posthypnotic action to so merciless a scrutiny that the effects may be neutralized. If such a person happens to be an insomniac, he will spend all night trying to figure out why he feels an impulse to fall asleep merely because this was suggested to him. With persons of this type, a simple way of overcoming such resistance is to supply them with a box of pills. Placebos will do, but the patient may discover that he has been tricked, so that it is best to prescribe a tablet containing iron or thiamine chloride which may possibly benefit his system. It is suggested to him, during hypnosis, that at a stated time he will take a pill, and that the pill will help produce the effect desired.

Sufficient emphasis cannot be placed on the importance of motivating the patient toward acceptance of a more rational therapy than symptom removal. A nondirective re-educational or analytic approach should be utilized wherever possible to insure the greatest permanency of results.

LIMITATIONS OF SYMPTOM
REMOVAL

Before Freud's monumental discovery of the economic significance of symptoms, suggestive hypnosis was employed indiscriminately for all types of functional and even organic conditions. There were varying reports as to its efficacy. Janet,[2] one of the most ardent devotees of therapeutic hypnosis, treated over thirty-five hundred patients. Follow-up studies revealed the surprising fact that lasting cures had been obtained in only seven percent of his cases, even though most of Janet's patients were hysterics.

Janet classified his patients into three groups. In the first group were those in whom response to hypnosis or to waking suggestions was complete, rapid and permanent. Here treatment consisted of an immediate attack on the symptom without psychologic analysis. Of the thousands of cases treated, however, only fifty-four responded sufficiently to fall into this group. Janet was aware of the seemingly miraculous nature of the cure in successful cases, but he justified this with the statement that he had accomplished as much for patients as could Lourdes at the saving of the cost of the journey. In the second group, which consisted of approximately one hundred and fifty cases, there were those patients who, though completely cured for one year, were influenced only by prolonged therapy, averaging from twice to three times weekly, for a period of three months. In the third group, hypnosis either had a temporary influence or no effect whatsoever, even after treatment had continued for the period of over a year. The effect of suggestion usually lasted no more than a few hours or a few days. Often the same symptoms removed during hypnosis would reappear, or, if a troublesome symptom were eliminated, another symptom would crop up to take its place. The bulk of Janet's patients fell into the latter group.

The most important objection to the indiscriminate use of symptom removal is that symptoms are surface expressions of deep fundamental conflicts. They are neither chaotic nor meaningless. On the contrary they appear to fulfill an important function in maintaining the psychobiologic equilibrium of the individual. They serve both as a vicarious means of gratifying forbidden impulses, and as a way of binding psychic energy which otherwise would be discharged as anxiety.[3] Thus they constitute for the individual an important means of defense and adaptation. To remove symptoms, therefore, is something like blowing away smoke, when one really wants to quench the fire underneath.

In suggestive therapy, because of the omnipotent position the therapist occupies in the mind of the patient, certain symptoms may be abandoned. Symptoms which are removed solely by prestige suggestion disappear because the patient has a need to comply with the commands of the therapist. The motivation to comply is conditioned by a wish to gratify important security needs through archaic mechanisms of submission to and identification with an omnipotent authority. So long as the latter motivation is greater than the gains the patient derives from elaboration of his symptoms, he will abandon his symptoms on command. And he will remain symptom free provided he continues to have faith in the omniscience and strength of the therapist. The patient may require constant demonstrations of the therapist's power and good will. More significantly the hostility generated by the dependency relationship—which is inevitably a part of such a relationship—may deflate the therapist's capacities in the patient's mind. This destroys the original motivation for the loss of symptoms and encourages a relapse.

As a general rule, no symptom will be abandoned, even

with strong hypnotic commands, which serves as a defense against intense anxiety, or as an important way of adjusting the patient to his life situation.   For instance, if a man develops a paralyzed arm as a defense against the fear of stabbing his wife, suggested removal of the paralysis will be so threatening to him that he will refuse to follow the suggestions of the hypnotist.

Another limitation of suggestive hypnosis is that a relatively large group of patients fail to respond to symptom removal because they are unable to regard the hypnotist as a sufficiently omniscient authority.   Those who doubt the capacities and power of the hypnotist will not feel the need to comply and will resist, and resist successfully, his commands.

There are, nevertheless, occasional patients, usually hysterics, whose need for an invincible and protective authority is so strong that they invest the hypnotist with supernormal powers and follow his suggestions, even to the yielding up of an important symptom.   To compensate for the latter, other symptoms may develop in different parts of the body which have the same dynamic significance to the patient.

Where a compensatory symptom is not developed, and where the patient's conflict continues in force and is not propitiated by the hypnotic relationship, the patient may become overwhelmed by anxiety which was hitherto held in check by his symptom.   His ability to cope with this liberated anxiety will depend on the strength of his ego and the residual defenses available for mobilization.   Where the ego is too weak to handle vast quantities of liberated anxiety, an acute excitement or psychotic shattering of the ego is possible.   The latter, though rare, must always be kept in mind before bludgeoning a patient with hypnotic commands to relinquish a symptom, which he believes has life-saving values for him.

The relapse rate among patients who have simply had their

symptoms removed by suggestion is greater than among those who have had a deeper form of therapy. Needless to say, the chances of helping a person in a permanent sense are much greater where one does a reintegrative kind of therapy that treats the source of the problem and permits the patient to develop ego strength and security within himself. In the latter instance, the person has the best chance of remaining symptom free even in the face of disturbing life situations and pressures. In symptomatic treatment, where no change has occurred in the ego strength, there is always the possibility of a relapse. This, however, is not inevitable because the patient's life situation may get less complicated, or the patient may, as a result of therapy, develop more adaptive ways of dealing with conflict and of getting along with people.

Another objection to symptom removal is that it is apt to eliminate an important incentive for deep personality change in those cases who have a potentiality for achieving this change. The inconvenience and discomfiture of symptoms incites the individual to inquire into the cause of his difficulty. If the patient is made too comfortable by removing his symptoms, he may lose the incentive to analyze their source. Where the goal in therapy is to achieve alteration in the dynamic structure of the personality, symptom removal or any other strongly supportive therapeutic method may act as a deterrent.

ILLUSTRATIVE CASE

THE FOLLOWING case of a patient with enuresis illustrates the technic of suggestive hypnosis, and demonstrates the need for a continuous study of the changing relationship between patient and doctor during psychotherapy even where the goal is symptom removal.

FIRST SESSION (May 13)

The patient presents a problem of enuresis since infancy which has persisted to the present day. He is unaware of any problems in his relations with people or of any other neurotic difficulties. He is a seaman and can spend but a limited amount of time in therapy. Because of the time element, the severity of the symptom, and the lack of insight into the broader neurotic aspects, an authoritarian approach aimed at symptom removal is decided on, with the secondary aim of bringing the patient to a realization of his deeper difficulties so that, at a later date, he can continue therapy. His reaction to the Rorschach cards indicates a slightly paranoid attitude. However, he seems cooperative and anxious to rid himself of the symptom of enuresis.

Dr. I should like to ask you a few preliminary questions before you tell me about your problem. How old are you?

Pt. Twenty-one. I'll be twenty-two in July.

Dr. And your marital status?

Pt. Single.

Dr. And your occupation?

Pt. I'm a merchant seaman.

Dr. Your education?

Pt. A year and a half of college. I intend to continue if that has any bearing on it.

Dr. Are you employed at the present time?

Pt. No, I'm not.

Dr. Your financial status? How do you earn a living now?

Pt. Well, my entire income is from when I'm sailing.

Dr. And who are you living with?

Pt. My aunt.

Dr. Now supposing you tell me your problem.

Pt. Well, the thing is I've never stopped wetting the bed, and it's been on, well ever since childhood. There has never been any let up, and I've been taken to people by my mother when I was younger. My guardian was a doctor, a practitioner, and they've done a number of things for me. I've been to a couple of doctors. Nothing has ever given me relief from it. I mean I've been circumcised and given tonics and things like that. But I mean I'm just getting to the point now where I figure I'm on my own, I mean I'm all alone now. I figure I might as well see what I can do by myself. Something that will satisfy myself anyhow.

Dr. I see. In other words, the problem as you see it is one of bed wetting that hasn't let up since childhood.

Pt. That's right.

Dr. And how bad is it? Can you tell me how many times a night you wet? Do you get up during the nighttime to go to the bathroom at all?

Pt. I do occasionally, yes. I mean it is not every night. And—well, I mean—it's hard to—

Dr. It is very difficult.

Pt. Yes; I mean like, for instance, I can't tell you one way or the other whether I think I will or not get up that night. I tried to narrow the wetting down to a certain thing myself, you know, to see what it could be that might be enhancing the condition, but I haven't been able to find anything yet. I mean even such things as a diuretic like beer, for instance, I mean sometimes I will and sometimes I won't. You see what I mean?

Dr. Yes.

Pt. And they had me, I mean when I was younger, do such things as not drink anything after supper, for instance.

Well that didn't settle it. Sometimes I would and sometimes I wouldn't.

Dr. And it puzzles you very much why this thing goes
on.

Pt. That's right.

Dr. Now, have you been able to connect it with any emotional state?

Pt. No. I'm a very nervous individual anyhow. I
always have been ever since I was a child.

Dr. Can you explain more about that to me? Nervous
in what sense?

Pt. Well I—I'm not at a point where I'm jumpy, I mean
where little things scare me and I jump at things. You
know what I mean? But it's that—like I can't sit still, you
know what I mean? I always have to be on the go. I get
trouble concentrating on things sometimes. I mean, for
instance, like sometimes something will happen as a surprise,
for instance, you know, and I'll get nervous and I'll urinate.
You know what I mean, things like that. And then sometimes I have to urinate, you know, and then something will
happen and take my mind completely away from it and I
lose the urge.

Dr. In other words, you can control it during the daytime, even if you have a full bladder.

Pt. You mean the flow of it?

Dr. You can control urinating, for instance, when you
have to urinate. It is possible for you to hold it back?

Pt. Oh, yes. Certainly.

Dr. Now let's get back to your early childhood. You
say you were a nervous child. Can you tell me more about
your childhood and your relations with children, your school
adjustment, and so on.

Pt. Well, my father died when I was five. My mother
was English and we went to live with my mother's sister and
her husband. There was my mother and her sister and my-

self, and there was my little cousin who is five years younger than I am. And—well as far as association with children I mean—I always had friends and things like that. I mean I never lacked for companionship and things like that, but I guess it was more my aunt that raised me.

Dr. What about your mother?

Pt. Well, she was a nurse and she was away from home. She was working twelve hour shifts.

Dr. Is she living now?

Pt. No. She died when I was thirteen.

Dr. What sort of a person was she?

Pt. Can you make that a little clearer?

Dr. Her personality—domineering—passive—quiet?

Pt. No. I wouldn't call her the aggressive type either. But, well, it always seemed to me she used to have the way about her that she seemed pretty well disgusted in general, you know. I mean, I don't know whether that is any help to you or not, but that is the one thing I can think of. You know, she used to be pretty well disgusted with things in general. I guess probably with the breaks she had in life. She'd been working pretty hard, and she was more or less helping my aunt along quite a bit because she wasn't happily married and didn't have much money, and I think she was pretty well disgusted, too, in me with my trouble.

Dr. Your mother?

Pt. Yes, and I know my aunt was.

Dr. And what sort of a person was your aunt?

Pt. Well, she was very, very domineering when I was young. I live with her now and I think I really love her; but at the time I used to pretty well despise her.

Dr. And did you play well with other kids?

Pt. Oh, yes.

Dr. Were you aggressive or did you act more like a retiring child?

Pt. Well, we used to—I don't think I was the leader type

in the group—but I was, we used to as far as I can see, play normally.

Dr. Did you fight a lot as a kid?

Pt. No.

Dr. Do you have any brothers or sisters?

Pt. No.

Dr. Your mother never remarried?

Pt. No, she didn't.

Dr. How did you feel when your mother passed away?

Pt. I don't know. I was just thinking about that today. Naturally I felt sorry, but the thing that hit me at first as soon as I heard the news, the one thing that came to my mind, was, "What the hell am I going to do," you know. I mean, I was only about thirteen at the time anyhow, and I've got an aunt out in Ohio that I didn't care for too much, and she was very good to me and all, and I knew that would be where I would end up. And that is where I did end up, and I don't think it was too much of a real hard blow to me.

Dr. When you went to school and into college, did you have any problems in your relations with people?

Pt. In college?

Dr. During your early adolescence and through college, right up to today. Do you have any problems in your relations with people?

Pt. No. I mean the friends I have I think highly of, and they think highly of me.

Dr. You get along very well with people? But do you get depressed at all?

Pt. Well, sometimes I'm depressed in that I stop to think that I, well, here I am all alone. Supposing I run out of dough, something like that. Who am I going to turn to, you know what I mean? Sort of a, not depression actually, it is sort of a feeling of insecurity, you know.

Dr. Yes, your aunt, she's alive?

Pt. Yes.

Dr. Would she take care of you in a pinch?

Pt. I think she would, sure.

Dr. In other words you have feelings, nevertheless, that you may be alone and that nobody will be around to help you?

Pt. That's right. And maybe the people that would help me, I wouldn't want to turn to.

Dr. Do you ever get panicky?

Pt. No.

Dr. What about phobias? Do you have any fears of any kind?

Pt. Hum?

Dr. You're not afraid of such things as elevators, closed spaces, open spaces?

Pt. No.

Dr. What about thoughts that keep recurring in your mind that frighten you? Frightening thoughts ever come into your mind?

Pt. You mean constantly? Over a period of time the same thing?

Dr. Over and over again.

Pt. Well, if there is anything, I guess it is not really prominent, or I'd think of them off the bat.

Dr. What about headaches or dizziness?

Pt. No dizziness, but frequently headaches which have let up since I got glasses.

Dr. What about stomach trouble?

Pt. No.

Dr. Impotency?

Pt. I beg pardon?

Dr. Impotency, any sexual problems of any kind?

Pt. Oh, no.

Dr. When did you start going out with girls?

Pt. When I was about thirteen.

Dr. And do you go out with girls now?

Pt. Yes.

Dr. Do you have sexual relations with them?

Pt. Yes.

Dr. And do you enjoy it?

Pt. Sure.

Dr. There is no problem there?

Pt. No.

Dr. Any homosexuality?

Pt. No.

Dr. Do you feel tense?

Pt. Yes.

Dr. What about insomnia? Do you sleep?

Pt. Yes, no trouble.

Dr. Any nightmares?

Pt. No.

Dr. Take any alcohol?

Pt. Some.

Dr. Do you get drunk often?

Pt. No. I think you can say frequently but moderately.

Dr. Sedatives? Do you take sedatives?

Pt. No.

Dr. Do you feel fatigued or exhausted or unable to work?

Pt. No.

Dr. You avoid people?

Pt. No.

Dr. Hate people or get dependent upon people?

Pt. No.

Dr. So that actually the only symptoms that you have are tension and this bed wetting?

Pt. Yes.

Dr. Now, can you give me your latest dream? When did you have a dream last?

Pt. I don't know. I was just remarking the other day that either I never dream or never remember them. I really can't remember my last one. Every once in a while, I mean,

I get an outlandish thing, I mean. They are absolutely funny.

Dr.   Suppose you tell me about it.

Pt.   I can't think of them, but I remember remarking about them at the time.

Dr.   Can you remember any dream?

Pt.   The only thing I do remember when I was young, quite often, I'd wake up, having just wet the bed, and I had been dreaming that I'd been standing at a toilet. I don't know whether that has any bearing on it, but that is one thing I do remember.

Dr.   Do you remember having any dreams as a child of a frightening nature?

Pt.   No.

Dr.   I see. So that the only dream you remember is standing at a toilet, and then the next thing you knew you were wetting the bed.

Pt.   That is the one I remember because that's naturally so closely associated with my condition and I do remember it.

(*At this point patient is shown the Rorschach cards to obtain an idea of his responses to instructured materials.*)

Dr.   All right. I'm going to show you some cards and I want you to tell me what comes to your mind when you see these cards. Would you move your chair around here? This is the first card.

Pt.   Looks like a pair of legs on the bottom here. This thing up here looks like some kind of a weird animal, like a bat, kind of gruesome.

Dr.   Yes.

Pt.   Do you want me to look at it that way?

Dr.   Any way you wish.

Pt.   I can't say that I can make much more out of it.

Dr. All right. Here's the second card.

Pt. Looks like a pair of clouded over eyes right there.

Dr. Like a what?

Pt. Looks like a pair of eyes, you know, clouded over like.

Dr. Where do you see the eyes?

Pt. Inside. Also it looks like something like a pheasant's tail. A couple of animal faces here snuggled together, puppies or something. This looks like an exploding bomb. Or else, I'd say, more like a ship being hit by a torpedo, something of that nature, you know.

Dr. All right, this is the third.

Pt. Looks like a couple of men in tuxedos pulling chairs away, two of them. Looks like a parrot sitting on a roost. A head of a fly. Do you want me to see this thing as a whole or in parts?

Dr. Makes no difference. Anything you see.

Pt. That's all I can see in that one.

Dr. All right. This is four.

Pt. This way it looks like an animal skin stretched out for drying, bear skin or something. I see some kind of animal, something I can't exactly put my finger on, with eyes there.

Dr. This is the fifth.

Pt. A butterfly. Looks like a caricature of a duck laughing, you know, sort of a cartoon version.

Dr. This is the sixth.

Pt. The thing that popped into my mind when I first looked at it, it reminded me of a design on an Indian blanket. This business right down through here.

Dr. Yes, inside there.

Pt. Looks like some weird-looking kind of head, facing straight ahead with black eyes.

Dr. Yes.

Pt. Looks like it could be, for instance, the top on one of those Eskimo totem poles, you know, those complex looking wings they had on them. I don't see much more.

Dr. This is the seventh.

Pt. A couple of young girls making faces at each other. Elephants facing outward.

Dr. All right. This is the eighth.

Pt. It looks like the, the whole thing looks like the shell of some crustacean, a crab or something like a museum specimen, you know, just the shell. Looks like a couple of things that look like raccoons, those here, head on the side. They almost look like they'd been drawn there.

Dr. Yes. This is nine.

Pt. The only thing I can associate these two orange things on top is a couple of seagulls. I see a couple of pairs of claws down here, long nails. This way these two orange things on the bottom look from here down like the chest and body of an eagle. I see a man with a beard there.

Dr. Where do you see the man?

Pt. Head, nose, eyes up here. I see a man's face here, too, looks like a handlebar mustache.

Dr. This is the tenth.

Pt. A couple of crabs on the outside here. A couple of strange looking animals here looking at each other. Something funny coming out of the top of their head there. It reminds me of the throat bone, the Adam's apple, you know. Up in here I see two eyes that look like two snouts, this thing in the middle here.

Dr. Your responses indicate that your personality functioning is fairly good. You could go deeply into your problems if you wanted to. But if you believe you have no time for that we can see if we can knock the props out from under the symptom and get control of the enuresis so it won't bother you.

Pt. Yes. I can't spend much time, got to get back to sea.

Dr. I see. You are going back to sea. You're not going to be around here long, so we'll try to knock the props out of this thing in as few sessions as possible.

Pt. I see, I won't be going away for a few weeks. Can you give me an idea how far apart these sessions will be?

Dr. They don't have to be every day. They could be twice a week, maybe.

Pt. I see. That would be fine.

Dr. Now the only problem is arranging time for you and I'd like to get started with you as soon as possible. We could meet tomorrow.

Pt. See you tomorrow.

Dr. Good.

SECOND SESSION (May 14)

In this session an attempt is made to control enuresis by building up an incentive which will counteract the purposeful nature of the symptom, whatever it may be, and the secondary gain. During hypnosis, the patient is conditioned to awaken upon a signal that develops prior to bed wetting. Utilizing his own symbols for fear and satisfaction, the desire is developed in him to get out of bed and go to the bathroom as soon as his eyes open. No attempt is made to investigate the symbolic significance of the enuresis since he has no motivation at this time to look for causes.

Pt. (*Patient coughs and fidgets about in his chair.*) I have a tickle in my throat.

Dr. Feel a little bit tense?

Pt. Always do when I'm in a doctor's office.

Dr. Have you had any dreams since I saw you last?

Pt. Yes, I had a dream last night. The girl I used to go with—just recently her father died—and I was over at the house there and she was there with her fifteen year old brother. The two of them live in the house together now. That's about all I can remember.

Dr. Do you see this girl now? How do you like her?

Pt. Haven't seen her in years. I mean, she's an old friend, that's all, and she's the first girl I had.

Dr. You don't remember anything more about that dream?

Pt. All I remember is that the two of them were living in

the house together, she, and her fifteen year old brother.
And he was doing the housework, setting the table and clean-
ing it off, like that.

Dr. Yes.

Pt. As far as I remember, I don't think I, I was entering
into what was going on. I was more the spectator.

Dr. All right, supposing now we discuss hypnosis. Supposing you tell me what you know about hypnosis.

Pt. Ah, very little.

Dr. You've never been hypnotized yourself? What
comes to you when you think of hypnosis?

Pt. Sort of a state of semiconscious coma, I think.

Dr. That is a very common idea, but actually a person
in hypnosis is just as wide awake as you are. It's merely
the ability to follow suggestions and commands without
forcing yourself. If suggestions are given to a person that
he is going to go into a coma, then he's going to assume the
state that you are talking about. But a person can be just
as wide awake, as a matter of fact, he can even have his eyes
open, and can remember everything and still be fully hypnotized.

Pt. I didn't know that.

Dr. Now, supposing you tell me what you would like
more than anything else in the world? If we could accomplish it for you here, something that you want more than
anything else in the world, what would you like? What's
the best thing that could happen?

Pt. Oh, you mean in the immediate present? Well, I
don't know. I think if I came across a good bit of money,
I'd like that more than anything else, right at this minute.

(*The desire to be given money or chance on it is probably indicative of his insecurity and feeling that he is unable to get it through
productive efforts of his own.*)

Dr. So that if you came across a good bit of money that
would be the best thing that you could think of? How about

yourself, as far as your coming here is concerned? What do you think you would like to have happen here between you and me?

Pt. Well, I, naturally the basic reason I'm here is to see what it is that's causing me to have this trouble that I've got. But I, even when I was a kid, when I'd been taken to doctors, I always knew myself that that wasn't going to do me a darn bit of good. And I actually do believe that the type of treatment that you are capable of giving will help me.

(*His hopefulness and faith in the therapy may be regarded as making him amenable to prestige suggestion.*)

Dr. And you'd really like to get over this thing?

Pt. Absolutely.

Dr. You really, sincerely want to get over it. If you do, you will be able to. Without any question you will be able to get over this thing, if your desire for it is very strong. Maybe there will be slips, but eventually you will build up that desire to a point where this thing just will not happen. And hypnosis will be able to get you to a state where you will be able to develop the power to control your bladder in the nighttime.

(*The aim here is to create an incentive for relinquishing the symptom that will grow stronger than the defensive value of the symptom or its secondary gain.*)

Now I'm going to give you an example of what hypnosis is. Hypnosis is the capacity to follow certain suggestions and to feel exactly what is being said to you. For instance, supposing you bring your arms up on the chair, just like this, and clasp your hands together. This is not hypnosis, this is just an example of what hypnosis is. Look at your fists and then close your eyes for a moment, and imagine a vise, one of those heavy steel vises, the kind that you tighten up with a screw. You know, the kind that you tighten up? Now, close your eyes and imagine that you are looking at this vise. And then begin to imagine that your hands are just like the jaws of that vise.   And then the screw begins to tighten, and as the screw tightens, the fingers become clasped together more and more firmly.   I am going to count from one to five.   As I reach the count of five, the hands will become clasped together very firmly, more, and more, and more.   So that at the count of five, the hands will be very firmly clasped together, just like that, as if they were the jaws of the vise; then, at the count of five, you will notice that it will be difficult or impossible to open your hands.   One, heavy; two, tight, tight; three, tighter and tighter; four, very tight; five, as tight as a vise.   And you'll notice that it's impossible to open your hands up no matter how hard you try.   It's very, very difficult.   They are clasped together, and the harder you try to pull them apart, the tighter they feel. Until, finally, I give you the command to open them, and slowly they open.   And now you'll be able to open them, just like that.

Now, another example.   Bring your hands down on your thighs and watch your fingers. I want you to become aware of everything your hand does. Watch your hands, particularly your right hand.   Keep your eyes fastened on your right hand.   Now I want you to become aware of every sensation, everything your hand does.   Perhaps you'll become aware of the feeling of weight of the palm of your hand upon your thigh.   Or you may become aware of the fact that you feel the pressure of your hand on your thigh. Perhaps you'll become aware of the feeling of tension in your hand, of muscle pullings, or maybe even sensations, tenderness in the fingers.   Or movement, yes, movement.

Just watch the fingers and see which one of them will move first.   Pretty soon one of them is going to start moving.   You don't know which one.   Pretty soon one of them is going to jerk a little bit, or move. It may be the middle finger, or the thumb, or the ring finger, or the index finger, or the little finger. One of those fingers will just move a little bit, or quiver, and you'll become aware of the movement in the fingers. Just keep watching. You don't know exactly when that will happen. Your hands remain absolutely still now, and pretty soon one of those fingers will jerk, will move. Or the spaces between those fingers will widen. And as you keep gazing at your hand, you'll notice that slowly the fingers will start moving apart, will start spreading apart, moving and spreading wider, and wider, and wider apart, spreading apart like that, just like that.

The spaces will begin to increase, and now you'll begin to notice something very interesting. The fingers are going to start feeling light. The hand will feel light and very slowly the hand will lift and rise in the air, just as if it's as light as a feather. Keep watching your hand; you'll begin noticing that the hand begins to feel light, very light, and that slowly it will begin to lift, a little bit higher, rising and lifting straight up in the air. It gets lighter and lighter, and now the fingers arch up on the trousers and move up, up, up. And the hand gets lighter, very light. And you'll begin to feel the arm getting lighter and lighter. Then the whole arm will begin to lift straight up in the air. It will rise and lift. Lifting higher and higher, and feeling light, just like that. And then it will suddenly begin to rise toward your face, rising and lifting, just as if it's just as light as a feather. It lifts a little bit more now, rising up, higher and higher. Slowly, automatically, the hand will lift, lift straight up in the air, straight up in the air. Higher and higher, moving, moving.

As you gaze at your hand, you'll notice that the eyes become heavy and tired. They blink and the hand gets light. You're to keep watching the hand and the eyes will begin to water, and your hand gets lighter and lighter, and the whole arm will begin to lift in the air, just as if it's being pulled up by a balloon. And the arm will rise and lift straight up, straight up in the air, till it touches your face. And as soon as it rises, the elbow will rest on the arm of the chair. Then the hand will change its direction and move straight up towards your face; slowly moving, and lifting, and rising, higher and higher and higher, lifting and moving and rising straight up in the air, rising higher and higher and higher. A little bit higher now. Straight up, up, up; lifting right up as if a balloon pulls it straight up in the air. Moving up, up, up, and as it moves up, your eyes get heavy; they blink, until you get sleepy, very sleepy. You're going to get so tired and sleepy and drowsy that your eyes will close, and you will go into a deep, restful, relaxed sleep.

Your eyes are blinking now. You feel very tired and exhausted, your breathing now becomes deep and automatic. And as you keep gazing at your hand, you become fascinated with the fact that it's beginning to move without any effort, moving up a little bit higher now than before. Rising and lifting a little bit higher, moving up, just like that; and it will continue to stay up there, a little higher in the same position, moving up, almost as if it's fixed there. And it continues to rise like that, lifting and rising straight up in the air. As you gaze at it, your eyes begin to feel heavy, just as heavy as lead, and you get tired and sleepy. Your arm begins to lift a little higher now. Rising and lifting straight up in the air, rising up higher and higher and higher, right up in the air, moving toward your face, straight up, up, up, straight towards your face.

Your eyes are getting heavier and heavier. They feel as if they are going to close, and you are going to feel very sleepy and tired. You go into a deep sleep. Your hand keeps lifting, but it must not touch your face until you go to sleep, until you feel as if you are in a deep, restful, relaxed sleep. Your eyes are closing, getting heavy. You're getting tired, you're getting sleepy, and the hand keeps moving up, up, up, slowly, rising, and lifting, moving straight up in the air. You're getting drowsier and drowsier and drowsier. You're getting very tired, everything seems to be heavy except your arm which continues to rise and lift. You are getting drowsier and drowsier. Your breathing is getting deeper and more automatic. It's harder and harder to keep your eyes open. They feel like lead now. They are getting tired, and you're getting tired. You are getting drowsier and sleepier. Your head feels like lead. It's getting heavier and heavier and heavier, and your eyelids feel like lead. They're going to feel so heavy that they close and you go into a deep, deep, restful sleep.

You listen to my voice now and pay no attention to other sounds. As you listen to it, you become very, very exhausted. You feel as if you want to go to sleep now. Let yourself go; go to sleep. The hand rises now, moves up towards the face, and the elbow rests on the arm of the chair so that you can support your head against your hand, the palm of your hand. Move the palm of your hand over, and just rest your head there, just like that. You go to sleep, and you get drowsier and drowsier and drowsier, as I talk to you. And you'll stay asleep until I give you the command to wake up. (*Pause*)

Now you'll notice that your left arm is going to get heavy, very heavy, just as heavy as lead, and I stroke it, and as I do it will become heavier and heavier, and more rigid, and more firm. As I pull it out in front of you, it will feel just as if it's made out of steel. You're going to feel as if it's extended right out, and can't move. I'm going to count from one to five. Imagine that you see a bar of steel in front of you. And as I count from one to five, the arm will feel just like steel. One, heavy, stiff; two, stiffer and stiffer; three, as heavy and stiff as steel; four, stiffer and stiffer; and at the count of five, it will become just as heavy and rigid as steel; five, it's so heavy and stiff and rigid that it feels just like a piece of steel. You'll notice that it will be impossible to lift it in the air, even though you try hard. The harder you try, the stiffer and heavier it will feel. And even though you try with all your might to lift it, the heavier you feel it to be, the harder it is to lift. The harder you try to lift, the heavier it will feel. And it's going to be stiff and rigid, just like that, until I give you the command for it to come down. (*Pause*) And now it slowly comes down to your thigh, slowly, just like that, and when I stroke it again, all the rigidity will vanish, and it will become soft again, just like that.

Now you go into deeper sleep, and when I talk to you again you will be more deeply asleep. (*Pause*) Now as I count from one to five, your body will become so heavy, you will not be able to get out of the chair. One, heavy; two, heavy, very heavy; three, rigid; four, heavy, very heavy, very heavy; five, your whole body is heavy, and even though you try to lift up from the chair, the harder you try, the heavier you feel. It's impossible for you to budge out of the chair. Even though you try and you make an effort, the harder effort you make, the more rigid and more heavy you feel. Continue to sleep deep. Now you're going to notice this, too: that it's impossible to talk even when you try hard. The harder you try, the more impossible it will be until I give you the command. I'm going to ask you your name now, and then you will be able to talk, to tell me your name just like a person who talks in his sleep. Now it will be possible for you to talk. What's your name?

Pt. John.

Dr. Good. Continue to sleep now, continue to sleep. Now as you sit there, I'm going to stroke your hand, and as I stroke your hand, your hand is going to start to get numb. The feeling will begin leaving your hand, and as I reach the count of five, it will be as if you are wearing a stiff, heavy leather glove. And as soon as you get the sensation that you are wearing a stiff, heavy, leather glove, as soon as you feel a feeling of numbness in your hand, you'll indicate it by your hand lifting about an inch. You are going to feel the hand getting numb, as if a band is around the wrist, as if a heavy leather glove is on your hand. You will have the sensation that you're wearing a heavy, leather glove on your hand, just as if you're actually wearing a leather glove on your hand. You indicate that to me by the hand rising up just about an inch. Feel, as you visualize this heavy, leather glove, as if there's a pressure on your hand such as a glove would make. As soon as you feel that indicate it by your hand rising up about an inch. (*Patient's hand rises.*) I'm going to prick this hand with a needle. Even though you may doubt that there is a numbness in your hand, you'll be convinced, after I prick your hand, that the sensation in this hand is less than in the other hand. This right hand is going to feel tender and this left hand is going to feel numb. Even though I poke the left hand with a needle very deeply, you will feel no real pain. You will feel pressure, but no real pain. And there will be a contrast to the sensation in your right hand which will be very tender and in real pain. I'll show you. I take your left hand and then I prick it with a pin very deeply. You notice the difference when I prick this other hand with a pin. You notice that difference?

Pt. I do.

Dr. Good, now as you sit there visualize yourself walking along with me on a street. We approach a church yard. As you visualize yourself with me approaching a church yard, indicate that to me by your hand rising up about an inch. (*Hand rises.*) Just picture yourself with me. We walk into the church yard and we look up at the church steeple. We notice a bell, and as you notice the bell moving, you get the sensation that the bell is ringing. Just as soon as you visualize that and get that sensation indicate by your hand rising. Your hand rises.

Now listen closely. Imagine that you are in a theater. Imagine that you are in the fourth or fifth row looking at the stage. And as you look up at the stage you notice that there is a fellow standing up on the edge of the stage watching actors who are behind the curtain. You notice that he has a sensation of horror on his face. A feeling of dread, a feeling of panic comes over him. You notice that he acts extremely frightened. Now as you watch him, suddenly the curtains of the stage open up, and you see what he is frightened of. A little play occurs on the stage in front of you and you see what he is frightened of. As soon as you see the action on the stage, indicate it by your hand rising up about an inch.... Your hand rises up. What did this man see? Tell me about it without waking up. What action was on the stage?

Pt. It looked like the doorman was beating up one of the actor's little babies.

Dr. Someone was beating up one of the actor's little babies. Was there anyone in particular doing that?

Pt. The doorman.

Dr. The doorman was beating up one of the actor's little babies.

Pt. A prop man.

Dr. One of the prop men. Now the curtain closes again, and you notice that this fellow looks happy suddenly, as if he's gotten the greatest thing in this world. It's as if all of his desires, all of his wishes, are gratified. You see an expression of extreme happiness on his face. It's almost as if he sees something that makes him extremely and intensely happy. And you wonder what it is that makes him so intensely happy, so gratifyingly happy. The curtain now opens and you see what makes him happier than anything in the world. No matter what it is, you're going to see action on the stage. As soon as you do, indicate it by your hand rising. Something that makes you intensely happy too. (*Patient's hand rises.*)

Pt. Looks like a lot of people standing around there, and people that are very fond of the guy standing up there.

Dr. People that are fond of the man standing up there.

Pt. They are standing there with their arms out like they're trying to welcome him, or something.

(*The rationale of this technic is first to teach the patient how to fantasy or dream on command, and second to get his own symbols for fear and happiness which will be used to intensify the conditioning process to be used later on.*)

Dr. Trying to welcome him. And he's extremely happy that he's accepted and that he's loved. As you sit there, you're going to listen to my voice and follow the suggestions that I give you. What you've seen, the fantasies, are virtually like dreams. Dreams are thought images in the drowsy state. When I give you a suggestion to dream, you will now be able to dream or to visualize yourself in the front row looking up at the stage like you've done. Or you will actually go into a sufficiently deep sleep to be able to dream. As you sit there, I want you to dream again. The same dream that you had last night. As soon as you've finished that dream, indicate it to me by letting your hand rise about an inch. (*Hand rises.*) Tell me about it.

Pt. There was the girl friend of mine and her young brother in a room. I watch. He's shaking out the table cloth, and she's quite the housewife now. Running around there fixing everything up. He's quite a help to her too.

Dr. He's helping her.

Pt. I think there's somebody standing there with me, a friend of mine is with me.

Dr. A friend of yours is there with you. Now I'm going to talk to you, and it will be possible for you to absorb the suggestions I give you. You have had a problem that has hurt you for a number of years. You've had a problem of bed-wetting. I'm going to give you a suggestion now that you have a sensation almost as if in bed, as if you've wet the bed, then dream a dream that is associated with bed-wetting. Let it come spontaneously, do not force it. Whatever dream comes up, let it come up, and tell me about it as soon as you've had it. (*Pause.*)

Pt. I get a feeling of shame and a feeling of being depreciated for the thing, for wetting.

Dr. You have a feeling of shame and a fear of being depreciated. Now listen to me. You will have increasingly a desire to overcome this shame, and this fear of depreciation. You will have a desire that will grow in strength, and will enable you to get to a point where your desire to control this enuresis, this bed-wetting, will be very strong.

You will do it in this way. When you go to bed at night-time, you will tell yourself that immediately upon having the sensation of wanting to bed-wet, you will have a dream. As soon as the dream begins to appear, which will be before the bed-wetting occurs, your hand will rise, this hand will rise to your face and will touch your face. As soon as your left hand touches your face, you'll open your eyes and you'll wake up. Or your right hand will rise up and touch your face. As soon as your hand rises up and touches your face, your eyes will open up. You'll be awake, you'll stand up and go to the bathroom and urinate. No matter what the reason for the enuresis is, no matter whether you have the desire to wet the bed or whether you do not have the desire to wet the bed, you're going to be swayed by the wish not to feel ashamed and not to have the feeling of depreciation that wetting the bed means to you. And that desire will become gradually so strong, that after going to bed, immediately before bed-wetting, a dream will come to you, and this hand, or this hand, will rise, will touch your face. Your eyes will open before the bed-wetting occurs, so that you will be able to get out of bed, walk to the bathroom and urinate. Do you understand me?

Pt. Yes.

Dr. Good. When you do get up and go to the bathroom,

a feeling of pride will come over you that will be just as strong as the sensation that came to this man when he was on the stage with the arms of people outstretched to him. You will have that same feeling. And that feeling will reinforce the desire that you have to control the bed-wetting. It will reinforce the desire to get to the bathroom. Being able to dream immediately before you have a desire to wet, to let your hand rise and touch your face so that your eyes open up and you go to the bathroom, will give you the same kind of feeling that came over this man when he looked and noticed these people having their arms outstretched to him. Do you understand me?

Pt. Yes.

Dr. At the same time, the desire not to bed-wet, the desire not to wet your bed, will become so strong that it will be just like the fear that overcame the man you fantasied on the stage when he saw the child being beaten with all the unfairness and the cruelty of that act. And the desire not to wet the bed will become extremely strong. It will be as if should you not wet the bed, the child will not be beaten. If you do not wet the bed, you will be able to prevent the child from being beaten. And that will reinforce the desire to get up and go to the bathroom. Now, as you sit there, I'm going to have you reproduce the sensation as if you feel you are about to urinate in bed. As soon as you begin to feel that, you immediately have a fantasy or a dream and your hand will rise, will touch your face, and as it touches your face, your eyes will suddenly open up and you'll awaken. You are going to have that sensation and dream, then your hand will rise, touch your face and awaken you.

(*Patient sleeps a while, then his hand rises, touches his face and his eyes open.*)

Pt. Hello.

Dr. What are you thinking about?

Pt. (*Coughs*) I don't think much about anything. I feel as though I just woke up.

Dr. Just woke up?

Pt. I say, I don't feel as if I'm thinking about anything. I just feel dopey like I do when I wake up in the morning.

Dr. Feel dopey as if you don't want to wake up in the morning?

Pt. I mean the way I do when I wake up in the morning.

Dr. Want to go to the bathroom?

Pt. That's funny, I do.

Dr. Good.

THIRD SESSION (May 16)

Patient has responded to the suggestions given him and has been able to control his enuresis for two days. An attempt is made to transfer control to himself so that he can function symptom-free in the absence of a doctor. There are still no indications as to the dynamic significance of the symptom of enuresis.

Pt. You know it's remarkable, but I haven't wet the bed since I was here. I woke up and I went to the bathroom.

Dr. You woke up and found that you had to go to the bathroom?

Pt. Yes, and it was really strong as though someone advised me to go. And then I had two ways to be; either to let it go on another day or start right off. So I got up to urinate. I would have liked to stay in bed, but I felt I was going to be uncomfortable if I did. Then the last couple of days I've been trying to, you know, stifle the urge. I found I can't wet the bed, I must get up.

Dr. All right, are you conscious of having any dreams?

Pt. No.

Dr. But in the past few nights you've noticed that you, without trying, suddenly find yourself awakened with a full bladder.

Pt. That's right.

Dr. And you go and empty your bladder and feel good after this. Was this automatic?

Pt. No, I'd lay there for a few seconds before I'd get up. Then I'd decide whether to lay there or get up. I mean, of course, it's a lot of annoyance, but I'd rather get up.

Dr. Fine, we're going to continue then, and you will be able to feel less and less annoyance with getting up. If you could get control of your bladder, would you be satisfied?

Pt. Yes.

Dr. You would. You seem to have the desire to overcome this problem, and with that desire, you will be able to overcome it and find it satisfying.

Pt. That's the reason I want to get to see someone like you. Because I think I was getting resigned about the whole thing.

Dr. Resigning yourself to it.

Pt. Yes, then I'd think of the circumstances, you know, and things like that, and I'd realize that it was something that I just had to get taken care of. And see, when I left here the other night, I ran into some friends of mine, and we went out to shoot shuffleboard and drink beer. And I considered that a pretty good test. I was interested to see what the outcome would be. As I went to bed, I made up my mind that if I had the desire to urinate, I would get up; and I did.

Dr. If you have a desire to have the gains continue, they will continue, with reinforcement produced by your coming here. I'm going to teach you the process by which the gains can be continued, so that you, yourself, can reinforce these suggestions by yourself.

Pt. How?

Dr. What I am going to do is transfer the control over to you. I'll virtually be doing that for you. So that even if I'm not around, you will be able to use the same sort of influence on yourself, to permit yourself to get to a point where you can exercise your own complete control over your bladder. You then won't be plagued by these difficulties.

(This statement of mine, as will be seen, constituted a threat to the patient. I was in no position yet to know how dependent he actually was and how he minimized his own capacities to do anything for himself.)

Now, just sit back in your chair and put your hands down on your thighs again, breathe in deeply and watch your hands. Watch everything your hands do, particularly your right hand. As you do, your breathing will get deeper and deeper, and you will fall into a deep, restful relaxed sleep. Your hand is going to start getting light, it's going to start to rise, it's going to rise, it's going to get lighter and lighter. Feel a movement in your hand. As you watch it, you'll get the sensation of the right hand starting to lift, the fingers will begin to lift up a bit as you gaze at your hand.

Your eyes are beginning to get heavy, very heavy. They're tired, and they blink, and at the same time your hand is light, and as it gets light, it begins to lift straight up in the air. It lifts and rises straight up in the air. It's moving towards your face now. As it moves toward your face, your eyes get heavier and heavier, and it's harder and harder to keep them open. They feel like lead. Your hand now rests against your face, and you rest your head against the palm of your hand and go to sleep. Go to sleep. Breathe in deeply and go to sleep, deeply asleep. The sleep gets deeper and deeper and deeper. You will sleep as deeply as you, yourself, wish. I'm going to ask you to sleep this way for a while, and then I'm going to talk to you further. *(Pause)*

Now, as you sit there I'm going to stroke this arm and as I do, the arm is going to start getting stiffer and stiffer and stiffer. I'm going to count from one to five, and at count five it will be so stiff that it will be as rigid as a board. One,

stiff; two, stiffer and stiffer; three, just as stiff as a board;
four, stiffer and stiffer; five, as stiff as a board.   As you sit
there and try with all your might to bend the arm, the harder
you try, the stiffer and heavier it gets.   And it will get heavier and stiffer until I stroke it backwards.   When I stroke
it backwards, it will come right down again to your thigh.
Now I stroke it backwards, and it slowly comes down again
right to your thigh, just this way.

   I'm going to talk to you now and it will be possible for
you to absorb the suggestions that I give you and to utilize
them.

   From your own experience, you know that whatever causes
your bed-wetting, it probably has served a purpose.   It may
have been that the bed-wetting occurred because you were
so firmly asleep that you didn't respond to the normal stimulus of a full bladder.   It may have been that the bed-wetting
was a means of resistence and of stubbornness.   It may have
been that the bed-wetting was something that you wanted
to do because you wanted to do it.   It may have been that
the bed-wetting was a protest that you were weaker than
you should be and hence should be helped.   Or it may have
been that the bed-wetting was a sign of your own aggression.
It makes no difference what the bed-wetting signified.   It
makes no difference what the meaning of the bed-wetting
was if it does have a meaning.   Whether it has a meaning
or whether it has not a meaning, you do know that what the
bed-wetting did to you was to make you feel shameful, to
sap you of your feelings of self respect, and, in the long run,
even though it may have served unconsciously another purpose entirely, it was something that you really did not want.
You wanted to give it up genuinely and honestly.   And
because you wanted to give it up, because you had the desire
to give it up, because you came to me of your own free will,
I was able to help you overcome it for a few days.   These
gains will continue with you.

You will have, when you go to bed, a desire to control your bladder. You may have gone out; you may have drunk beer the way you did the other two nights, or you may not have drunk beer. You may have drunk before you go to bed or you may not have drunk before you go to bed; but before closing your eyes, I want you to have the desire to say to yourself, "I am not going to wet the bed tonight." You want to have that desire, don't you?

Pt. Yes.

Dr. You will then say to yourself each evening, when you go to bed: "I do not wish to wet the bed. I will wake up as soon as I get the signal to go to the bathroom." And you will have the desire to do that, and that desire will come from you, yourself. You, yourself, will have come to the conclusion that you desire it. And when you go to bed, and when you go to sleep, no matter whether you sleep soundly or whether you sleep firmly, no matter if you've drunk or haven't drunk, as your bladder fills up and immediately before you have the desire to urinate, a dream will come to you, or a thought will come to you, that will make your hand, either your right hand or your left hand, want to rise up and touch your face. And when your hand touches your face, you will wake up and your eyes will open, the way they did the other night.

Perhaps you may feel a little bit stubborn, and you may want to feel stubborn about getting out of bed. But in spite of the fact that you feel stubborn about getting out of bed immediately, unconsciously, without thinking of it, you'll weigh the two alternatives. Wetting the bed will be exactly the same thing to you as that image you had of the boy being beaten. It will signify the horror and shame of it.

And it will embody within it all the thoughts you've had about how you had not wanted to wet the bed. And not wetting the bed will come to mean to you that same feeling of pleasure and acclaim as when you saw the people extending their arms toward you, applauding you and being sympathetic and warm toward you. You'll have these as an association to the bed-wetting. And they will reinforce your will and desire to overcome the bed-wetting. That desire will increase, and get bigger and bigger each day, and you will want to control it, you will have a desire to control it. It makes no difference what happens, you'll still have the desire to get up. Possibly you may not have the desire to get up and go to the bathroom, but still these forces will make you want to get up and go to the bathroom. No matter what happens, they'll continue to operate.

You must never get discouraged, if it doesn't happen consistently. You must never get discouraged. You must fight all the harder, if you have any slips; you must fight all the harder, so that there will not be any. Your feelings of self respect, of being a real person, of being able to feel as good as anybody else, of being a person in his own right will come to the fore and make you want to go ahead and not wet the bed, make you want to control your bladder, the way you did the last two nights. And the more you are able to control it, the more firmly imbedded will this control be. And no matter how stubborn you may want to be, you'll be able to express your stubbornness in another area. For instance, it may not be necessary, if you don't want it, for your hand to rise up and touch your face. And if you don't want your hand to rise up and touch your face, you still will be able, immediately before the bladder fills up, to get a signal that will open your eyes. Do you understand me?

Pt. Yes.

Dr. Now, I am going to begin to transfer control over to you, so that you can do the things I do for you. I am going to teach you how to put yourself to sleep and give yourself suggestions to reinforce those I've given you.

(The desire here was to create self control and permit the patient to function symptom-free without needing a doctor to give him suggestions. As will be seen later, his dependency needs conceived of my attempt as tantamount to abandoning him and caused a return of the enuresis temporarily.)

The reason I want you to do this is that it will help you control the bed-wetting better. You will have a desire to control that and to reinforce your desire. You'll get better and better. Controlling it will make you feel more self confident, stronger, happier. You'll feel happier and happier and happier. As the days go by you'll gain more and more self respect. I want to teach you how to do the same thing for yourself, so that when you leave here, after the course of treatments are over, even if you get an emergency call to go away from town tonight, you'll be able to put into practice what I have taught you. As you sit there, I want you to be able to put yourself to sleep and to give yourself the same suggestions I've given you. It may take time before you learn this technic, but I will help you perfect it. It will be possible for you to put yourself to sleep. I want you to sleep for a while. Then I will say: "Now," and you will begin counting from one to ten. Your right hand will slowly get light; it will rise, it will touch your face, your eyes will open at the count of ten. Then say to yourself: "Go into a trance," and you will put yourself to sleep. You'll be able to fall into a deep sleep, and as soon as you fall into a deep sleep, you're going to say to yourself: "I'm going to control myself. I wish to control myself. I will not wet the bed. I do not have a desire to wet the bed. I will be able to control my bladder no matter what it means, no matter how stubborn I want to be, no matter what; but I will be able to control my bladder, and I will not wet the bed."

Then as soon as you've told yourself that, give yourself the suggestion that you have a feeling in your bladder as if you want to urinate. It will stimulate a dream or thought that will make your hand rise and touch your face. As soon as your hand touches your face, it will make your eyes open. Do you understand me?

Pt. Yes.

(*Patient mumbles to himself: "Go into a trance," and his eyes close. Then slowly his arm lifts again and he awakens.*)

Dr. How do you feel?

Pt. Groggy.

Dr. A little groggy. Now if any problems come up, if you feel that there is any other thing besides this enuresis that bothers you, I want you to mention it to me. There may be reasons for this bed-wetting. There may not be; it may just be a bad habit. If there are any reasons for the bed-wetting, we may have to tackle them. If you become aware of other problems besides the bed-wetting, and if you have a desire to go into other problems, bring them to me and we'll go into them.

Pt. All right.

FOURTH SESSION (May 19)

After controlling bed-wetting for several days, the patient slipped up one evening and had enuresis. A dream which followed this slip indicates that he feels like a defeated person and that his enuresis is, at least in part, a sign of resignation, hopelessness and passivity. To bring him to a point where he can see that his urinary symptom has a meaning and serves a function, an attempt at interpretation is made. Furthermore a strong directive effort is made to create in him a motivation to explore and to correct deeper personality problems. This effort is to provide him with the beginnings of insight to offset, as much as possible, a relapse, and to prevent the development of other symptoms to take the place of the enuresis.

Pt. So I slipped up Saturday night. I don't know why.

Dr. You were here on Friday. What happened Friday night?

Pt. I was all right. Well, Saturday was the first time in several days.

Dr. First time in several days that you slipped up. And what about Sunday night?

Pt. No, I didn't wet.

Dr. We have to consolidate the gain. I told you you might have a slip, and that it wouldn't make any difference.

Pt. You know, I almost feel as if it was my own fault because I didn't more or less make up my mind that—I was tired when I went to bed Saturday night. I just wanted to, you know, I dropped off to sleep involuntarily, you know. The other nights I more or less put my mind to it and made up my mind that I would get down out of bed.

Dr. So that we have to tackle the thing of making up your mind before going to bed.

Pt. Yes.

Dr. Well we'll have to use every experience, to learn something from it. For instance, you wet the bed on Saturday night. We should learn something valuable from that to help you. You do have a desire to overcome this thing; you want to overcome it, and I'm very much convinced and so are you that you can overcome it, aren't you?

Pt. Yes.

Dr. It is natural for any person when he goes to sleep to want to stay in bed. It is understandable that when a person goes to bed, he resents getting out of bed. You probably resent that too.

Pt. I believe I do somewhat. I mean, I say to myself that I don't, but maybe actually when I'm in bed half awake, I don't want to get up.

Dr. Yes. How do you look upon that slip? You're not upset by it?

Pt. No, because I don't expect you to go mumbo-jumbo, and I'm all through with it, you know what I mean. And naturally it depends a good deal on myself, too.

Dr. Yes. On both of us. And I'm going to help you to help yourself. Now each night when you go to bed, you do say to yourself: "I'm going to watch myself and control the wetting." The chances are what happened Saturday night is that you went through all the motions and woke up, but probably you were so sleepy that you didn't care, and you closed your eyes and went to sleep again.

Pt. That might very easily have been. Because I— another thing, the more nervous I get, the more frequently I have to urinate, and Saturday I was in a funny frame of mind, unsettled, and I didn't know what I wanted to do.

Dr. Maybe we can work at that. Maybe we can, as a result, settle your nerves, because you do see that there is a link between how nervous you feel and the fact that you have to go to the bathroom more frequently. Did you have any dreams since I saw you last?

Pt. I did have one dream last night. I can't remember it too distinctly, but well, yesterday I was thinking quite a bit about the time I spent in Cuba. I mean, I have been going back and forth to Cuba for about eight months, and I know quite a few girls down there and quite a few people. And I dreamt last night I was with a girl. She had on an evening dress. She was of Cuban or Spanish descent of some kind, you know. But she was speaking with a Brooklyn accent, and I was dancing with her like, and she seemed very distracted as though she was expecting something. I mean I'd be dancing with her, and she'd go away and come right back, and she'd be looking around like this, and all of a sudden a bell rang or something happened at the door, or something, and she went off. And I woke up and I had to urinate at that time.

Dr You had to urinate right at that time when you woke up.

Pt. Yes.

Dr. So in the dream there is a situation in which you're

dancing with a Spanish girl, who has a Brooklyn accent. She looks around almost as if she is distracted, not paying attention to you. A bell rings and she goes away, and you have the impulse to urinate. Can you tell me your ideas about Cuban girls? Do you like them or what?

Pt. Yes, uh-hum, I mean I had quite a few affairs with them. And then I know a couple of decent girls, you know, respectable girls, quite a few, and I thought quite a bit of them and they thought quite a bit of me. I mean there is one girl down there who comes from a very fine family and was in love with me. I used to like her, but there was never any real emotion for her, I mean.

Dr. I see. How do the Cuban girls stack up against the American girls?

Pt. Well, they are nice as a change, but not as a steady diet. I much prefer the American girls to them.

Dr. Is it easy to get to know these Cuban girls? Are they easy to know?

Pt. Because an American down there has got everything on his side, because as a rule any Cuban girl down there thinks much more of an American than they do of their own people. I mean they pride themselves on being able to speak English just so they can come in contact with Americans.

Dr. And an American girl is she different in her whole approach towards men than the Cuban girl?

Pt. I don't know.

Dr. Would you say the American girl is a little more standoffish?

Pt. I think so, yes.

Dr. How have you been able to rate with American girls?

Pt. Well, I like them, but the thing is I've gotten myself so that the ones that I do like, that I did care for, well, sometimes I didn't get along with them, or else I'd lose interest in them, or else I'd find girls whose company I'd like—

the type who were looking for a husband, you know—and I decided, I mean, I don't want to get involved with anyone right now, because I have too much to do ahead of me now. I mean I go around with girls and things and enjoy myself, but I don't have any very really close association with any one girl. I have had, but not too much very recently.

Dr. I see. How do they accept you? How do the girls like you? When you find a decent girl, and it is pretty hard to make the grade with her, how does that work out?

Pt. Well I usually say the heck with her.

Dr. You say, "The heck with her."

Pt. I mean I—I'll tell you the truth—the last time I think I was ever really fond of a girl that I cared for, I mean that I really liked, but I couldn't make out with her. I felt pretty bad about it for a while, but I mean, of course, I got over it. And she made pretty much of a fool out of me.

Dr. She did?

Pt. Yes.

Dr. What did she do?

Pt. Well, I mean, I guess I more or less made a fool out of myself. I mean she was running around on the side like and—

Dr. She was going out with some other men?

Pt. That's right.

Dr. That must have hurt.

Pt. Well, it did, yes, because she was sort of hanging onto me and hanging onto them at the same time, one of those things. I was about seventeen at the time. It was one of those things I thought I'd never get over. (*Laughs*)

Dr. It hit you kind of hard to think that she preferred another man in addition to you?

Pt. At the time, yes. I knew I was making a monkey out of myself and still I went right ahead and did it.

Dr. Maybe you felt you didn't rate with her so much?

Pt. That's right.

Dr. How do you feel about women in general? Do you think you are ever going to get married?

Pt. Oh, absolutely.

Dr. What sort of girl would you marry if you had the chance, I mean if you were to pick the right one? What standards, what ideals do you have?

Pt. Well, I want somewhat of a soul-mate type, you know. The thing that I don't see in a wife is what my aunt out in Ohio is always telling me I should look for. Somebody who can cook, and somebody who can sew, and keep the house clean, and things like that. I mean naturally that's important, but as far as I'm concerned, it's not primary. Somebody whose company I can enjoy, I mean, the kind of an association where sex would be secondary. I mean, I don't, I can't see marrying a woman just because she appeals to you physically or anything like that. But I don't know, I don't think I've ever met anybody yet that I would actually want to take for a wife, probably because I never looked at a girl as being a wife of my own. Because I've never been in a condition and under circumstances where I could look for a wife. But I look at girls now more as friends and companions.

Dr. Perhaps your circumstances have been such that when you found a girl that you felt you really liked very, very much, you felt that maybe they just didn't like you. Have you known women that you felt were just exactly the type that you would have liked?

Pt. Yes.

Dr. Can you recall which?

Pt. Well, do you, are you speaking of like in any particular way?

Dr. You see the reason I bring this up is that the dream seems to indicate certain things about your relations with girls. Here you are dancing with a girl, and it is almost as if in dancing with her you are being close to her. She is looking around as if she is not interested particularly. And then a bell rings, and she just goes away and leaves you flat. Then you have an urge to urinate. It is almost as if you feel, "Here, by God, I'm being left flat. What's the use? I might as well give up. I might as well just urinate in bed and the hell with it." You see what I'm driving at?

> (*An attempt is made here to get the patient to see that there is a dynamic cause for his enuresis, even though the nature of the cause cannot be defined exactly.*)

Pt. Yes. Well I did get up at that time.

Dr. I mean the association between the feeling of despair and urinating.

Pt. I see what you mean, yes.

Dr. And resigning yourself, saying: "I'm a jerk and girls leave me and what's the use. So there is no sense in my getting up out of bed. Might as well go ahead and do this." There may be a link that may be very important in showing you the sources of this thing, giving you a kind of courage not to be so nervous and get over this business of urinating in bed. You see what I mean?

Pt. I get you entirely, sure.

Dr. Because, you know, here you were brought up in an environment—you were brought up mostly by your aunt weren't you? You were brought up in such a way that you probably didn't develop a normal attitude towards yourself. You never got the feeling that you were a pretty good guy, who rated and could have anything mostly that he went after. There is a good possibility that left a scar on you, so that you felt you were inferior to everybody else. You're smiling now.

Pt. You know why I'm smiling, Doc, because the last time I was up here, you asked me to talk over any problems I had when I came in this time. So I've been thinking about them over the week end, you know, and I couldn't think of any definite problem. Just personality traits that I can recognize in myself, and I wrote them down, figuring, you know, so I wouldn't forget them, and there were a couple of things right here that you mentioned.

Dr. Supposing you repeat them to me.

Pt. I wrote them down, so I wouldn't overlook anything 'cause they were fresh in my mind. You take a look at them, yourself.

Dr. All right. Let's see, I'll read what you've written. "One, nervousness. Two, tense drawn up feeling. Three, lack of ability to really concentrate. Four, feeling of insecurity, living from day to day and not really belonging in any home unit. Five, meager self respect. Six, quite often rely on elaborate and convincing excuses to cover up my shortcomings and unwilling to take my medicine. Seven, feel that I have never actually grown up emotionally. This is something I would find it hard to discuss beyond the original statement."

In other words here you have the very things we're talking about. A general feeling of nervousness, tenseness, a feeling that you can't really concentrate, a feeling of insecurity, a feeling of not belonging, of not having anything that you can rely on, not being a part of any home unit. And then meager self respect, and on the basis of your meager self respect, feeling what's the use, you'll fail anyways, and then relying on elaborate and convincing excuses to cover up your shortcomings. Then a feeling that all this is going on, and it is the sort of thing a kid would do, and you don't feel particularly grown-up.

Now a thing like this very often happens to a fellow who is brought up so insecure that he feels that life hasn't got a great deal to offer him. On the one hand, he wants to get himself in a dependent position with somebody who will take care of him, and on the other hand he feels that if he does that, then he's really going to be like a little boy. He doesn't want any part of that. So on the one hand, he wants to get dependent, be little and be taken care of, and on the other hand, he resents that, since that is not what he really wants. He says, "I don't want to be a kid again. I want to be grown-up."

Pt. That is exactly the way I feel about it. I mean it is more or less taking the words out of my mouth.

> (*Patient apparently recognizes poignant personality defects, although he sees no connection between them and his enuresis, and sees no solution for them. An attempt will be made to motivate him for deeper therapy.*)

Dr. The reason what you wrote is important is that I want you to be helped not only in overcoming this urinary problem, but helped to overcome your nervousness, tenseness, and lack of ability to concentrate; helped to grow into a stronger person, which is part of a bigger problem. Just to recapitulate about your symptom of wetting the bed. Wetting the bed is usually the result of a lot of other things that go on in a person, and the average fellow who has this symptom has the feeling of nervousness and tension, not knowing what the blazes is happening to him. But all this is part of a bigger pattern in which he feels he is not secure. There are two common ways of getting security. One is getting linked up with a stronger person who will take care of you, and the other one is growing up and being able to stand on your own feet, being able to be a man and doing things in your own way, plotting your own life.

Now everybody has both of these in a combination. When a child develops, he's little, he's got to be taken care of, he can't do things for himself. Somebody has got to take care of him; he's got to have his needs supplied by somebody, usually the parent. Out of this security, he wants to grow up emotionally and stand on his own feet. If he has no security as a child, he usually does not want to grow up.

Now something happened to you. I don't have to tell you
that you were an insecure kid, and that you just never got
that amount of affection, that amount of tenderness, that
amount of love that made you feel as if you were secure and
you knew where your security was going to be the next minute. Your father died when you were little, your mother
was always busy at work and died when you were thirteen.
You were brought up by an aunt you really didn't like.
You must have been very insecure. You never were convinced anybody liked you. Isn't that so?

Pt. That is absolutely so.

Dr. So that right now you're left with that scar. It's
almost as if emotionally you are seeking to make up what
should have been present when you were little. You may
have a tendency to want to get yourself dependent upon
somebody, to make yourself part of a home unit, as you say.
You never had the feeling that you belonged. Life seems
like a very hollow, empty shell. You've felt depressed, as
if you are not a part of anything. But more importantly
you've felt as if you're licked, that you'll never get what
you want. Why? Because you never had it. But inter-
estingly, you may not even want it right now, because what
you may seem to think you want is a dependent kind of
relationship, but inside of yourself you may think that's a
trap. "That is what a kid does. I don't really want
this at all. It is just that I must fill up an emptiness inside
of me, a need."

Then the other thing of wanting to stand on your own feet
and wanting to be aggressive and assertive, but then feeling
you haven't got the stuff; like saying: "I'm neither fish,
fowl nor herring. I'm nothing. Why struggle? Why
get up at night time and urinate? What's the use? It
doesn't make any difference anyway." You get the angle?

Pt. Yes. It sort of strikes home.

Dr. So that what we have to do really is work at what

is behind this bed-wetting. We can get it cleared up in a short time, but it is important that you straighten out the emotional problems that are behind it. You'll get to a point where, when you go to bed, you'll very deliberately say to yourself, "Come what may, under any circumstances, I'm going to get out of bed, and I'm not going to collapse in helplessness and wet my bed." But more important, we've got to correct this helplessness inside of you, this insecurity, that makes you feel that life isn't worth a damn thing. We've got to correct the notion that it is no use going on the next day.

Pt. You know, it's this feeling I get, Doc, I mean, to start I'm not stupid, I mean, I know that. It's been proven to me, like I took a superior rating on my I.Q. test. I was commissioned in the Maritime when I was nineteen. I made Chief Purser when I was twenty, and I was on a scholarship up in college. You know how I feel? I feel as though I'm full of potentialities, and it is just some thing that won't let me go ahead, just sort of pulling me back.

Dr. Almost as if there were something pulling you back.

Pt. That's right.

Dr. Well, we've got to try to find out what the heck this thing is that holds you back. Maybe we will be able to get clues to that, so that you'll be able to correct this feeling of insecurity within yourself, and establish good kinds of relationships. Because, you know what happens to a person who has this type of problem? They get themselves tied up with people and form the wrong kind of relationships. For instance, supposing you go and find a woman and you feel she is the right sort of woman. You believe you'll be part of a family unit, and then you make yourself act little, be just a child to her. You become her little boy.

Now when that happens, you're likely to find that you get mad at her for letting you become a little boy. And you resent it very much because you don't want to be a little boy.

You're a grown man, and you've got a lot of good stuff in you. You've got a lot of drive, and you are a masculine person. But your emotions tend to make you feel as if you are not. They make you feel that you want to be little. There may be a link between the feeling of not being satisfied, giving up, and bed-wetting. You are smiling now.

Pt. It strikes home.

Dr. All right, now, supposing you go to sleep for me. Supposing you put yourself to sleep as you sit there. You know how to do that. Keep telling yourself that you're getting drowsy and tired. Watch your hand, and slowly count from one to ten, and as you go from one to ten, very slowly, you will notice that your hand is getting lighter. It will begin to lift a little. It will rise straight upward toward your face, until it touches your face, and just as soon as it does that, your eyes will suddenly get heavy, you give a sigh, doze right off and go to sleep. When you're asleep, and your hand has reached your face, I'm going to give you suggestions that will enable us to get more of an idea of what goes on inside of you. (*Pause*)

You're counting from one to ten; your hand rises and touches your face. Now you're asleep, and as you sit there, your breathing will get deeper and deeper and deeper, and you go into a very deep, restful, relaxed comfortable sleep. As you sleep, you're going to find it possible to follow the suggestions that I give you, because you know that they are going to be of help to you.

As you sit there, I'm going to stroke your left arm. When I stroke your left arm, you'll begin to notice that it gets stiffer and stiffer. When I count from one to five, it will be so stiff that it will remain frozen. It won't budge. One, stiff; two, stiffer and stiffer; three, stiff as a board; four, stiffer and stiffer; five, just as stiff and rigid as a board. Even though you try to move it, it will remain exactly as it is, until I give you the command to bend it. It is getting heavy and stiffer and stiffer.   Now it is going to lose its rigidity.   Slowly it comes down.   Just like that.

You are going to notice something very interesting. Imagine that you have a boil on your finger, right over here, and imagine that you go to a doctor to have the boil opened since it causes you a lot of pain.   The doctor injects novocain right around your wrist, like this, to create a wrist block, to create anesthesia in your hand.   As you sit there, imagine that the hand gets more and more numb, and that the feeling leaves your hand.   Imagine that the feeling leaves your hand.   I'm going to count from one to five.   At the count of five, you'll have a sensation of wearing a stiff heavy leather glove.   Then I'm going to poke the hand with a needle, and you'll notice that it will be numb, so numb that you will not feel pain.   One, two, three, four, five.   I'm going to jab this now, and you'll notice that there will be a distinct difference when I poke this left hand as compared with this right hand. Do you notice that?

Pt.   Yes.

Dr.   Now listen carefully to me.   When you came to see me, you had a symptom of bed-wetting which you wanted to get rid of.   It was very uncomfortable, it made you feel small and hopeless.   Through the medium of suggestion we were able to control that symptom so that right now, under the proper circumstances, if you have the will and the desire to control this symptom, you will be able to do so.   Do you understand me?

Pt.   Yes.

Dr.   You will at nighttime, then, give yourself the suggestion that come what may, even if you don't want to get up out of bed, even though you may feel that things are hopeless, that you are nervous and irritable, you still will get up and go to the bathroom.   You will go to bed with the idea that immediately before your bladder gets filled up, either a dream or a sensation will cause your eyes to open, and you will then want to get up and go to the bathroom. Perhaps your hand will rise and touch your face, but if you don't want your hand to rise, it will not have to rise. Going to the bathroom to prevent wetting is something that is important for you. Not going to the bathroom will be symbolic to you of being a beaten person. But going to the bathroom will make you feel like an acceptable, lovable person. You will have no desire to be a beaten person. You will improve until you can control your bladder, even if you decide to wait until the morning before going to the bathroom.

Now let us examine why you had that slip on Saturday. On Saturday you told me that you felt very shaky, nervous and unstable. Now what seems to have happened was that something occurred within you or outside of you that made you feel weak and inferior, as if there was no use. The fact that you felt this way probably made you feel that in spite of your desire to get out of bed and not wet, it didn't make any difference anyway. Do you follow me? (*Patient nods.*) In other words, what actually seems to have happened to you was that you resigned yourself to the belief that you were a beaten person and that it didn't make any difference anyway. So what was the use.

I'm going to give you some very, very strong suggestions, because this seems to be one of your chief problems. If you follow these suggestions, then you will be able to control bed-wetting, because we will then be able to control its cause. Because of what happened to you when you were a child, you never had the feeling that you got the proper amount of tenderness, or love and understanding. You became insecure and felt that nobody liked you, even though your aunt and other people were demonstrative toward you. They still did not instill in you sufficient security for you to feel you were a likable person. You interpreted this lack as being a beaten person, and your wetting the bed may have been indicative of the fact that you felt like a beaten person.

So that nowadays, the moment you feel you have quality or worth, as if you're an intelligent person, you suspect it. However, it does make you want not to give up, not to wet the bed, not to collapse, at least for a short while, even though you suspect it is not so. You always feel like a beaten person, because you never had the type of upbringing that really made you feel secure.

So what does a person do who has a problem like this? He would like to belong. He believes he must get security through other people, maybe even by getting the kind of mothering he never got. But he feels somehow inwardly he may not rate this thing, that maybe people won't like him. He may feel that a worth while woman, perhaps, won't like him, and then he begins to feel a little resentful of that and gets embittered. You have problems in your relations with women that may be like that.

I'm going to give you a strong suggestion in addition to that of controlling the urination. I want you to look into and examine all the facts in your case, to see if it isn't true that you have felt so insecure that you want a dependent kind of relationship with someone. I want you to inquire to see if automatically you feel you are going to be rejected because you're not worth while, because you feel as if you're a beaten person. I'm going to suggest to you that you do those things that will make your estimate of yourself grow. Inquire into yourself and see if what you actually experience now is not a product of your upbringing, a product of your training, a product of the fact that when you were little, you felt you didn't get the proper amount of love.

I want you to examine all the facts to see if you aren't really a different kind of person now than you were then. If you do that, you may be able to feel more self confident, stronger, and more able to be on your own, more capable of making the grade with any kind of girl, Cuban or Brooklyn. However, it is going to be a struggle, because this thing cannot be overcome in a period of a few weeks or so. But if you see that your ideas are due to misconceptions on your part, if you understand that, then you will have a chance to correct your difficulties. You must not give up. You must tackle this thing no matter how long it takes, in order to develop an entirely different attitude towards life, towards people and towards yourself. You must test your idea that you are a beaten person and see if you are not really a very likable and acceptable person. You will be likable and acceptable if you, yourself, think so. Because if you do, people will respond to you positively. But if you feel that you are a beaten person inside, you're likely to become antagonistic and automatically feel that people think you are a beaten person. It will all originate from within yourself then. I want you to think that over and see what you feel to be true, so you can correct the conditions that start your bed-wetting, that make you feel like a beaten person, that make you feel helpless.

The reason this is important for you is that you want to lead a normal life. If you solve your problems, you will feel you can have a nice relationship with a worth while girl or with people in general. You then will feel capable of leading an entirely different kind of life. There will be no need for you to run away, no need for you to retreat. You will be able to choose a type of work that will bring you into relationship with people whom you really like. You may even be able to find a girl friend who is the right sort of a girl for you, who merits your love.

> (*An attempt has been made here to create the incentive in the patient to work more deeply with his personality problems by showing him that his urinary symptom is merely a by-product of more fundamental issues. Even though he may not accept the need for more therapy at this time, the hope is that he may come around to it later on.*)

I'm going to give you a strong suggestion then that you become able, not only to control the urination, but to tackle this whole estimate of yourself, and develop a more hearty

respect for yourself as a human being.   You understand me?
And do you want to do that?

Pt.   Yes, I do.

Dr.   I think it is excellent for you to want to do that, because it will give you a more permanent cure.   Because we
can control this urination, but as long as you feel like a
beaten person who doesn't rate, you're always going to say,
"What's the use?"   And you'll have slips.   Mind you, every
time you have a slip, every time you wet your bed, you should
go over what has happened to you during that day.   You'll
see that there are reasons for it.

I'm going to give you a strong suggestion then in two directions.   First, at nighttime, before you go to bed, you must
tell yourself you are not going to let yourself wet your bed.
The moment you get any kind of sensation or a feeling that
you are going to wet your bed, open your eyes, and even
though it is hard to get out of bed, even though you don't
want to get out of bed, you will force yourself to get up, go
to the bathroom and relieve your bladder.   Then you will
be able to go back to your bed and sleep comfortably.   The
second suggestion is that you will want to understand yourself better, the causes for this thing, and want to search
yourself and your reactions to consolidate your gain.

You will be able to do this by yourself, when the proper
time comes.   Right up to this time I'm going to help you
with it.   But, as we go along, you will develop more and more
strength within yourself.

I'm going to count now from one to five.   At the count of
five, you'll have a sensation as if you have to go to the bathroom.   As soon as you get that sensation, or just before you
get that sensation, your hand will rise, touch your face, your
eyes will open and you'll wake up.   One, two, three, four,
five.   (*The patient's hand rises, touches his face and his eyes
open.*)   How do you feel?

Pt.   Sleepy.

Dr. Now what do you think of all I've been talking about?

Pt. Well, I think you've been telling me just what I've been trying to tell myself. I mean things I just couldn't grasp, because I was so close in my own self.

Dr. And you've got to lick this thing, don't you? There is no reason why you can't lick this thing. You've got to lick it, not only from the standpoint of controlling the symptom, urination, but from the standpoint of your personality. It is a shame that a fellow like you just drifts around and does not permit himself to feel what you should feel about yourself.

FIFTH SESSION (May 22)

The patient's response to the last session is indicated in a dream in which he regards self sufficiency as a heroic gesture totally outside his immediate grasp. He craves a dependency relationship. It is apparent from the material that comes up, that his enuresis is a symptom that serves many purposes. Particularly it is an expression of his feelings of helplessness with a plea for support from a good parental figure. Because of the short-term nature of the therapy, an attempt is made to create an attitude in the patient in which he feels secure and lovable as a grown-up person who can control his bladder. The positive dependent relationship is used as a means of getting the patient to abandon his symptom. The hope is that the auxiliary insights he has gained in therapy will permit him to grow emotionally to a point where he wants to be self sufficient and assertive in his own right, and does not need to gain security through the agency of another individual.

Pt. I don't understand it. I wet again on Wednesday.

Dr. Well, supposing you bring me up to date. You were here last?

Pt. Monday.

Dr. And on Monday night?

Pt. I was O. K.

Dr. And Tuesday?

Pt. O. K. but not on Wednesday.

Dr. Monday was O. K., Tuesday was O. K., but Wednesday was no good.

Pt. That's right.

Dr. Perhaps we can find out something important about why you wet. As you remember we discussed the fact that there are reasons for a thing like wetting. Did you dream?

Pt. Yes, here's the dream, Doc. I was so damned sure when I went to sleep last night that I would get up if I had to. I was tired. I was out shooting shuffleboard and drinking beer. I wasn't intoxicated, I didn't even feel it. I woke up once early in the morning, but this happened at night, and I was pretty tired when I went to bed. I, I don't know how you feel about it, I think the thing for me to do now is to, not to try to press too hard the good your treatments are doing me, until I get a little confidence in myself.

Dr. Absolutely.

Pt. Because, ah, well, Tuesday night I was out with my cousin. We went out shooting shuffleboard in a tavern, and I came home and I was perfectly all right.

Dr. Well, something happened to you; something happened to you so that, on Wednesday, yesterday, your feeling about yourself suffered. Something happened to you that made you feel as if you were less than the person you actually want to be. And what happened to you?

Pt. I can't understand it. I, you see, yesterday, about noontime, I came over to New York and went to a movie. Then I went home, had supper, went up to a friend's house and helped him fix up his motorcycle. I came back and decided I wanted to shoot shuffleboard. And, ah, I got home about two o'clock in the morning.

Dr. You got home about two o'clock in the morning. What about the dreams since I saw you last?

Pt. Yes, gee, Tuesday night I had three crazy ones. I remembered, which is unusual, because I don't usually remember what happens. You want to hear about it? Well, the first one was kind of vague, and I remember walking. It looked like a plantation home, you know. It was very dark and gloomy, trees and shrubs. And there were three elderly knights sitting around a round table on the porch. And I walked up there with a package, a couple of packs of chewing gum. I was sitting on the table in front of me, like this now. I was sitting there with my hands on the table holding them like this. And this one fellow started telling some kind of a weird story. They were elderly men and I knew that there was a clarinet playing in the back. It sounded like it was coming from the house, and it had sort of almost like a human voice quality at times. That's as much as I remember about that one.

But the second one I had was: there was this other fellow and myself, and we were scheduled to put on a performance, at some time in the very near future, which consisted of jumping out of an airplane. It was from a parachute, from the, what I considered at the time, the phenomenal height of one mile. And, ah, this was supposed to be done in some kind of a suit. It looked to me like a diver's uniform, you know, without the helmet on. And we had a distance to travel before we got there where we were going to put on this show. Everyplace we got to, there was a lot of people around, you know, to celebrate, and we're on our way passing through their town. We got off a boat, and went through the town. I don't remember if I actually jumped with the parachute, or whether I just imagined what it would be like if I did, but I could feel myself jumping out. You know, the thing wrenching, and counting to ten, you know, as I'm coming down. One, two, three, four, five like that. I was dreaming it, and I think that's about when I woke up there.

But the third one is the beaut. I was dreaming it. (*Laughs*) The other one was little Annie Rooney in the funny papers. Anyhow she's a little orphan, and there's this cruel woman runs an orphan home, Mrs. Meaney. And she's always chasing her, you know, trying to get her back to the orphan home. Well, I dreamt that Charlie Ruggles, the movie actor, was going to adopt me. (*Laughs*) And this Mrs. Meaney was after me. And there was Barbara Stanwyck sort of protecting me, too, you know. I could see myself laying on the lawn and hiding behind a bush. And she was staring around there trying to distract this woman. And I was old as I am now, I mean, in the dream. He was going to adopt me, to keep me, keep her from dragging me off.

> (*One might speculate that the dream is a response to the last session. The elderly men may symbolize myself pronouncing truths which sound weird to the patient. Being self sufficient is anathema to him at this time and is symbolized as doing something heroic like jumping from an airplane. In the third part of the dream, he identifies himself with the orphan in the comic strip, "Little Annie Rooney," who escapes Mrs. Meaney (possibly his aunt and other parental figures toward whom he has felt ambivalent) and is rescued by Charles Ruggles (possibly myself, with whom patient may envisage the idealized type of dependency relationship).*)

Dr. And where did Barbara Stanwyck come into this thing? She was going to adopt you, too?

Pt. No, she wasn't. Charlie Ruggles was going (*laughs*) to adopt me, but she was more or less just helping me out, you know. Hiding me.

Dr. She was helping you out, hiding you from this Mrs. Meaney?

Pt. That's right.

Dr. And in the first part of the first dream. There were three elderly men sitting there, you said, and while they were talking, you didn't believe anything they said?

Pt. I really can't remember.

Dr. Well what was it that they were talking about?

Pt. I don't remember, but it was some kind of a revelation, it sounded, you know, as something you could imagine one of the old prophets sitting there discoursing on, you know. And I don't remember just what it was about, but I think that was the frame of mind they put me in, that it was something like that.

Dr. And what this man said was, was it true? Did you feel it was true?

Pt. I believe I did, yes.

Dr. Then in the second dream, you were supposed to begin a performance of jumping out of an airplane, and people were cheering you as you went by.

Pt. Yes, on our way over there, you know, as if this was that they were going to prove to me that I was a pretty good guy.

Dr. And then in the third dream, you are going to be adopted by Charles Ruggles.

Pt. Yes.

Dr. So in the first dream an elderly man makes certain revelations to you. In the next dream you are supposed to do something quite heroic, quite a brave thing. And in the third dream you're taken over and adopted—just like a little boy—taken care of. Last time we had been talking about your feeling alone and helpless, wanting a kind of relationship in which you were taken care of. Have you thought any more about being alone? Have you thought any more about being without anybody to turn to?

Pt. No, as a matter of fact, I've felt less alone than before.

Dr. You felt less that way.

Pt. I mean I felt like I, I can look at a thing myself and say, "What the hell, you're a grown guy now."

Dr. Well, do you recall what we were talking about last time?

Pt. Oh, yes.

Dr. All right, supposing you give me an idea of what I said to you then. And what you feel is true.

Pt. You mean about the fact that I have two traits in

my personality? One, that I want to be alone and independent on my own, feel like a grown man. The other that
I've got, I want somebody to care for me and want to have a
feeling that I'm dependent on somebody, that somebody is
there to care for me.

Dr. Yes.

Pt. Is that what you meant? I'm sure it's so.

Dr. Well, now, the dreams that you had on Tuesday
night seem to be indicative of those two things. The revelations you listened to, may have been what I said to you last
time. I'm a combination in the dream of the three men
making revelations to you, a little boy. And the revelations
may refer to the content of the other two dreams. One, the
second dream, if you're strong, if you're independent, if you
do something pretty brave, heroic, like jumping from an airplane, people will applaud you. Two, the third dream,
making yourself dependent upon somebody, being a little
boy, which is diametrically opposed to the other thing.

Now something maybe happened to you Monday or
Tuesday which possibly made you feel you were a little boy,
something maybe happened that either undermined your
self confidence or made you feel something as if there was no
use. As if you said, "I never will be able to be independent,
it's something like jumping out of an airplane. It's so
damned far away, I've got so far to travel, I've got so great
a distance to go, I don't know if I'll ever be able to jump out
of the airplane." And still the other part, you may feel is
dangerous for you, too. You don't want any part of being
anybody's little boy. It is like being adopted again and
being taken into an orphan asylum and being treated in a
very summary way.

So here you have these two opposite things working in you
at the same time. Part of you wants to be the little boy,
part of you really wants to be adopted and wants to be taken
care of. It's understandable why that's so, because you had
been a very insecure kid, all your life. That's the part that

may sabotage your desire to control this bladder business, the bed-wetting.

Supposing you tell me how you get along with other people. First, with your men friends.

Pt. Swell.

Dr. You don't feel inferior to them?

Pt. No, as a matter of fact my cousin was telling me the other day—my cousin is my best friend, you know, of my own age, he was the one that introduced me to all these fellows when he was going to school, and I've been palling around with them for years now—and he told me one day, he said that they actually consider me superior to them. I get along swell with them, I mean, they think I'm a swell fellow, and I think they're great guys, too.

Dr. How about girls?

Pt. I do really think I do have kind of a feeling of inferiority. I believe I do. I've had a good number of pleasant associations with girls, have had girls fall in love with me and things like that, girls I like. But it's more so recently that I feel more distracted, more. Makes me feel as though It wouldn't want to take the emotional responsibilities of having a girl, do you know what I mean?

Dr. As if you don't want to take the emotional responsibilities of having a girl friend?

Pt. That's it.

Dr. Well, what would that involve for you?

Pt. Well, the thing is that I figure this way. There'd be certain things I'd have to say, certain promises I'd have to make, and things like that. I've got years ahead of me yet before I can ever think of closing up the thing the way it should be and marry. And that, well quite often I go to a girl and ask her why I lose taste for her, you know. I mean, somehow I'll go all out for her one hour, and then suddenly something better will come along, or I'll get tired of it and just close it off.

Dr. So that you don't really want to be tied down?

Pt. No.

Dr. Do you think that's the big thing?

Pt. That is probably the big thing.

Dr. So you don't want to get yourself involved in the situation where you'll be tied down, and the other thing is that you don't know if you'll make the grade or not.

Pt. That's right, doctor.

Dr. When did you go out with a girl last?

Pt. Oh, a couple of weeks ago.

Dr. Couple of weeks ago.

Pt. I stayed up there two days. I'd get up in the morning and she'd rush around. "Why don't you eat something? Why don't you have some of this?" You know, fussing and fuming at me.

Dr. And you don't want to get into a situation like that with any woman?

Pt. Not particularly.

Dr. To get yourself tied down. Well, you are a young fellow, and there's no reason in the world why you should get yourself tied down if you don't want to. On the other hand there's no reason why you shouldn't go out with girls if you want to. Do you feel powerless to be able to resist them if they insist that you marry them?

Pt. Yes.

Dr. But you don't really feel powerless, if you really want to avoid getting yourself tied down, you can tell them that, can't you?

Pt. Sure. Well the way I feel about the thing, I'd go to a lot of trouble to save somebody's feelings, if you know what I mean.

Dr. That you feel powerless to cope with some women?

Pt. I never thought too much about marriage. I mean it's sort of in my relationships with the girls I've gone with as a forerunner of marriage.

Dr. Well what about your occupation. Is seamanship the sort of thing you want to do all the time?

Pt. Absolutely not. I don't. The only reason I'm
doing it was because, well, I did it during the war, and the
only reason I stuck in it as long as I have now is that I was
just saving some money to go back to school, you see.

Dr. You are going back to school? What course are
you going to take?

Pt. I'm going to take up business or finance. I like that
kind of work. I worked for a, in a steamship office as a
paymaster, and I like that kind of thing. When I went to
school at first, up in Michigan, I wanted to be a doctor. My
mother was a nurse, and I was brought up in that atmosphere, you know, and I thought I'd like it. She liked the
idea, too. On my own I'd never have the money for it, and
it would take a good deal of time to get through. I've developed a distaste for it because I had to do that kind of thing
too during the war.

Dr. There is no reason why you can't go ahead with your
education, especially as you get a clearer idea about yourself.
Your life has apparently been ruled by diametrically opposed things that have caused you to veer from one to the
other and get nowhere. You will be able to handle your life
a great deal better, and you'll be able to see that you've been
going around in circles as we go on. There's nothing wrong
with you basically. Now if you can tackle this thing and see
it through clearly, it's going to mean a great deal to you.

As far as the bed-wetting is concerned, I think we have a
better idea of what it means. It is a sign to you that you
are just a wash-out, so it doesn't make any difference to you
if you do wet. Also it may be a means of asking for support
out of helpless feelings.

We are going to control this bed-wetting, so that under no
circumstances will you permit it to get the best of you. No
matter what the meaning of this thing is, you'll wake up and
open your eyes. You won't close them and go to sleep again
— which is probably what you did when you slipped up—
until you've gone to the bathroom. Even if you have to

walk in your sleep, you'll get up and go over to the bathroom. And that will be important for you to do. Later on you may not have to go, but can retain without wetting. We'll reinforce those suggestions, and then I want you to try it on your own after that. Call me up once in a while and tell me how things go.

Now, in the event you'd like to work out more concretely what this is all about, I mean how you function and other aspects of your personality, you will require a different type of therapy along psychoanalytic lines. Psychoanalysis costs a lot of money, but I will try to find a therapist whose fees are not too high. I hope you will be interested in wanting to go ahead with your personality development. As far as the enuresis is concerned, the chances are that it will get less and less, and it will probably disappear completely. But that you've got to correct this personality difficulty, too, in order to be well completely goes without saying.

Pt. You know, doctor, if you're thinking of switching me over because of your high fee, I mean that's—doesn't matter.

Dr. I don't want to switch you over. When we've controlled the enuresis, you can decide what you want to do.

Pt. I mean, that's entirely secondary with me, I mean the low cost.

Dr. I won't switch you over, unless we talk things over and decide between us that is what is best. All right now, supposing you go to sleep now. Just watch your right hand now, and as you gaze at it, you'll begin to notice that it will slowly move. And as you keep watching it, your hand will get lighter and lighter and lighter. It rises now, and you are asleep. Supposing you sleep for a while, and when I talk to you next you will be more deeply asleep. (*Pause*)

Listen carefully to me. A person carries within him every memory and every experience that he's had in all his life. It makes no difference how far back we want to go, there is in the mind an imprint of every experience the person has gone through. The fact that you can't remember it, doesn't mean that it's not there. You, yourself, have noticed, for instance, that sometimes you forget certain things, and then all of a sudden they pop into your head. You've noticed that, haven't you?

Pt. Yes.

Dr. Now you have to ask yourself, where can these memories go? They are a part of your unconscious mind, and they're there all the time. There are many, many things in your past that are really not forgotten. Perhaps there are some which are important to you. I'm going to give you a suggestion now to go back back into your life to a point when you were a little boy. It is possible to turn back time like the pages of a book. As I talk to you, you'll feel yourself getting little. You'll feel yourself getting smaller and smaller and smaller. You'll feel yourself getting so tiny and so small that you feel just like you did when you were six years of age. I'm going to count slowly from one to five, and at the count of five, I want you to have the experience of being a little boy. As soon as you have that experience, whatever day you happen to go back to, indicate it by your hand rising. One, you're getting very little now; your head gets little, your arms get little, your legs get little; you get tiny, very tiny. Two, you are getting littler and littler and littler; you're getting smaller and smaller. Three, tinier, and tinier still. Four, smaller and smaller and smaller. Five, very, very tiny. And now as you feel yourself getting small, as soon as you feel that you are exactly six years of age, indicate it to me by your hand rising. I'm somebody that you know and like and you are exactly six years of age. As soon as you feel that you are six indicate it to me by your hand rising. (*Hand rises.*) Your hand rises. How old are you?

Pt. Six.

Dr. What grade are you in?

Pt. Second.

Dr. What's your teacher's name?

Pt. Miss Maden.

Dr. Do you have any friends in the second grade?

Pt. A few.

Dr. Can you, can you give me their names?

Pt. John, Tom.

Dr. Well, now, as you sit there, tell me something about your parents.

Pt. My father's dead.

Dr. How long ago did he die?

Pt. Six months.

Dr. Six months ago. How do you feel about that?

Pt. I don't know.

Dr. What about your mother? Is she alive?

Pt. Um.

Dr. Does she take care of you?

Pt. My aunt.

Dr. Your aunt takes care of you. Do you like your aunt?

Pt. No.

Dr. What did she do to you?

Pt. I'm always getting hell for something.

Dr. You're always getting hell for something. Are you afraid of her?

Pt. Yeah. She got a new baby.

Dr. What about that new baby?

Pt. I feel like it's a strange little animal.

Dr. You don't like that baby?

Pt. No, no.

Dr. Do you feel that she pays any attention to you, now that she's got the baby?

Pt. Yeah.

Dr. But you don't care for that baby, anyway. All

right, now as you sit there, how about bed-wetting at night?
Do you wet the bed at night now?

Pt. Uh huh.

Dr. You wet the bed. Well when did you start the bed-
wetting? How long ago?

Pt. I think I never stopped.

Dr. You never stopped; you wet all the way through.

Pt. I think so.

Dr. Now, as you sit there, I'm going to ask you, as a little
boy, to dream. And I'm going to ask you to dream the same
kind of dreams you have while you're bed-wetting, or before
you're bed-wetting, if you have any dreams. If you don't
have any dreams, then you won't dream, and you'll show me
that by your hand rising. If you have dreams, dream the
same kind of dreams that you have. If you don't have any
dreams, the hand will rise. Go ahead. (*Pause.*)

Pt. I used to dream.

Dr. I can't hear you, talk a little louder.

Pt. I used to dream now. I was scared or something.
Somebody was blaming me, or someone that I was afraid of,
the teacher or someone.

Dr. That somebody was blaming you, or that you were
afraid of something?

Pt. I don't know. Somebody made me do things that
I didn't want to do. I had to do what they said.

Dr. They made you do things you did not want to do?
All right, now I'm going to give you another suggestion.
When you grow older, when you wake up, you're going to
start getting over that fear of being blamed and feeling you
have to do everything they want you to do.

That fear started because you were little and your aunt
was big, because you were small and your teachers were
large, because you felt like a little boy. I'm going to give
you a strong suggestion that you feel I like you and you can
trust me. You're going to feel I like you and I want to help

you. Also you can be yourself. You don't have to be a baby to have me like you. You will feel I will like you even if you act like a big boy. You will feel I will like you more if you are a big boy and don't wet.

(*Here the positive relationship is being utilized as a means of getting the patient to abandon a symptom to gain love and approval. There is a strong possibility that the patient's enuresis is the product of a feeling of helplessness, a resignation to this helplessness as well as a desire for it, in order to win support from adults around him. Genetically it may have started as protest against the coming of a younger sibling, with a desire to return to the status as a wetting infant on a dependency level. The enuresis, therefore, probably occurs in relationship to a parental figure, either as a plea for support on the basis of infantile helplessness, or as aggression against the adult for curbing, frightening, abandoning and infantilizing him. Since the therapy is, because of lack of time, on a short-term basis, and since the patient, at this period, regards self sufficiency as a threat [as evidenced in his dream], establishing a relationship with me on a dependency level, and utilizing the relationship to remove the symptom may be all that can be accomplished at this time. Whereas previously enuresis served to win love and support on the basis of helplessness, my aim is to make abandonment of enuresis a condition that will win my acceptance of him. At the same time the hope is to orient him toward self sufficiency, and this may require further treatment later on.*)

Now you will begin to grow up again, you get older and older, until you are the same age as today. You are deeply asleep. I'm going to ask you soon to open your eyes and still be asleep. I will then show you a red bottle. As you watch it, it will change color to green. A person is capable of opening his eyes even if he is asleep. You will be able to open your eyes and you still will be asleep. I'm going to show you a red bottle, and as you look at this red bottle, you will be able to see the red color turning into green. As soon as you see the red color turn into green, your eyes will become heavier and heavier, and then will close. I am going to show you a bottle now. Here is a bottle. Open your eyes and as soon as you see the red bottle turning into green, your eyes will close and you'll go back to sleep. (*Patient opens his eyes and is shown a bottle with red medicine. He blinks his eyes, then slowly closes them.*) Did you see the color change?

Pt. Yes.

(*The reason for this suggestion is merely to test the depth of hypnosis and to see if any resistance has been stirred up as a result of previous suggestions, which resistance might be reflected in a refusal to conform with the present suggestion. Should resistance have been manifested, I would suspect the patient might resist my therapeutic suggestions, and I would then have to discover the reason for the resistance.*)

Dr. Now go to sleep very deeply again. I am going to give you a suggestion that you dream. As soon as you've had a dream, you'll suddenly wake up, but you will not remember the dream until I tap on the side of my table this way (*knock, knock, knock*) three times. The dream will then pop up into your mind. Tonight, before you go to bed, I want you to give yourself a suggestion that no matter what happens, no matter how you feel, the moment you have the urge to go to the bathroom, the instant before you even have a desire to go to the bathroom, before you wet yourself, one of the hands will rise up and strike your face, hard enough to arouse you. You will feel if you control your bladder from now on that you are the kind of person who deserves those things you want from life. It will be possible to control your bladder. Do you understand me?

Pt. Yes.

Dr. I am going to count from one to five, and at the count of five start dreaming. As soon as you've had the dream, open your eyes and wake up. But do not remember the dream until I tap on the table three times. At the third tap the dream will suddenly pop into your head. One, two, three, four, five, start dreaming. (*Pause. Then patient opens his eyes and rubs them.*) How do you feel?

Pt. O.K. Sleepy.

Dr. Feel sleepy? What comes to your mind?)

Pt. It's a blank.

Dr. What now? (*Taps made on table three times.*)

Pt. A dream, I could see eyes looking at me. Almost look like my own. I see this lighted parapet, you know, it was all inside of some place where the window had a stained glass. Something like you'd probably see in a tower of a castle. I was looking at it from the inside. That was the only source of light coming through there. I never had a dream like that before.

Dr. Eyes staring at you?

Pt. Yes.

> (*It will be remembered that the patient saw a number of eyes in his responses to the Rorschach cards. No paranoid manifestations have been in evidence, although these might be latent. It is possible that they are a symbol of a feeling of being watched which reflect his guilt over inner desires or demands. The watching eyes possibly are both those of authority and, as the dream indicates, his own conscience, at being in a forbidden castle, which may have something to do with secret gratifications he envisages, perhaps through the medium of the therapeutic relationship.*)

Sixth Session (May 23)

> Patient has responded favorably to my manipulation of the transference. A strong directive effort is made to get him to control his symptoms, and he spontaneously mentions that he is beginning to feel more respect for himself.

Pt. Hello.

Dr. How are you?

Pt. Fine. I didn't wet. But I'd like to tell you about the last time. I mean, it impressed me very strongly. I remember the dream I had. And I remember the talk we had at the beginning. Not too much about it, though. I don't want to be transferred to another doctor.

Dr. I don't want you to feel that you are going to be transferred to anybody else. I want you to feel that I want to work with you, if you really get hold of this thing and learn to control yourself, to control your bladder. I'll work with you even later on if you decide to come back to correct the deeper personality problem. The money angle doesn't count, that is, if it's a matter of your not being able to afford it. You can still come to see me and we'll work something out. But you have to show me that you are very sincere about wanting to work this thing out with me. The first step is controlling your bladder and utilizing the suggestions that I give you constructively.

Pt. Absolutely.

Dr. I think it's very, very necessary that we continue because you have been a very insecure kid all your life and the basic thing is correcting the insecurity.

Pt. I remember your saying something about that from my dream.

Dr. The one where you're back in the orphanage and running away from Mrs. Meaney? Now your mother actually went away from you, didn't she? She left you and went to work out of necessity. She left you in the care of your aunt. And that aunt may be something like this person in the dream who wants to bring Annie Rooney back into the orphanage. It so happens that your relationships with women are likely to be such that on the one hand you'd like to have a motherly kind of relationship with them, and on the other hand it would bring up the fear of getting yourself back into the same pickle you were with your aunt.

Pt. Yes.

Dr. And get yourself tied down so you wouldn't be able to do what you wanted to do. But still the fact that you just didn't get enough love and security such as you wanted would make you demand it from someone else. Maybe an older man who would be able to take care of you the way your aunt didn't. The last part of the dream is that you were adopted by an older man.

Pt. You know, it's a funny thing. I didn't like my aunt, but when I joined the Merchant Marine, I more or less established myself back there with her. Until I went into the Army I actually despised her. But right now I think the world of her.

Dr. I see.

Pt. I mean she's, ah, I mean I think I'd, if she ever passed away now, I'd feel worse than I did when my mother did. But at that time when I was staying with her before I was thirteen, I had absolutely no use for her at all.

Dr. Now it's important that you understand all this, because ultimately you've got to see yourself as an independent person. You've got to get to a point where you really feel within your soul that you've got value and strength. If you straighten yourself out, your relations with women will improve. Then if you meet a girl you like, you're not going to get tied down and feel your independence will be taken away from you, the way you did when you were little. Because that's apparently what happened to you.

Do you want to go to sleep for me now? Just sit there and relax yourself. Watch your hands, just watch your hands. Look at the right hand, and it will slowly get light, and then lift in the air, and you'll go into a deep sleep. Keep gazing at it, and as you gaze at it, you'll get drowsier and drowsier and drowsier. Your eyes will get heavier and heavier, and your arm will begin to lift. As it touches your face, you'll be in a deep, restful, relaxed, comfortable sleep. Go to sleep now, go to sleep, sleep, sleep. Your hand continues to rise and you get very drowsy, and tired and you'll go into a deep, restful, relaxed, comfortable sleep. Now you're asleep. (*Pause.*)

I'm going to stroke your arm again, and it gets rigid, very, very stiff, so stiff and rigid that it will not budge. I'm going

to count from one to five. At the count of five, the arm will
have gotten so stiff and rigid that it will not budge. One,
stiff; two, stiffer and stiffer; three; four; five—rigid and stiff
and firm, and even though you try with all your might to
move it, it remains exactly as it is. The harder you try, the
more rigid it is, until I, myself, stroke it backwards, and then
slowly it begin to come down. Slowly it comes down, just
like that. And you'll go into an even deeper, deeper, more
restful sleep. When I talk to you next, you'll be more deeply
asleep. (*Pause*)

As you sit there, I'm going to give you the suggestion that
you imagine yourself to be at home. You sit in front of the
radio. You go over to the radio and you turn it on. Can
you see yourself at home, in front of the radio?

Pt. Yes.

Dr. Turn it on, and the radio begins to play a song. As
soon as you hear that song, indicate it by your hand rising
up about an inch. The hand rises up. What song was
that?

Pt. Tommy Dorsey's theme song.

Dr. Good. Now, as you sit there, we have to go even
further into this problem. You can see that it is possible
for you to control this tendency to bed-wet, can't you?
(*Patient nods.*) And you know you can do it and must do it.
No matter what the significance of the bed-wetting is, no
matter whether it means that you just want to feel yourself
completely helpless and taken care of, or whether it means
you don't give a darn about anything or anybody, it's extremely essential for you to be able to control it.

Now I am going to work with you, so that you will be able
to control it. And I'm going to help you not only control it,
but to achieve a better life so that you are more secure.
You've been extremely nervous and jittery all your life as if
you sometimes were about to jump out of your skin. I want
you to feel that it's not necessary for you to be that nervous

and jittery, because you will be able to get that security that will make it possible for you not to be nervous and jittery.

You felt that you never had the kind of love, the kind of affection, the kind of understanding that you wanted. We're going back now, we're going back into your early life where you will be able to see and to experience how insecure you've been. The last time you came here, we went back into your past life, and I explained to you how a person never quite forgets anything that's happened to him. You're going to be able to go back into your life to a period when you felt very insecure. And I'm going to give you the suggestion that you begin to feel as if you hear the ticking of a clock. That will take you back, back, back to a time when you felt very insecure, no matter when that time was. As soon as you feel yourself to be back there, indicate it to me by this hand rising. Your hand rises. How old are you?

Pt. Thirteen.

Dr. You're thirteen years of age. What's happened?

Pt. My mother died.

Dr. Your mother died. How do you feel?

Pt. Confused and don't know what's going to happen next.

Dr. You feel confused and don't know what's going to happen next. Who's taking care of you?

Pt. My mother's sister.

Dr. Do you feel like crying?

Pt. No.

Dr. But you feel very insecure.

Pt. Um, hum.

Dr. Now, go back, back, into your life to a point where you're even littler than before. I want you to go back to a point where you're six years of age. You're six years old now, and the next time I talk to you you'll be exactly six. And then I'm going to ask you to open your eyes. Even though your eyes are open, you'll be asleep. I'm going to put a pencil in your hand and it will be possible for you to write. It will be possible for you to draw; you'll be exactly six years of age. You just sit there and the next time I talk to you, you'll be six, exactly six years of age. (*Pause*)

Now you're exactly six years of age. Very slowly, even though you're asleep, your eyes will begin to open when I give you the command. Your eyes will begin to open, and you still will be asleep, you still will be asleep. You hear the ticking of the clock now. So long as you hear that ticking, even though you have your eyes open, you'll still be asleep. When you wake up, you will not remember what happened. You hear that ticking? (*Patient nods.*) Now slowly open your eyes, but stay asleep. You're six years of age, exactly six. Now sit up. I'm going to give you a paper and I want you to draw a picture of a man. (*Patient draws a childish picture of a man and prints under it, "I want daddy."*)

I know you want your daddy, but he has gone away. I know you feel you've got to do what your aunt wants you to do. But remember that you can do things for yourself, too, and when you grow up, you're going to feel that you can do things for yourself, even if you didn't have a daddy around.

Now I want you to grow up. I'm going to count from one to five, and at the count of five, be back there in the doctor's office, grown up. One, two, three, four, five. You're still asleep, you're asleep, continue to sleep. You are going to get so deeply asleep now that you will be able to open your eyes and still be asleep.

I now put a pencil in your hand, and your hand will write automatically as if some force pushes it along. Pay no attention to what your hand writes. (*The patient writes a jumbled line: c s r g l s i s l a r w. He then looks at it and then translates it as "Charles Ruggles is L.R.W."* (*my initials*). *Apparently he identifies Charles Ruggles in the dream with me.*)

Close your eyes, and sleep deeply as I talk to you again. It's extremely urgent that you control your bladder. I know that you feel quite insecure, as long as you have no othe
r

way of making yourself secure through your own resources. You will be able to get that eventually. But now you feel that you come to me and I will help you. Of course I will help you, and then you will begin to feel stronger in yourself, too, so you can have strength in yourself. One way is to better yourself in every possible way. What about education? What would you like to be when you get educated?

Pt. Ah, business or a doctor.

Dr. You want to be a doctor or you'd like to get into business of some kind. Like what?

Pt. Into a corporation of some sort.

Dr. Do you have a plan as to the kind of educational program that you can follow? (*Patient nods.*) You do. Good. You've talked it over with the college advisors? (*Patient nods.*) Fine. What class will you start in?

Pt. The second year.

Dr. You'll start in the second year college. Very, very good. I want you to feel that I want to help you overcome this wetting problem, and also help you achieve maturity within yourself, security within yourself. I want you to feel that our relationship is one that doesn't have to terminate when you leave here, that I will still be your friend after you've gone, after you stop coming to see me as your doctor. You understand that, don't you? (*Patient nods.*) I'd like to have you understand it that way. I want to help you solve this problem so that you can gain security within yourself. I want you to mobilize every effort, every force to conquer your difficulty.

I want you to overcome this symptom of bed-wetting. That will give you more respect. At nighttime when you go to bed, automatically without any concentration or any effort, in spite of any resistance that may occur, you're going to control that bed-wetting. It will be impossible for you to wet that bed. Immediately upon having the desire, you'll open your eyes, get up and go to the bathroom. Or else you'll control the bladder. Even if you have an occasional slip, it will not matter. You will continue to improve. You will try to figure out what caused the slip. It's extremely necessary that you control your bladder. You must continue to do this until you establish a habit pattern in which you automatically stop bed-wetting. You've been able to stop it now and to go days without bed-wetting. You can stop it. You must stop it.

Now I'm going to give you a suggestion that you have a dream. As soon as you have had the dream, wake up automatically. But you're not going to remember that dream until I tap on the desk three times. When you hear the third tap, you'll suddenly remember the dream. In other words, have a dream, and then as soon as you've had the dream, wake up. Your mind will be a total blank. It will be as if you just woke up from sleep. You won't remember anything. When I ask you, "What do you remember?" you won't remember a thing. But when I tap on the desk this way (*rap, rap, rap*) you'll suddenly remember the dream. Then you'll tell me the dream. As soon as you've told me that dream, you're going to be extremely happy, as happy as you've ever been in all your life. You'll feel as if you'd like to dance—exuberant, joyful, very, very happy. You won't know exactly why, but you'll feel an emotion of happiness that will well up in you. Now have a dream rapidly, then wake up. (*Pause—then patient opens his eyes.*) Hello, how do you feel?

Pt. O.K.

Dr. What do you remember?

Pt. Well, nothing except writing something on a paper.

(*Rap, rap, rap*)

Pt. I remember something else now—a dream. I was sitting in a church. It was in the afternoon and the church wasn't crowded. There was somebody playing an organ there, light streaming in the direct pattern of the window, into the darkness of the church.   There, ah, there was some one in some sort of clerical garment arranging things on the altar.   I was feeling more or less in rest and peace, sitting there very relaxed and in a concentrating mood.

(We may speculate this dream refers to the hypnotic situation,)

Dr.   Felt as if sunshine was coming in through darkness, and that everything was at peace.   Was that the end of the dream?

Pt.   Yes.   No other action there, just the dream of that feeling that I had.

Dr.   How do you feel now?

Pt.   I feel as if I were walking out in sunshine.

Dr.   And what feeling is that?

Pt.   I just feel like strutting around and being active.

Dr.   Just for exercise?

Pt.   No, just for the heck of it, you know.   Moving around, see what's going on.   You know you get the feeling sometimes that you've got to get out and walk and swing around your arms, especially on a nice day.

Dr.   Happy, sort of?

Pt.   Um hum.

Dr.   Have you had periods of happiness very much?

Pt.   Not really exalted happiness.   Pleasant moods and things.   It never affected me in such a way that it would be a permanent thing that I could hold onto.   All of a sudden things would happen, you know, to give me a temporary feeling.

Dr.   What are you thinking about now?

Pt.   I wasn't thinking much of anything.   It just happened to pop into my mind that a couple of girls are giving a party next Friday, that I'm going to.   It just came across my mind.

Dr.   You haven't got a steady girl friend?

Pt.   Oh, no.

Dr.   Is there any reason for that?

Pt.   I never cared for one.

Dr.   You never cared for one.

Pt.   I mean, I always like to go around, but not be tied down.

Dr.   You'd like to be a free lance, capable of doing what you want to do and not be tied down.   Well, of course you're a young fellow and that's your privilege.   All young fellows feel that way, but you may possibly be afraid of getting yourself involved for fear of getting yourself tied down like "Little Annie Rooney" was tied down.   (*Pause*)   Do you feel that you're getting any good out of coming here?

Pt.   Absolutely.

Dr.   In what way?

Pt.   Well, I sort of feel that I'm getting a little more confidence in myself for one thing.   I always felt the feeling, as I said, of self respect wasn't strongly based on anything.   I mean probably just an outgrowth of something that really isn't anything as far as the people I'm associating with goes. What I mean is, such a thing as lack of self respect that I have is, I am beginning to see, not something that anybody else is particularly aware of.   I mean, I'm not inferior in their eyes.

Dr.   It's just inside of you, you are getting to believe.

Pt.   Yes.

Dr.   Well, I'm very, very glad you see that.   It gratifies me a great deal for you to feel that you're getting more self respect.

SEVENTH SESSION (May 26)

The patient's enuresis continues to be under control even though a dramatic shift has occurred in the character of his relationship to the therapist.   He questions the value of dependency and seems more motivated toward self sufficiency.   A change in technic along less authoritarian lines is attempted in the hope of enhancing self growth.

Dr. How many days is it now that you've gone without wetting?

Pt. The longest I've gone.

Dr. It is?

Pt. Um hum.

Dr. Very good. Have you had any dreams?

Pt. The only dream I had was last night. It was very short. I was dreaming that I was with my cousin at some kind of a bar or something, and Gus Lesnevich, the heavy-weight prize fighter, was down at the end of it, don't you know.

Dr. Yes.

Pt. My cousin knew him, and he was talking to him. He looked like a fat slob, the fighter did, when he was standing down there drinking, you know. There wasn't anything more to it, it was just that.

Dr. Just that you were kind of disappointed that he was drinking, and was fat, and wasn't the way you wanted him to be?

Pt. No, he didn't look at all what I know him to be.

Dr. He's a pretty good fighter isn't he?

Pt. Oh, yes.

Dr. Anything more come to your mind?

Pt. No.

Dr. Have you been thinking any more about what we've been talking about?

Pt. Yes, I have. I was getting myself into the frame of mind where I actually believe that there's no such thing as not being able to help it. You know, the condition, I mean. But after all, I mean, if I can wake up now, there is no reason why I can't at any other time. And knowing the things that I do now, I mean—after all there is a signal, and as far as I can see there's no excuse for doing it.

Dr. How do you figure out that it's been going on all this time before you came to see me, if there is no reason for it?

Pt. Well, I don't know.

Dr. Maybe you felt that you just didn't give a darn about things.

Pt. It might have been, very easily might have been it. Because I said just before I came here I was getting into a state of mind about the thing. This is the first time I've ever actually put my mind to it, and really wanted to do something about it. See, when I was a kid, they, before I was sixteen, figured by the time he's sixteen, he'll outgrow it. And after that, I didn't. And they didn't know what to do about it. I went to a couple of doctors after that with no results.

Dr. How has the nervousness been since I saw you last?

Pt. Well, I think I've calmed down quite a bit. My aunt spoke about it the other day. Everything was rush, rush, rush. Everything I did was under pressure, and it was to meet a deadline, you know. And I've been able to sit still, and take things a lot easier than I was before. And that's not my own opinion. I know because my aunt mentioned it, spoke about it the other day.

Dr. Do you resent being with your aunt?

Pt. No.

Dr. Do you think you can take her more calmly now, and not get yourself too tied down to her?

Pt. Yes.

Dr. And not get yourself so that you feel that you've got to do what she says without questioning it?

Pt. Absolutely.

Dr. Well that's extremely important.

Pt. Because, ah, she, she doesn't regulate my way of doing things of life at all any more. The only thing she does is she's always looking sometimes to give you advice, things that she knows I'm doing wrong. She knows that I'm old enough to know what I'm doing. She knows that I know the difference between right and wrong and things like that.

Dr. She's the one you didn't care for much?

Pt. That's right. I used to, I felt pretty lousy toward her when I was a kid. As I said, right now she's the grandest person I know.

Dr. You certainly don't want to go back into a kind of relationship with her that you used to have when you were a kid, do you?

Pt. Oh, absolutely not.

Dr. It would be very destructive for you. The thing is you are making a very concerted effort to better yourself at this point. You are going to go back to school, at least you are going to get started in September, and you are going to put this thing across, and lick the problem that you have. We're going to work this thing out together no matter how long it takes. I want you to feel that if you have any kind of problem, you can come to me and we'll work the thing out. It would be very destructive to you to go back to your childish relationship with your aunt. It is necessary for you to liberate yourself.

Pt. Well, I mean, you see the way I am with her now. I don't have to explain what I'm doing, or let her know where I'm going and things like that. I can do things on my own, take things upon myself, you know. I'll talk them over with her, because I like her, and I feel like that I belong there more than I do any place else, the way you talk things over with any parent. But I mean, I don't let her regulate me. I mean she's the type of woman who has a marvelous sense of humor, and we can have a lot of fun with her, I mean, she's the kind that I'd just as soon take out walking in the afternoon and take her to a movie because I enjoy her company.

Dr. Fine. Supposing you go to sleep now. Sit back, relax and start going to sleep.

Pt. Before that I want to tell you I am a lot better.

Dr. You mean as far as the wetting is concerned? There's practically none of it now.

Pt.   It's only been twice since I've been here.

Dr.   We've just got to continue that.

Pt.   Because, as my aunt said, you must be doing me some good because it used to be every night.   Shall I sleep now?

Dr.   All right, do you want to look at your hands?   Start breathing in deeply, breathe in regularly, and very soon your eyes will get heavy.   Your hand slowly begins to lift and rise, your breathing gets deeper and deeper, and you get sleepier and sleepier, until finally you go into a deep, comfortable, relaxed sleep.   Keep watching your hand and very soon it will begin to lift, up, up, up, and get lighter and lighter, and as it rises your eyes get so heavy and tired, you go into a deep, restful sleep, a very deep, restful sleep.   You will go into a very deep, restful, relaxed sleep.   Lean your head against the hand, go into a deep, deep, restful, relaxed, sleep; go to sleep.

Now, listen closely to me.   No matter how long it takes, get into the deepest state of sleep possible, so deep that you have a dream.   The dream that you have will be exactly the same dream that you had the other night, but if you left something out, it will be more complete.   As soon as you have that dream, continue to sleep, but tell me about it without waking up.   (*Pause*)

Pt.   Well, I was there with my cousin, and this guy Lesnevich was down around the corner, the corner of the bar. And my cousin Joe was between he and I, and there were some fellows on the end of the bar directly opposite from Lesnevich there.   And my cousin was talking to him as though he knew him.   I didn't recognize him at first, because he didn't look at all what I know him to look like.   He was fat and pudgy, and he wore glasses, and he was standing drinking beer.   And these guys on the other end of the bar looked like the type that were bookies, or the type that hang out in sports arenas, and pool halls and all.   I didn't pay much attention to the guy because, I don't know, I didn't feel

like being one of the mob and hero worshippers or whatever
you call them.

Dr.   Were they hanging on to him?

Pt.   Beg pardon?

Dr.   The fellows, they were sort of hanging on to him, hero
worshippers?

Pt.   No, they were on the other end of the bar directly
opposite him.   And they were sitting there as though they
knew him, and there was no great treat for them to see him.

Dr.   I see.

Pt.   And I was, didn't pay much attention to them, you
know.   They all looked like the, ah, typical autograph
hunter type.

Dr.   Anything more in the dream?

Pt.   No, I remember it was in the afternoon, there was
light coming through the windows.

Dr.   The light coming through the windows, could it have
been something like the light that came through the windows
in other dreams you've had here?   You remember all the
dreams you've had with light coming in the window?

Pt.   I guess so.

Dr.   That has a certain significance to you we may be able
to understand better.   There is then an indication in this
dream that you don't like to be a hero worshipper, and that
a fellow like Gus Lesnevich whom you admired, you kind of
devalue now.   Maybe you made him a little bit pudgy so
that you wouldn't have to worship him so much.   There's
a type of personality, the hero worshipper, who doesn't find
any real values himself, but has to go smelling around somebody else.   You don't like to be that kind of a fellow do you?

Pt.   Oh, no.

Dr.   You don't like to just go smelling around and depending upon anybody else.   Do you?

Pt.   No, sir.

Dr.   And that dislike probably conditions the dream.

Now listen to me. In dreams the person an individual dreams about, is usually somebody very important to him. The dreamer's attitude is reflected in the dream in the kind of person dreamed about. In other words right at this moment you may not want to get yourself in a position where you will hero worship anybody or get yourself bound down.

I'm going to give you a suggestion as you sit there that you have another dream that will clarify for you the meaning of the dream about Gus Lesnevich. Now let this dream come up automatically almost as if you were sitting in the front row of an audience looking up at the stage and seeing action in front of you. Just don't direct it, just let it come up and as soon as you've seen the action, or you've had enough of a dream that explains the Lesnevich dream, tell me about it without waking up. (*Pause*)

Pt. I can see Lesnevich up on that stage there. He's coming out and he's got his fighting togs on. He's got his gloves on. And, ah, someone walks out of the right wing, and he sort of takes him all around to show him off. He takes him around his arm and sort of brings him up to the front of the stage. And this guy Lesnevich looks very much out of place there because there is very beautiful scenery around the stage there, a lot of girls who look like chorus girls in very elaborate costumes. And it is like some very fancy, exclusive night club. And it don't seem to make any direct pattern around there, sort of milling around the back of the stage there.

Dr. No, he doesn't belong there really.

Pt. He looks extremely out of place. Kind of naked standing there.

Dr. A ridiculous figure.

Pt. Um, hum, well, not ridiculous in view of his accomplishments.

Dr. How do you tie that up? What does that mean?

What meaning does it have to you?   Does anything come to you when you think about that?

Pt.   I don't think anything that I've really concentrated on, except coming here.

Dr.   What have your thoughts been about me?   What ideas have come to your mind, when you've thought about coming here and about myself?

Pt.   Well, I more or less explained to you that I should have known the things I learned, but I just couldn't put my finger on them.   They are things that I felt, but didn't understand.

Dr.   Have you had any different kind of attitude towards me, since the last time I saw you?   Were you in any way led to feel that this thing wasn't going to be the thing you planned it to be?   In other words is there a possibility your attitude towards me may have changed like towards Lesnevich in the dream?

Pt.   Oh well, I have a great deal of respect for you, I mean, in fact I, in view of the fact that I thought you could help me, I know you must be the tops of your profession.   But the last time I left here I was a little worried that I wasn't exactly reacting to these treatments the way I, the way you wanted me to.   I mean as though I was remembering things that I shouldn't remember.   And I had difficulty sometimes following certain suggestions you made to me.   I mean certain things that you'd say such as when we were walking down the street into a church yard, the bell was ringing, I could see and hear those things perfectly, turning on the radio and things like that.   But certain things I really had difficulty imagining those things.

Dr.   And you thought you weren't doing right?

Pt.   That's right.

Dr.   Well then, we must correct this misconception.   In the first place a person sometimes feels that it is necessary for him to follow every single suggestion.   Well, that isn't the case. There are some things that the person is more adept at, that a person responds to more. There are some people, for instance, who in a visual sphere are very astute and can see things under hypnosis. Other people in an auditory sphere are very keen and can hear things. You may possibly be able to show responses in one direction, but not be able to show them in another. It always happens in hypnosis that there is a selectivity of suggestions. It has to be that way. You must not comply automatically. You have to retain a sufficient amount of independence within yourself to be able to feel like a free agent. You see what I mean?

Pt. You mean it's all right for me to resist doing things if I want?

Dr. It's very necessary for you to do so, because what we're shooting for is that you will be able to liberate yourself from this feeling that you are a helpless, no good person, a fellow without value, a person who can't make the grade. You'll gradually be able to relate yourself better to people if you retain a certain amount of independence. Also, your relationships with people will take a different turn if you don't make yourself so dependent on anybody that you're like "Little Annie Rooney," all hemmed in by a witch.

(*The dream seems to be a transference dream which indicates a new attitude toward me and toward himself. In the dream a prize fighter [apparently identified with myself] does not seem so glamorous a figure as the patient once imagined. In view of the existing dependent relationship on me, one may assume this is a reflection of the patient's hostility toward me for not being so omnipotent a personage as to satisfy the patient's fantasies of a powerful paternal authority. It may be argued, that since he was able to resist successfully some suggestions during the trance, I lost face, and his confidence in me was shaken.*

That these assumptions are not correct is evidenced by the fact that there has been no relapse of the enuresis, no reactive depression, and no search for another, more powerful therapist. Indeed the patient feels better than he has ever felt before; he is much more independent with his aunt and with his friends. A more

*likely explanation is that he is starting to doubt the values of a
dependent relationship, and is beginning to experience satisfaction in self sufficiency.   Thus he has not the exclusive motivation
to comply with every suggestion I give him.   He tests his capacity
to resist and is successful.   His desire to retain his symptomatic
improvement and to please himself rather than me probably has
prevented a relapse of the symptom.*

*The case illustrates the fallacy of the blandly accepted dictum
that suggestive hypnosis creates dependency and crushes self
sufficiency.   It shows that the patient's needs and demands for
growth are stronger than any attempt to keep him on a dependent
level.   It shows also that suggestive therapy, wisely utilized, may
motivate the patient toward self growth.   More surprising is that
so dramatic a change in motivation could have occurred in so
short a time.   The night club atmosphere and presence of girls
in the dream may point to his desire for a heterosexual relationship rather than a relationship with a paternal figure.)*

Dr.   Once you become more independent, your relations
with women will be better.   You will not feel they want to
take your freedom away from you.   It's true that if you get
to the point where you marry, that your freedom will be
somewhat circumscribed.   You'll have to stay home more
than before.   But it is not true that you have to give up all
your independence.   That's destructive for you and would
be destructive for anybody.   We're striving for a liberation
of yourself as a person, and that liberation can come right
here.   As soon as you feel that you have the right to make
certain decisions and certain choices, or to resist some suggestions in hypnosis, you will begin to develop strength of
character.

What we have been doing is working on control of your
bed-wetting.   That is part of the problem.   The other part
is even more important, gaining self respect.   You should
get yourself so conditioned that automatically, even though
you may not want to get out of bed, even though you may
desire to stay right there and wet the bed, you will not want
to because it is important for you to feel grown-up.   You'll

either be able to control your bladder, or you'll be able to get up and go to the bathroom, one of the two. I'm going to give you suggestions that this thing eventually will come to pass within yourself. And I'm going to couch my suggestions in terms of your own ability to gain the control of this thing, so it will not occur under any circumstances. You will be able to control it and not only control it, but be able under all circumstances to make yourself sufficiently strong so that other problems will be mastered too. And that's the point we're shooting at ultimately—to liberate you and make you a free person, so that you can carry on your relationships with other people in a satisfying way.

The result will be that you will not be nervous, shaky, or tense. You'll be more relaxed. You'll take things in your stride more. You'll feel more and more self confident. I'm going to invite you, if you wish at any time in the future after we've finished with our treatments, to feel free to come here and talk things over with me until you feel that you've got the mastery within your own self to make your decisions and choices, and feel you don't need the aid of any other person.

Now as you sit there, I think it extremely important that you understand fully the role that you play here. You must not feel that you've got to comply with everything. It is not necessary.

I'm going to count from one to five. At the count of five, I want you to have another dream. No matter what that dream is, let it come. As soon as you've had it, tell me about it after waking up. One, two, three, four, five. (*Pause, following which patient awakens.*)

Pt. There are a lot of seemingly unrelated things. I see a steeple raising through the water making an awful churning foam. Seems like alligators coming through the water with their pointed noses just above the surface all reaching for something. Looks like pointed gliders of airplanes raising in the water at certain places. Looks like on the edge of a stream or pool, or whatever it is, and a guy is standing up in a tree, looks something like Tarzan, dressed something like Tarzan.   And there he sort of passed over a bunch of, like a handful, of beautiful flowers, something I couldn't name. I've never seen them before.   And then it happened to pass over like it happened to me last night.   My cousin and I were out with a couple of nurses from the Medical Center, and I couldn't get over how beautiful those buildings were down there.   They were the most massive structures I've ever seen and really impressive looking structures there. And it seemed like a sort of nostalgic feeling being down around the hospital atmosphere again, because I've done that thing during the war, and in the Merchant Marine.   I was a medical officer and was originally interested in medicine, and I've got a sort of warm feeling about the atmosphere.

Dr.   You do like medical work?

Pt.   Yeah, I do and I don't.

Dr.   What don't you like about it?

Pt.   What it will take to get there.

Dr.   The time element?

Pt.   The time.

Dr.   And the money?

Pt.   That's right.

Dr.   How far, how many years of college do you have to go?

Pt.   I'd have at least six or seven years before I'd get a degree.

Dr.   In medical school?   Well, you're still a young man. You may, perhaps, after all, decide that it may be a worth while investment for you.   But irrespective of the pros and cons, it's something that you must decide for yourself. What you do must be in line with something that will give you gratification later on, rather than in terms of how long it's going to take.   It's extremely important that you do those things that you feel ultimately will be good for you.

And if you calmly and deliberately, through your own efforts, decide that you want to go to medical school, the amount of time isn't going to be so terribly important. You will, in the long run, be better off. But if you, yourself, decide, after thinking it over, that you do not want to go, you'll be able to decide against it. It's up to you entirely.

Pt. That's what I'll do, think it over.

Eighth Session (June 5)

The patient continues to be free from enuresis. In addition he shows signs of increased self esteem. He is anxious to begin work and decides he has gained sufficient help from therapy, at this time, to warrant his stopping treatments. Therapy is accordingly terminated.

Pt. I was O.K. since I was here last.

Dr. It's been quite some time now.

Pt. It was a week ago last Wednesday.

Dr. That is about ten days.

Pt. Yes.

Dr. How is everything going with you?

Pt. Fine.

Dr. Any dreams?

Pt. No, but I happened to have a funny experience Monday night. I woke up and my eyes were wide awake, and I felt like somebody was nudging me, and I almost, I felt like I was on the verge of saying, "Damn it, I'm on my way up. I'm getting up." It was as though I were dreaming that someone was saying, "Get out of bed. You got to go." And I did wake up, you know, and I was almost going to say out loud, "I'm getting up." The same thing happened Tuesday night, but not quite as strong a feeling.

Dr. Was there any resentment on your part?

Pt. No. I woke right up wide awake and got right out of bed and went to the bathroom.

Dr. How is the nervous tension?

Pt. Well, I think I've calmed down quite a bit.

Dr. You do feel calmed down quite a bit?

Pt. Another thing I've noticed—I don't know whether it has any bearing on it—but for as much as over a month while I wasn't working, if I was out with some friends or something, you know, about eleven o'clock at night, I usually wouldn't bother going home. I'd go some place else and look for a little excitement or something, you know. I wouldn't get home until two o'clock in the morning or later. Recently I just as soon come back and not go looking around.

Dr. Recently there hasn't been this need then to go searching for excitement, possibly because you feel a little more stable. And perhaps you feel that life is making a little more sense to you.

Pt. Could be. Because I know if I don't have to get up in the morning, I never go home and go to bed. There was something I'd have to sit and watch and take part in, you know, and feel that I was getting a little excitement, you know.

Dr. Do you have any other thoughts before we go on to hypnosis?

Pt. Well I think I'll go when I'm through up here, go down to the shore and get a job before school starts.

Dr. I will stop with you only on one condition, that you feel you can call on me when you, yourself, see fit to do so. You can rest assured that I will help you if you wish. You might even want to drop me a line and let me know how things go with you. If you want to talk things over with me on any score—your education, what life means to you, girl friends, anything—come to see me, and we'll work things out.

Pt. Fine. You know, I don't know whether it makes any difference or not—but you know how we were talking and we more or less established the fact that quite often I feel inferior and a jerk as far as my relations with women goes, you know. Well, Sunday night my cousin and I went down to Jersey City Amusement Center to see his girl friend, you know, she's a good friend of mine too. She wasn't there so we met a couple of her girl friends there and we took them out. And that, I think, was the first real date I've had since I've been coming to you. And I did feel different, changed, you know what I mean, as far as what I'd do, how I'd act, how I'd feel after. I mean I felt after as though I didn't feel inferior, didn't feel as though I'd been acting as a jerk or something like that. As a matter of fact, when we spoke to this girl whom we had originally gone down to see, who wasn't there, she was saying that the girls were saying what a wonderful time we had down there, you know. A lot of baloney like that, but I mean, as I said before, when I left that night, I felt a little different.

Dr. You really feel some changes going on inside of you?

Pt. Absolutely.

Dr. I think it is quite important for you to get started and do some work. But if you like, you can come to see me once in a while. I'd like to see you, too.

Pt. Well, I'd like to stop in.

Dr. I'm going to show you the cards again and then you tell me what you see. After that we'll get right into hypnosis.

Pt. You know I believe I've got this bed-wetting licked. I almost feel that it would be the expected thing not to, and I just naturally just won't.

Dr. And it is with increased assuredness and confidence.

Pt. I mean, I don't really have to. I don't think too much about it.

Dr. You just accept it. I'm going to show you the cards again. Tell me exactly what you see. This is the first card.

Pt. I can see the figure of a woman from the hips down right there. Here is some kind of a raccoon faced animal with his head like this.

Dr. This is the second one.

Pt. I still see the same things. Looks like a pheasant's tail hanging up like. This looks like an exploding bomb or a torpedoed ship. Looks like a couple of puppy dogs with their noses together.

Dr. This is the third one.

Pt. Guys with tuxedos on pulling chairs away. A butterfly and two parrots sort of on a ridge with their heads bent over. A fly's head.

Dr. All right, this is the fourth one.

Pt. Looks like the head of some crustacean animal or something. Looks like lobsters' eyes.

Dr. All right. Now this is the fifth one.

Pt. Looks like the beak on one of those duck-billed platypuses. The two light pieces on the end here sort of look vaguely like a profile of an alligator with his jaws open.

Dr. All right. Here is the sixth one.

Pt. Looks again like the top of one of those Eskimo totem poles with a peculiar head on top. Some sort of pelt spread out to dry.

Dr. This is the seventh.

Pt. Couple of chubby faced youngs girls with their hair up, sort of pouting expressions on their faces. Heads of elephants.

Dr. This is the eighth card.

Pt. This still looks like a preserved specimen skeleton of some animal like a crab or something, something like you'd see in a bottle in a museum. Raccoons on the side here. They look as though they are stepping over here, over there, to that. Looks like a side view of the same face. Well, I guess that's all I can find in that one.

Dr. O.K. This is the ninth one.

Pt. A couple of sea horses facing toward each other. Looks faintly, except for the eyes, like a profile of a walrus looking type of animal—tusk here—mustache. Looks something like a version of King Neptune with a seaweed beard, clothes, something the likes of which I've never seen. Seems to have weird, distorted, nonseeing eyes. Not much more to it.

Dr. And this is the last one.

Pt. A couple of crabs down here. A couple of sad looking animals looking at each other with plants growing out of the top of their heads. It doesn't look too much like it, but it reminds me of it. Throat bone. Looks like the head of a rabbit and behind it two figures—can't see it too distinctly, but I can see the eyes, the face, the nose. Right in there where those two dark spots are, they look like faces of a man that are carved into a rock. They seem to be looking to the right upward on this side and to the left and upward on this side. This looks like a rear left side view of a shepherd dog laying on its right side. I still see these things as animals.

(*The responses to the Rorschach cards show no remarkable change, but productivity is increased.*)

Dr. Thank you. It seems to me now that we look at this whole picture that you kind of resigned yourself to a stalemate, before you decided you wanted help. You perhaps felt that relationships with people weren't too important for you. With girls you didn't want to get tied down, because you didn't want to get yourself involved too deeply with them; or else you felt that you were inferior and didn't know if they'd accept you. So that you were sort of going around in circles. I wonder if you have a different attitude now.

Pt. I think so. I mean I feel as though I have. It's not the kind of a thing where you crawl for years and then decide you are going to walk. It's not a thing I can notice as strongly as that, but somehow I kind of feel a little difference there, as I explained to you before.

Dr. Yes. Well now, after all you came to me first on May 13 and this is not so long. It isn't a long time when you've got your whole lifetime behind you. But at least you can get a clearer picture, a blueprint of what's been happening to you. How many times have you been here now altogether?

Pt. I believe this is the eighth.

Dr. This is the eighth time. We will go ahead and reinforce under hypnosis everything you've learned, so that you can go forward. Now the main thing is, as you know, and as I've pointed out to you, that eventually you're going to be able to liberate yourself from all the things that have kept you hemmed in and have wanted to make you a little boy without any value. You are going to liberate yourself eventually from the fear that you're going to be thrown out and not liked, that you are different from other people. You'll be able to feel as good as anybody. You're making your own choices and your own decisions now, and feeling that what you decide is the right and proper thing. Finally, you're going to try to achieve your own ambitions and go forward with your education. You happen to be a clever fellow. You haven't had a great deal of formal training, but you can always get that. You've got the basic resources and intelligence. You can go ahead.

All right, now do you want to lean back in the chair and put yourself to sleep. You know the technic. (*Patient puts himself to sleep.*)

Now I'm going to give you the suggestion that you dream how you feel about yourself at the present time. Go ahead and dream and tell me the dream without waking up. (*Pause*)

Pt. Well, I feel like I've got a reasonable amount of intelligence and culture. I can get along with people and make friends. The friends I do have, they pretty well accept me. I still have, ah, I'm not too sure of myself as far as force of personality goes.

Dr. You're not too sure about yourself, about the ability to have your way?

Pt. Not too much of it as far as influencing people.

Dr. As far as being able to influence people and be a leader.

Pt. That's right.

Dr. Well, there are definite reasons for that as you know. All your life you felt you had to depend and lean on somebody. The kind of life that you had, the insecurity that you felt, the rejection that you actually experienced, made you feel as if you were perhaps more dependent than the average person. You never developed within yourself a feeling that you had the right to develop your own resources and strengths, to develop the capacity to be a leader rather than a follower. If a person is dependent and feels rejected, then he will naturally feel that he hasn't got much on the ball, won't he? (*Patient nods.*) And that is exactly, it seems to me, what has happened to you. Now in certain circumstances have you ever tried to assume a leadership role?

Pt. Yes, I have. I mean I've more or less quite often had people look to me for advice and leadership and things.

Dr. How did you take that?

Pt. Well, it seemed to me to be a kind of thing that I was expecting, but still it was more like a surprise, you know, that somebody would come to me and look for it in that way.

Dr. It made you feel almost as if they didn't know you as well as you knew yourself?

Pt. That's right.

Dr. And gradually as you work this problem out, you will be able to assume more and more of a leadership role. But you must start feeling better about yourself. Now I want you to visualize yourself as you did the first day you came here, when you imagined you were in the first row, or the first few rows of a theater, and you looked on the stage and noticed a fellow up there. He had a very fearful expression on his face and he was afraid. This time you again see what it is that this man is afraid of, the worst thing that can happen to a person. He sees the worst thing that can happen to a person. Watch the curtain open up, and you will be able to see exactly what he saw that frightened him so, that caused the frightened expression on his face. (*Pause*)

Pt. He seems to be looking off the stage and there is a guy, a young man in his twenties. The man seems to be very, very despondent over something, and he is sobbing and weeping and putting his head on his arm and laying it down. It seems to be something dreadful has happened to him, and it horrifies this man to see him in this condition.

Dr. Now listen closely. As you sit there, you are going to have a dream. I'm going to tap on the desk here three times. With the third tap, suddenly you'll have a dream that will explain what it is that this twenty year old man is sobbing about. It will come automatically without any effort. You'll suddenly see a picture in front of your eyes. Describe it to me exactly the way you see it. (*Three taps.*)

Pt. He seems to feel cast out. As you tapped that third time, he seemed to fling himself around in defiance of people who were standing around him. He still had that crying, sobbing look on his face as though he were saying, "For God's sake, leave me alone."

Dr. He felt like an outcast.

Pt. Well, as though he were being persecuted for something. As though he seemed to feel that he didn't have anything ahead of him, and from now on the road would be down.

Dr. There was nothing ahead of him at all?

Pt. That's it.

Dr. Now listen to me. Look at the stage again, and you'll see this time the man with a smile on his face, as if something marvelous, the greatest thing in the world, has happened to him. The most marvelous thing in the world has happened to him. As soon as you see the man this time, the curtain will open up, and you'll see what it is he's looking at. You will notice what it is that has made him so ecstatically happy. Go ahead.

Pt. I don't know whether I can see it as you want me to, doctor, but what I can see off that stage is a man who seems to be sitting on the edge of a trunk with one foot up on it, resting his arm on his knee. He's got a very pleasing at-peace-with-the-world look on his face. And people coming by and speaking to him, passing the time of day, and he has time for everybody. He nods to them, "How do you do," and he is a very suave looking fellow, very pleasant, very charming. But he seems to be thinking that he's got things of his own that he can rely on, what he has to do and what he's driving for, that he can be nice to people. He can enjoy himself with people, but that is just a side track, that the things that he himself does in his mind are what he wants, as though he is not a terrifically impressionable type.

Dr. That he is self reliant.

Pt. That's it.

(*Comparing this fantasy with the one produced with the same stimulus at the start of therapy, one gets the impression of a changed attitude towards himself.*)

Dr. Now listen to me. I'm going to reinforce the suggestions that I've given to you before. You will be able, under any circumstances, no matter where you are, or what you do, to control this bed-wetting, no matter when you go to bed, no matter how much you've drunk, no matter where you've been. When you go to bed, the moment you feel a sensation of a full bladder and the desire to wet the bed, before you have had a chance to, your eyes will suddenly open. Your hand may or may not rise and touch your face. Your eyes will nevertheless open, and you will then desire to get out of bed and walk to the bathroom. Or else you'll be able to control your bladder and still not wet. Another thing, it is important that you continue working on your deeper problems for which you may need further help now or later.

I am going to give you now the opportunity to decide whether you want to interrupt treatments with me now, and go ahead with your plans to get a job, or whether you want to continue with me further. I'm going to leave that up to you entirely. I will wake you up by counting from one to five, and at the count of five your eyes will open. Then I'm going to tap on the side of the chair three times, and with the third tap your mind will have been made up. You, yourself, will make up your mind as to whether you want to go on your own now, or whether you want to continue still coming to see me. You, yourself, will decide that whichever way you want. I'm going to count now from one to five. At the count of five open your eyes. One, two, three, four, five— open your eyes and wake up. (*Patient awakens.*)

Dr. How do you feel?

Pt. Fine but sleepy. (*Three taps.*) The thing that bothers me is, doctor, I got a lot of confidence in myself when I'm home, but I feel funny, for instance, if I got stuck over-night at somebody's house, I feel that I'd be all right, but, I mean, when I think of the circumstances, if I ever did slip up at a time like that.

Dr. How do you feel about it? Do you want to continue coming here for a while longer or do you want to go out on your own?

Pt. Well I, it's kind of hard to say.

Dr. How would you like to try this. Supposing you do sleep away from home, and we go ahead with treatments. Come back next week and we'll see how things go when you are sleeping away from home, whether this confidence in yourself continues. Can you do that? Is it possible to?

Pt. What I would like to do is stop now, and if I go down to the shore, take a job there. There would be times when I'd work nights and be free during the day and come back later—in say a week or so after I've been down there, if things are not satisfactory, if I wet or things. If that would be satisfactory to you?

Dr. Absolutely.

Pt.   Well, I'll keep in touch with you, doctor.

Dr.   Good.

Pt.   It was very nice knowing you, and I'm sure you've helped me quite a bit, you can see that yourself.

Dr.   Yes, well you can feel that yourself.

Pt.   Sure.

Dr.   Goodbye.

Pt.   Goodbye, doctor.

REFERENCES

[1] ERICKSON; M. H.: Hypnosis in medicine.   M. Clin. North America.   May, 1944, pp. 369–652.

[2] JANET, P.: Psychological Healing.   Vol. 1. New York, Macmillan, 1925.

[3] FREUD, S.: The Problem of Anxiety.   New York, W. W. Norton, 1936.

Part Two

HYPNOSIS IN PSYCHOBIOLOGIC THERAPY

PSYCHOBIOLOGIC therapy is the name given to a variety of technics, chief among which are guidance, reassurance, persuasion, desensitization, re-education and reconditioning. Psychobiologic therapy aims at a regulation of the patient's life, and a restoration to effective functioning, after factors which have led to the disorder have been studied, and a careful assay made of the individual's assets and liabilities. It is particularly applicable where the therapeutic objective is not a drastic reorganization of the personality structure, but a rapid return to social functioning by elimination of detrimental forces which retard mental health.

Psychobiologic therapy is a far more rational form of treatment than simple symptom removal by prestige suggestion. It even has, in some cases, certain advantages over analytic methods. It is a briefer form of treatment and sometimes can, in an incredibly short period, restore a patient to an emotional equilibrium, symptom-free and capable, because of the knowledge he has gained, of avoiding pitfalls that have hitherto created anxiety. Additionally, the patient may learn to utilize his assets to best advantage and to get along far better than he ever has before. By showing him how to avoid difficulties in his relationships with people, it may relieve him of much anxiety, tension and hostility. Acquainting him with his character weaknesses, and guiding him to organize his activities around them may make his life more tolerable. Helping the person to discover positive qualities within himself may raise to some extent his pathologically low estimate of himself. While the dynamic sources of the individual's emotional problem are not tackled directly as in psychoanalysis, the relationship with the physician may inspire curative forces that influence personality growth.

On the other hand there are some serious disadvantages to psychobiologic methods as compared with psychoanalysis. It is a more superficial form of treatment and hence concerns itself more with effects than with causes. It is less capable of producing the drastic reorganizations of character and personality such as develop in those cases which respond successfully to psychoanalysis. Finally, as in symptom removal by suggestion, the elimination of discomfort in a relatively short time may prevent the patient from achieving the motivation to inquire more deeply into his inner conflicts.

In spite of these disadvantages, psychobiologic methods are eminently useful in many cases. There are patients who because of limited time or finances are unable to enter into a long-term therapeutic procedure. There are others whose motivations militate against deep therapy. Exposing them to a nondirective or analytic approach serves merely to confuse them. There are others, as prepsychotics, psychotics and extremely dependent people, whose ego strength is diminutive, and because of this they may be harmed by the intense anxiety aroused in an analytic type of treatment. In such cases psychobiologic therapy is valuable. Even though manifest neurotic difficulties continue in force, life becomes more tolerable and the person adopts a more constructive attitude toward reality. Furthermore, if the relationship with the patient is studied carefully, and utilized wisely, it may be possible to prepare the patient so that he can accept the need for a more incisive inquiry into his difficulties. An analytic approach may then be more capable of achieving success.

THE INITIAL WORK-UP IN PSY-
CHOBIOLOGIC THERAPY

A THOROUGH investigation of both the patient's problem
and his personality is essential in psychobiologic
therapy in order to determine which technic would be most
effective. This usually involves an inquiry into the individual's life history, a physical examination, and psychologic
testing. A psychiatric social worker, clinical psychologist,
internist and psychiatrist can function together as a team
here in making a proper psychosomatic study.

The character of the complaint, the history of its development, and past and current attitudes toward it are discussed
thoroughly with the patient. All available sources are ex-
plored, with the help of a psychiatric case worker if necessary,
to determine hereditary, constitutional and experiential elements of importance in explaining the patient's reactions.
The patient's social, sexual, work, educational, and recreational adjustments are investigated, as are his interests,
ambitions, habits, cravings, and conflicts. Since the therapeutic objective is the retraining of unhealthful attitudes,
and the elimination of immature reaction patterns, it is essential to obtain as clear an idea of the patient's personality
in operation as possible.

A physical examination is important not only in detecting
existing organic conditions, but also as a psychotherapeutic
measure. Many persons resent the physician's assumption
that no physical disorder exists when he has failed to make
an examination. A physical check-up helps reassure the
patient, and inspires confidence in the competence of the
doctor. In psychobiologic therapy there is no objection to
the physician, who will treat the patient psychiatrically,
doing the physical examination, as there might be in analytic

therapy. It goes without saying that x-ray and laboratory facilities are utilized where indicated.

Psychologic testing, particularly projection tests, as the Rorschach, Thematic Apperception Test, Goodenough and Expressive Handwriting, yield data as to personality resources and liabilities, existing anxieties and conflicts, and the nature of the patient's defenses against anxiety.

The initial work-up is invaluable in estimating the best type of therapy to utilize at the start, the prognosis and possible duration of treatment, and permits of a much more scientific approach to the patient's problems.

THE INTERPERSONAL RELATION-
SHIP IN PSYCHOBIOLOGIC
THERAPY

THE DIFFERENT technics employed in psychobiologic therapy presuppose a relationship of the physician to the patient that varies from strong directiveness, as in guidance therapy, to a more passive permissiveness, as in confession and ventilation. In most cases the relationship is essentially authoritarian.

Success in therapy is associated with acceptance of the physician as a wise or benevolent authority, and an effort is made to establish and to maintain a positive relationship at all times. Because resentment and hostile attitudes oppose the incorporation of therapeutic suggestions, it is essential to avoid establishing a neurotic transference. Hostilities are therefore dissipated as soon as they arise, and an attempt is made to win the patient over to a conviction that the physician is a friend who will help him at all times. Once a good relationship with the patient is established, the physician provides the patient with "education in living," with practical ways of overcoming his personality liabilities and of enhancing his assets.

Unless an analytic approach is combined with psychobiologic therapy (which presupposes that the physician has been personally psychoanalyzed and has secured training in an accredited school for psychoanalysis), no real attempt is made to analyze the interpersonal relationship. Indeed, as has been indicated, an effort is made to avoid the development of a neurotic transference. This is contrary to what we would do in psychoanalytic technic. Whenever the patient begins to evidence irrational attitudes toward the physician, therapy is interrupted, and through discussion and clarification, the patient is brought back to a reality level, in an attempt to restore the original positive physician-patient relationship. This may be difficult in some instances, since the patient will always try to involve the physician into his neurotic structure. Much skill may be required to break up the transference as soon as it starts developing, but unless this is done, the physician will find himself in the midst of an emotional cataclysm he may be unable to control.

Not all physicians are able to do psychobiologic therapy. A general liking for people, and a desire to help others is essential. Forcefulness of personality, and an ability to inspire confidence are other important qualities. The ideal attitude toward the patient is that of a good friend—sympathetic, kindly, but firm. The physician must be so constituted as not to derive sadistic satisfaction out of the patient's submission, nor to resent the latter's display of aggression or hostility. He must not succumb to excessive blandishments of praise or admiration.

A noncondemning, accepting attitude, shorn of blame or contempt, secures best results in psychobiologic therapy. The neurotic individual has impulses and attitudes which can incite irritation; but if the physician is unable to avoid getting emotionally stirred up, he probably will be unable to do constructive work with the patient. His irritation cannot usually be concealed by a judicious choice of words. Of course the physician cannot help disliking certain patients, for one reason or another; but if he is unable to analyze and to dissolve this dislike, he had best refer the patient to some other therapist, since no good psychotherapy is possible where dislike exists, in spite of all efforts to be objective.

The attitudes of the physician are important because many of the patient's reactions are the result of how his neurotic impulses have been regarded by others. Withdrawal tendencies and aggression may be conditioned by the hurt he has experienced in his past contacts with people. At the start the patient will expect the same kind of rejection or condemnation from the physician that he has received from others. The noncondemning, sympathetic attitude of the physician injects an entirely new element into the situation that can start a process of rebuilding the patient's confidence in people and in himself.

As the patient begins to realize he is not condemned or criticized for his symptoms and reactions, his attitude toward the physician assumes a quality significantly different from his other relationships. He begins to feel accepted as he is, and a warmth toward the physician develops which paves the way for constructive therapeutic work. The patient begins to accept the physician as an ally. He identifies with him and incorporates some of his standards and values. He feels a unity with the doctor which gives him strength to abandon some of his customary maladaptive patterns. This "rapport" is akin, in part, to what an infant feels toward the omnipotent parent.

The physician need not be flattered by the praise and love showered on him by the patient for there is a strong neurotic element involved. An objective attitude on the part of the physician is mandatory, respecting the patient's feelings, but keeping aloof from any other than a professional relationship. Should the physician trangress these bounds, the result may be disastrous to the patient. Certainly all therapeutic work will cease.

The female patient may become furious with the physician, accusing him of spurning her in turning down her amatory proposals. Where this happens, it is essential to remind the patient of the professional limitations to the relationship, and to explain that she is bound to develop loving feelings toward one whom she has taken into her confidence. The physician must convince the patient that the entire purpose of therapy would be destroyed if he reciprocated, and that her welfare dictates that no involvement occur.

The male patient may attempt to shower the physician with gifts, to invite him out to dinner or golf. To accept these offerings means that the therapeutic objective will in all probability be jeopardized.

Psychoanalysis has taught us that such positive manifestations on the part of the patient often are smoke screens behind which lurk intense hostility. This is especially the case in those patients who have never dissociated love from hate as a result of disturbed relationships with early authorities. A desire for an intimate relationship with the physician can be a manifestation of resistance against further therapy, and for practical purposes should be regarded as such.

The interpersonal relationship between patient and physician in psychobiologic therapy is thus, as in any other form of psychotherapy, the core of the therapeutic process. It must be studied constantly by noting the patient's verbalizations, his dreams and behavior patterns, and therapy must always be adapted to the current trends in the relationship.

TECHNICS OF HYPNOSIS IN PSY-
CHOBIOLOGIC THERAPY

HYPNOSIS is remarkably effective as a catalyst to the various technics used in psychobiologic therapy. Guidance, reassurance, persuasion, desensitization, re-education and reconditioning gain reinforcement with its use. There is scarcely a patient who does not show the most gratifying response to the combination of methods. The reason for this is that the trance state expedites the positive relationship so necessary in psychobiologic therapy. It permits a more rapid development of feelings of confidence and closeness than if the relationship were to develop spontaneously. An increased faith in the therapist caused the patient to respond more forcefully to persuasive and re-educational influences. In addition, the hypnotic experience has the unique quality of convincing the patient that something definite and important is being done for him immediately.

The patient is introduced to hypnosis as rapidly as possible, generally at the second or third session, as soon as some idea of the patient's difficulty has been obtained, and a partial study of his problem made. It is best not to delay trance induction because as the patient begins to elaborate on his illness, he may start developing resistances to therapy. Should a more complete study of the problem be essential before therapy is started, the patient may be told that he is being taught the technic of hypnosis, so that it can be used later on. As a general rule, some therapy can be employed even at the start.

In such therapies as guidance, persuasion, confession and ventilation, reassurance and re-education, a light or medium trance is sufficient. Suggestions are made both during hypnosis and in the waking state. Should a posthypnotic amnesia develop spontaneously during a trance, the patient may be enjoined to remember the discussions under hypnosis. In reconditioning and in the creation of experimental conflicts for purposes of desensitization, a deep or somnambulistic trance with posthypnotic amnesia will be required. Once the patient is trained in hypnosis, the total period of trance need not last any longer than twenty to twenty-five minutes. The first twenty minutes of the interview may be spent in discussing on a waking level the patient's problems and experiences. Following this hypnosis may be induced, and after the interruption of the trance, five or ten minutes may be spent advantageously in summarizing the discussion.

As has been stated, the chief value of hypnosis is its effect on the interpersonal relationship with the physician. The various psychobiologic technics may be employed both on a waking and trance level. During hypnosis, the patient should be urged to carry suggestions over into the waking state. Although the patient is not so active as in the analytic technics, an effort should be made to get him to participate in the hypnotic discussions. He may be requested to repeat the suggestions made to him and to outline his reactions to them. At all times it is important to follow the trend of his relationship with the physician, particularly by observing his dreams.

In order to utilize hypnosis most effectively, it is necessary to understand how to apply the various psychobiologic technics, a discussion of which follows.

HYPNOSIS IN GUIDANCE

G UIDANCE presupposes a more or less complete acceptance by the patient of the authority that is vested in the physician. Most patients, at least at the start, come to therapy with this in mind. The neurotic person feels spiritually helpless. Life makes no sense, and it is natural for him to look to some authority for help in order to solve his problems. Many psychotherapeutic methods embody guidance and advice until the patient is able to free himself from his turmoil. At this point the technic is altered to a less authoritarian approach in the hope that self development may proceed to where the individual can fulfill himself and plan his own life.

Hypnosis can aid guidance therapy materially, the physician commanding the patient during the trance to comply with suggestions. The patient often experiences a security in the hypnotic relationship that parallels the child's attitude toward a loving adult who protects, advises and guides him into paths to avoid the pitfalls of life. The patient, consequently, may assume the role of the demanding infant who depends on the parent for love and support.

Forms of Guidance

Guidance may take the form of active direction involving the patient's health, education, employment or difficulties in his relationships with friends, relatives or marital partner. It may concern itself primarily with the correction of faulty attitudes toward sex, marriage and children. It may involve environmental manipulation or provision for outlets in hobbies, recreations and social activities.

The extent to which the patient is permitted to make his own decisions varies with the patient's condition. In extremely helpless and dependent persons, and those suffering from psychotic or prepsychotic states, the physician may be forced to play the role of a completely directive authority. He may actually have to plan a daily routine, since the patient may be so obsessed with his inner problems as to allow his habits and daily routines to lapse. A balanced day may have to be arranged for the person, relating to the time of arising, working hours, rest periods, activities, and sleep. The extent to which this program is prescribed will, of course, vary, and in very severe cases it may be essential to account for every hour of the day. Patients who are unable to make their own decisions may, under hypnosis, be directed to follow the program outlined. In some cases, as in psychotics and prepsychotics, the only thing that can be accomplished in psychotherapy is to create in the patient the feeling that he has a kindly powerful person on whom he can depend, and who, in the event of an emergency, will help him master the situation.

Schemes of guidance along these lines have been outlined by Payot,[1] Barrett,[2] Vitoz,[4] Eymiew,[5] and Walsh,[6,7] details of which can be obtained by reference to the works written by these authors. In general, the daily regimen is planned for the patient so that he has no time for idleness and destructive rumination. In some plans of guidance the patient is enjoined to review his daily accomplishments at the end of the day, outlining his successes and failures.

Such complete control of the patient's routines is rarely necessary. Most frequently guidance is directed toward a local problem which disturbs the patient and interferes with his adjustment. This presupposes a careful study of the immediate life situation in order to discover and to correct an existing environmental difficulty; or where the latter is irremediable, to help the patient cope with it.

Guidance suggestions must always be made in such a manner that the patient accepts them as the most expedient and logical course of action. It may be essential to spend some time explaining the rationale for the outlined plan until the patient develops a conviction that it is what he really wants to do. The patient always should be led to feel that his wishes and resistances are understood and respected by the physician.

There are some patients whose personalities are so constituted that they resent a kindly and understanding authority. Rather they are inclined to demand a scolding and commanding attitude without which they seem lost. Such patients appear to need a punitive reinforcement of their conscience out of fear of yielding to inner impulses over which they have little control. Individuals overpowered by homosexual drives, or psychopathic personalities who act out their conflicts and fantasies, feel most stable in a relationship in which they are subjected to inflexible rules and prohibitions. For example, a patient with a homosexual problem who had failed to get any relief whatsoever out of two years of psychoanalytic therapy, responded to three sessions of directive guidance therapy and hypnosis with a complete loss of anxiety and a return to satisfactory functioning. It was apparent that he wanted to stop engaging in homosexual affairs and sought a prohibitive but understanding authority, which role I successfully played.

At the start of therapy, it may be advisable to respect the needs and demands of such personalities, but an effort must always be made later on to transfer the disciplinary restraints to the individual himself. Unless such an incorporation of prohibitions is achieved and becomes an integral part of the individual's conscience, he will demand a greater and greater display of punitive efforts on the part of the physician. To complicate this, when he has responded to dictatorial demands, he will burn inwardly with resentment and hate for the physician, and feel a tremendous contempt for himself for being so weak as to need such pressure.

One way of conducting the guidance interview is to avoid, as much as possible, giving direct advice, but rather to coach it in such a manner that the patient himself believes he has made his own decisions. Furthermore, all advice should be given in a nondictatorial manner, so that the patient feels he may or may not accept the advice, in accordance with his own judgment. There are times, of course, when it is necessary to take a firm stand with some patients, but this should be done only in exceptional cases where it is necessary to protect them against yielding to a dangerous impulse.

The sicker the individual the more he will need active guidance and direction. How long the supportive relationship will have to be maintained will depend on the strength of the ego. In general, as the patient gains security and freedom from symptoms, he will want to take more direction and responsibility into his own hands. Even those persons who offer resistance to assertiveness and independence, may be aided in developing a motivation to be more independent. This may require considerable time and patience, but in most instances it can be achieved. The physician then must shift his technic to a nondirective form of counselling in which the patient is taught that he has the right to make his own choices and decisions and to determine his own values and goal. Ultimately the hope is that he will feel inner strengths with which to master the stresses of life without external help or guidance.

Among guidance approaches which act as adjuncts to hypnotherapy are environmental manipulation and externalization of interests.

Environmental Manipulation

There are some environmental difficulties so disturbing that the individual may be unable to live with them. These may be directly responsible for much of his emotional turmoil. Sometimes the patient is so bound down to his life situation out of a sense of loyalty or out of a feeling that he has no right to express his demands, that he tolerates his condition as unalterable. He may be unaware of the tension and resentment generated, and he may blame his difficulties on situations altogether different from those actually responsible.

The physician may have to interfere actively where the environmental situation is grossly inimical to the best interests of the patient. This usually implies work with the patient's family. It is rare that a patient's difficulties are limited to himself. As a rule his family is also involved. The various members may require re-education, desensitization and other forms of psychotherapy before the patient shows a maximal response to treatment. Indeed the cooperation of the family is not only desirable, but in many instances indispensable. A psychiatric social worker can render invaluable service to the psychiatrist here.

Difficulties arising out of undernourishment, shabby physical attire, bad housing and other consequences of a subminimal budget standard may be completely outside of the patient's control. The sense of futility, tension and unexpressed rage will not be abated by any psychotherapeutic procedure until the material difficulties themselves are relieved. In such instances a community or private agency may have to render assistance. An individual who is living with a brutal or neurotic parent or marital partner may be unable to achieve mental health until an actual separation from the home is brought about. Persons subjected to domineering parents who resent the individual's self sufficiency may feel that their plight is hopeless since compliance seems to be a condition for security.

The physician, through the medium of a social worker, can materially help such problems by simple environmental manipulation. This is particularly the case where the people with whom the patient lives are capable of gaining insight into existing defects in the family relationship. Such factors as favoritism displayed toward another sibling, lack of appropriate disciplines and proper habit routines, the competitive pitting of the child against older siblings, overprotective and domineering influences of the patient's parents or mate may sometimes be eliminated by inculcating proper insights. The correction of sources of discord and tension frequently is rewarded by disappearance of anxiety.

Situational treatment, while admittedly superficial, can have a definite therapeutic value, and may permit an individual to proceed to a more favorable development. Often family members become so subjectively involved with the problems of the patient, so defensive and indignant about them, that they are unable to see many destructive influences that exist in the household. An honest and frank presentation of the facts may permit intelligent people to alter the situation sufficiently to take the strain off the patient.

It must not be assumed, however, that all situational therapy is successful even when gross disturbances exist in the household. Frequently the family is unable or unwilling to alter inimical conditions because of severe neurotic problems in other members, or because of physical factors in the home over which they have no control. Here the social worker, through repeated home visits, may start interpersonal therapy which may bring the family around to accept the recommendations of the psychiatrist. She may, in specific instances, render material aid to the family or assist in the planning of a budget or home routine. Direct contact of the social worker with the family will almost invariably reveal that others need attention or therapy. Often this treatment is necessary before any change can be expected in the patient.

Another function that the social worker can fulfill is to make available to the individual the various church, school and neighborhood recreational facilities. Persons with emotional problems frequently become so rooted to their homes out of a sense of insecurity that they fear outside contacts.

Establishing a relationship with the patient and introducing him to groups outside the home may start a social experience that becomes increasingly meaningful for him, helping to release forces that make for self development.

In cases where the destructive elements within the family are irremediable or where the individual is rejected with little chance of his eventual acceptance, it may be necessary to advise him to take up residence elsewhere. Temporary or permanent placement in a foster family or rest home may be essential. Although there is evidence that temporary placement rarely has an effect on deeper problems, placement in a rest home with kindly and sympathetic adults may serve to stabilize the individual who has not yet suffered structural defects in his personality. The most significant factor in placement is the meaning that it has to the patient himself. If he regards it as another evidence of rejection, it can have an undermining rather than a constructive influence. Instead of getting better, he may regress to more immature patterns of behavior. Above all the patient must be adequately prepared for placement and should look forward to it as a therapeutic experience rather than as a form of punishment.

In certain instances placement in an institution has definite advantages. In alcoholic individuals and those subject to drug addiction, an institution may provide the only environment under which hypnotherapy is possible. In hypomanic reactions, hospitalization may be one of the ways of protecting him against the consequences of his compulsive behavior. In patients suffering from very disturbing hostile tendencies, hospitalization may remove them from sources of temptation to aggression, thereby lessening their anxiety at the same time psychotherapy is employed. In neurotic illness associated with physical disability, as anorexia, persistent vomiting and other grave hysterical and psychosomatic complaints, hospitalization may provide the best medium in which to treat the patient. In depressions and excited reactions, institutionalization may be mandatory.

The process of hospitalization itself may put a halt to a tremendous amount of tension that results from intrafamilial conflicts. The patient is provided then with a chance to start psychotherapy under the most favorable conditions. Restriction of visits on the part of relatives who have a traumatic effect on the patient is more practicable in a hospital than in any other environment. They are usually satisfied with the explanation that the patient needs complete relaxation. Patients who refuse to go away on a vacation when they need a complete change of environment and absence of emotional strain often will accept hospitalization as something they are unable to refuse, since this implies the recognition that they are ill. Hospitalization thus can strengthen the bond between the physician and patient. It may convince the patient that the physician realizes he has an illness that is not imaginary, and that he is not malingering. The patient's morale may thus be partially restored, particularly where it has been undermined by his friends and relatives.

The Weir-Mitchell treatment of complete bed rest, isolation from all visitors, and overfeeding depended to a large degree on the removal from inimical environment. In this therapy there was a reproduction of the parent-infant situation in which support and sustenance were offered through the good graces of the protecting, all-wise physician. The relationship with the physician was probably therapeutically more important than the rest and dietary regime, and many of the "cures" reported were undoubtedly due to the psychotherapeutic effect of the treatment itself.

It must be recognized that the patient may use hospitalization as a means of re-enforcing his neurotic drives. He may welcome admission to a hospital as a sign that he has been grievously injured by his family or the world. He may seek to collapse completely in the helplessness of a bedridden patient, and he may even resent leaving the hospital. Hospitalization must consequently be prescribed only where indicated, and not as a sop to the patient's neurosis. It is essential to appraise what possible effects hospitalization may have before resorting to it.

Caution must also be exercised in effecting drastic and permanent changes in the work or home situation, and thorough study of the patient is essential before one is justified in advising anything that may recast his entire life. This applies particularly to problems of divorce and separation. For instance, a woman came to see me for advice regarding her relationship with her husband. She complained about his coldness, lack of understanding and even viciousness toward her. Marriage to him, she claimed, had been a tragic nightmare for her. He was distant and hostile. Her lawyer had advised divorce, but she wanted professional advice before starting proceedings.

It was obvious after several interviews that the patient's marital relationship was destructive to her. It was apparent also that both partners were using the relationship as a vehicle for their neurotic fears and expectations. The patient had always been an extremely dependent person with few resources of her own, and had in her girlhood lived in fear that she would never find a mate. This thought filled her with despair and resentment. Accordingly she accepted the first man who proposed to her, although she was not sure they loved each other. As time went on she grew fond of her husband, but she was never convinced that he loved her. Signs of his rejection seemed apparent, and she made more and more inordinate demands on him, responding with anger at his inability to live up to her expectations.

The husband, on the other hand, reacted to his wife's hostility by a sullen withdrawal, and finally by impotence. Immersing himself in work, he paid less and less attention to his wife.   The patient interpreted this as a sign that he was finding romantic interests outside of the home which increased the tension between the two.

Several interviews with the husband helped clarify for him the meaning of his wife's emotional problem and the role he played in it.   His own guilt feelings were alleviated by this understanding.   Spontaneously he began to spend more time in pleasurable pursuits with his mate.   A re-educational approach with hypnosis helped the patient master some of her neurotic patterns, particularly the incessant demands she made on her husband.   The ultimate result was a satisfactory adjustment between the two, and even though the patient continued to have feelings of rejection, she began to doubt their validity, and she refused to permit them to create further marital discord.

Many patients seek advice from the physician while on the crest of a wave of resentment which compels them to desire separation or divorce.   Mere encouragement on the part of the physician serves to translate these desires into action. The physician should therefore always be chary of giving advice that will break up the marriage until he is completely convinced that there is nothing in the marital situation that is worthy of saving, or until he is sure that the relationship is dangerously destructive to the patient and that there is no hope of abatement.   This precaution is essential because the patient may completely bury, under the tide of anger, positive qualities of his mate to win sympathy from the physician or to justify his own resentment.

Where the physician lets himself be swept away by the patient's emotion, and encourages breakup of the home, many patients will be plunged into despair and anxiety. They will blame the physician for having taken them so seriously as to destroy their hopes for a reconciliation.   It is advisable in all cases, even when the home situation appears hopeless, to advise the patient to attempt the working through of his problems in his present setting, pointing out that his mate may also suffer from emotional difficulties for which treatment will be required.   The patient therefore will not only help himself, but also his mate.   Whatever positive features exist in the relationship will be saved.   It is wise to get the patient to talk about positive qualities possessed by the spouse instead of completely absorbing himself with the latter's negative characteristics.

In marital problems, it is often advisable to interview the patient's mate even though it is to be expected that the latter will be antagonistic out of a conviction that he or she is being blamed for everything.   Experience shows that whenever a marital difficulty exists, no one party is completely responsible.   A patient, in working through her tangled relationships with her husband, frequently becomes aware of the fact that she actively antagonizes him by inordinate expectations, by nagging and by resentment of which she may be unaware.   On the other hand she may find that in submitting herself to her husband without qualification, he has lost respect for her.   The ability to make demands and to stand up for her rights, may produce a wholesome change in her husband's attitude toward her.   Change brought about in the patient through therapy is reflected in improvement in the partner, since marital difficulties are usually the product of an active relationship between the two.

Where a partner has done something that offends the pride and standards of his mate, a changed attitude toward the provocative incident may prevent its recurrence.   For instance, where the husband has been unfaithful, and the wife has become aware of his infidelity, her immediate reaction may be a desire to break up the home.   While infidelity should not be condoned, the patient must be shown that she may have been in some measure responsible for a turning of her mate's interest elsewhere.   She may be reminded that while she has been grievously hurt, her emotion, expressed explosively, will serve merely to drive her husband further away from her.   Actually the infidelity may be a passing fancy which has no lasting significance to her husband.   A changed attitude toward the situation may produce a better understanding between husband and wife when they realize that failings on both their parts have been responsible for his meandering.

One must not assume that environmental correction can help all patients.   In many cases environmental difficulties, while accentuating the patient's problems, are only precipitating factors.   The basis for the individual's maladjustment here is his personality structure, which has so many inharmonious elements that inner conflict is incessant, with little relationship to outside circumstances.   As a matter of fact most people have a tendency to objectify their problems by seeking out conditions in their environment that can justify feelings of rage or tension.   For example, if a person has a problem associated with the fear of being taken advantage of by others, he will find evidences of this in any situation in which he is involved.

In a relatively large number of persons, environmental correction has little effect on the existing emotional upheaval. Here the difficulty has been structuralized in such a widespread character disorder that problems in interpersonal relationships seem to perpetuate themselves endlessly.   Indeed the individual seems to create situations to which he can react in his customary destructive manner.   More confounding is the fact that he may need a disturbing atmosphere for proper functioning.   He may, for instance, seek to be victimized by others in order to justify feelings of hostility that could otherwise not be rationalized.   In cases such as this the correction of environmental stress, without a corresponding alleviation of inner conflicts, may produce a crisis, with depression or psychosomatic illness due to an internalization of aggression.   One of the most discouraging discoveries that the physician can make is that in liberating a patient from a grossly disturbed environment, he finds that the latter immediately involves himself in another situation equally as bad as the first.

A safe rule to follow is to remedy gross environmental defects with the patient's consent and cooperation, at the same time that he is brought to some realization of his existing personality difficulties. The effects of environmental manipulation must be studied constantly and changes made in the treatment plan in accordance with the patient's reactions.

EXTERNALIZATION OF INTERESTS

Neurotic patients often become so absorbed in their own inner problems that external reality begins to lose its meaning. If in such cases interest can be directed toward games, sports, hobbies or recreations, attention may be channeled from the self into constructive external outlets. Many interests can be exploited in this effort, such as woodwork, needle craft, weaving, rugmaking, gardening, bridge, chess, table tennis, handball, quoits, swimming, golf, riding, dancing, dramatics, drawing, painting and sculpturing. There are countless other hobbies and recreations that may be utilized to divert attention from inner tensions and anxiety.

Occupational and recreational therapy are important adjuncts to other forms of psychotherapy. The chief difficulty is getting the patient sufficiently interested. Outside activities usually have little significance for the patient, since he may be so completely wrapped up in his illness or in a rigid routine that he will regard all hobbies or sports with disdain.

If the patient's initial resistance can be overcome, he may find certain phases of a suggested diversion so fascinating that his interest will automatically be maintained. Indeed, he may devote himself to the activity with the same avidity

with which he exploited his neurosis.   Alcoholics and compulsion neurotics, for example, become so intrigued with a
hobby that they may become completely absorbed.   This
substitution is, of course, far more wholesome and less destructive than the exploitation of their neurotic interest.

Occupations or diversions in which the patient evinces
some interest should be chosen at the start.   A survey of his
prevous activities is important.   Should he have no interests, it is important to guide him so he will develop some.
The physician may discuss with the patient the need for a
new interest, and he may suggest a hobby or group of
hobbies.   It is best, however, to leave the choice up to the
patient, himself, since a hobby of the physician's choice may
fail to satisfy vital needs.   Or the patient may lose interest
in it after a short time and then chide himself for another
failure.

Considerable resistance may be encountered in getting the
patient to act upon the physician's suggestions.   Hypnosis
may sometimes be helpful here by stimulating the patient to
activity through posthypnotic suggestions.   One patient
who had refused to get interested in a hobby was given a
detailed account of stamp collecting.   Suggestions under
hypnosis that he read a small book on the subject stimulated
him to start a collection that gave him enjoyment he never
before believed possible.

Patients who have built a wall of isolation around themselves to avoid social contacts may also be helped on occasion
by posthypnotic suggestions.   If the patient responds
favorably, he will find himself automatically engaged in social
diversions from which he derives a tremendous amount of
enjoyment, and which he could not have brought himself to
try through his own efforts.   The initial breaking through
of his defenses may suffice to enable him to repeat his experience spontaneously.   In the case of a patient who had
refused to leave her house or to go to the movies because of

lack of interest, she found herself unable to resist a posthypnotic suggestion to attend a neighborhood movie. This one incident sufficed to break her resistance against plays and movies.

A most effective hobby is one that provides an acceptable outlet for impulses the person cannot express directly. The need for companionship, assertiveness, the ability to give and to receive affection, the desire to be part of a group, to gain recognition, to live up to certain creative abilities and to develop latent talents may all be satisfied by the hobby interest.

External activities can provide compensations which help the individual to allay some of his inferiority feelings. Instead of concentrating on his failings, he is encouraged to develop whatever talents and abilities he may have. For instance, if he is proficient as a tennis player, or has a good singing voice, these abilities are encouraged so that he feels he excels in one particular field. Whatever assets the individual has may thus be encouraged. In very dependent people, especially, occupational therapy can serve as an aid to self expressiveness.

Some patients harbor within themselves strong hostilities of an unconscious nature, with needs to vanquish, defeat, and to overwhelm others. Hostility may have to be repressed as a result of feelings that he will be rejected or punished if he expresses rage or aggression. In extreme cases even ordinary forms of self assertiveness may be regarded as aggression. As a consequence, the person may have to lead a life of detachment to avoid giving expression to what he considers forbidden impulses. In such patients hobbies that do not involve competition will be more acceptable at first. The ultimate object is to interest the patient in a hobby that does have a competitive element. The patient may come around to this himself. For example, one patient chose photography as an outlet principally because it involved no contact with other people. Gradually, as he became more expert, he exhibited his work to his friends, and, finally, he entered his pictures in various photographic contests. Later on, with encouragement, he learned to play bridge, which acted as a spur to an interest in active competitive games and sports.

The ability to express hostility through activities that involve the larger muscle groups permits a most effective expression of unconscious aggression. Boxing, wrestling, hunting, archery, marksmanship, fencing, and such work as carpentry and stone building can burn up a tremendous amount of energy. In some individuals the mere attendance of games and competitive sports as baseball, football, and boxing has an aggression releasing effect. It must be remembered, however, that this release is merely palliative, because it does not touch upon the dynamic difficulties in the life adjustment of the person that are responsible for the generation of hostility.

Many other impulses may be satisfied through occupational or diversional activities. Hobbies can foster a sense of achievement and can help the individual to satisfy a need for approval. Energy resulting from inhibited sexual strivings may gain expression sometimes by an interest in pets or naturalistic studies. Frustrated parental yearnings may be appeased by work with children at children's clubs or camps.

One must expect that the patient will try to employ his hobbies as a means of re-enforcing the neurotic patterns by which he adjusts himself to life. If he has a character structure of perfectionism, he will pursue his hobby with the goal of mastering intricate details. If he is compulsively ambitious, he will strive to use his interest as a means to fame or fortune. The same holds true for any of the other character traits he may possess.

Most patients gain temporary surcease from neurotic difficulties during the period when they are working at a new interest, and their illness will become exacerbated when their hobby has failed to come up to their expectations. However, the hobby may open up new avenues for contact with others which will neutralize this tendency.

Neurotic difficulties are associated with profound disturbances in interpersonal relationships that tend to cause the individual to isolate himself from the group. The pleasure he derives in social activities does not compensate for the tensions and anxieties incurred by his mingling with people. Occupational therapy, hobbies and diversions give the person an opportunity to participate with others in a project of mutual enjoyment. Pleasure feelings radiate to those with whom the patient is in contact, and help lessen his defenses against people. They may even lead him to find values in a group.

Man is a social creature and needs to interact freely with other persons. Without this interaction he becomes ill. Neurotic patients feel inferior, lonely and rejected. They have a general fear of people. One of the strongest forces towards health is identification with the group. Because of the strong barriers the patient has built up against people, it may be very difficult to convince him to visit his friends and to participate in group activities. He realizes, of course, that there are many pleasures he can obtain from group experiences, but he dares not take a chance. Through the medium of a hobby or a sport, he may be helped to get closer to others. He may then have a chance for identification with a group. He may also be able to win praise and recognition for his own contributions to the group endeavor.

Once the patient has established a social contact, he may find sufficient pleasures to tempt him to continue. He will usually take more interest in his external appearance. It is to be expected that he will manifest his customary character defenses and hostilities. But the beneficial sublimations he obtains, will more than compensate for his discomfiture.

In some instances, it may be possible to convince the

patient to engage in activities of a social nature, such as community endeavors or work that contributes to the general welfare of the community. This can create in him a feeling of active participation with others, and a conviction that he is really doing something creative and altruistic.

LIMITATIONS OF GUIDANCE THERAPY

The superficiality of guidance treatment must, of course, be acknowledged. One does not start this type of therapy under the illusion that any deep change will occur in the underlying conflicts or in the dynamic structure of the personality. Conflicts are usually whitewashed, and the person is encouraged to adjust to his problems rather than to rectify them. The patient may be taught many methods by which he can avoid emotional blind alleys. He may learn how to correct some environmental defects or to adapt himself to circumstances that cannot be changed. However, where guidance is not supplemented by other therapies calculated to render the person self sufficient and independent, fundamental difficulties in interpersonal relationships will probably not be changed.

Guidance therapy is dependent upon an irrational attitude that the individual has toward authority. There is over-evaluation of the capacities and abilities of the authoritative person to a point where any utterance or suggestion becomes a mandate, any banal remark dogma. As a result the individual may suspend his reasoning abilities and his rights to criticize. He may be completely dominated by feelings of awe, fear and reverence.

It goes without saying that under these circumstances any doubt that crops up relating to the strength or wisdom of the authority invokes strong insecurity. Hostility and guilt feelings, if they develop at all, must be rigidly repressed for fear of invoking counterhostility or disapproval. One may recognize from such irrational patterns the same attitude the child expresses toward the omnipotent parent. Actually the emotional helplessness of the neurotic individual resembles to a strong degree the helplessness of the immature child, solution for which is sought in dependency on powerful parental figures. The neurotic person thus recreates in the physician the original authority he invested in his parents, and he will seek from him the same type of love.

There are many destructive seeds in guidance therapy. The very essence of the relationship is self abasement, and one of the immediate consequences is an inner paralysis of the self with the incapacity to be self expressive and assertive except so far as these meet with the consent and approval of the physician. Furthermore, the individual has to maintain an image of the physician as infallible. Should the latter display any human frailties or lack of invincible qualities, the faith of the patient may be shattered, precipitating helplessness and anxiety. An interruption of therapy and a return of symptoms may be consequent. The patient may then attempt to master his anxiety by again annexing himself to another person who possesses those magical and godlike characteristics that he believes are essential for his security. The life history of such dependent individuals demonstrates that they have flitted from one physician to another, from clinic to clinic, from shrine to cult, in a ceaseless search for a parental figure who can guide them to paths of health and accomplishment.

Some patients for these reasons will resent guidance, even though they feel too insecure within themselves to direct their own activities. Others will reject guidance because of previous conditionings in relationship to an authority who has been hostile or rejecting, or who has made such unreasonable demands on them as to thwart their demands for pleasure fulfillment. Acceptance of advice may be tantamount to giving up one's independence or may mark one as inferior.

In spite of its disadvantages, guidance may be the only

type of treatment to which the patient will respond. Most persons seek guidance at the start because they feel helpless in the grip of their neurosis. They have neither the motivation nor the strength to work with a technic that throws the bulk of responsibility on their shoulders. Where the physician utilizes guidance as a temporary measure, working toward motivating the patient to accept insight into his problems, he will achieve more gratifying results in therapy. As soon as a good relationship with the patient is established, the physician should shy away from any attempt to force the individual to comply. The patient must be shown that the physician does not desire to impose any edicts, but rather that he wishes to work cooperatively with the patient, presenting certain impressions to him for what they are worth. The patient, himself, may then decide to act on these suggestions or to reject them as he sees fit. A considerable amount of activity and cooperation on the part of the patient will be necessary. He may resent this at first, but eventually he will learn that he gains strength from making his own decisions.

Unfortunately there are some patients who never develop in their personality growth to the point where they can take over the reins of their own destiny. So strong a resistance to self assertiveness exists that they can function only when they have a parental figure on whom to lean, who can prod them on in their daily accomplishments. In such cases it is essential to try to get the patient to be as self sufficient as possible.

In some guidance approaches, where it is apparent that lack of motivation and ego strength make a more scientific form of therapy impossible, the patient is guided toward religion. An attempt is made to convince him that he will be aided in gaining health by kinship with the divine being, since in union with God, the soul need not struggle alone. It can draw sufficient strength from this relationship to conquer evil thoughts and impulses, to crush dread and fear, to achieve confidence and faith in living. This help is to be gained through faith and prayer.

Certain individuals are made immensely more comfortable by this religious type of therapy, which has advantages over pure guidance in that the patient gets his doses of reassurance through his own efforts of prayer and through participation in church activities. In religious therapy also, the patient is not in a position to dispute the powers of God as he can with the physician, whom he may discover to be less infallible or masterful than he desires.

HYPNOSIS IN REASSURANCE

SOME REASSURANCE is necessary in all forms of psycho-therapy. The patient often voices doubts concerning his ability to get well or to gain relief from neurotic suffering. Many fears embraced by the patient are the product of false ideas gleaned from friends as misinformed as himself. Other fears are the result of the patient's own fantasies or irrational thinking. Sometimes they are caused by lurid stories that have no basis in fact. For instance, in early life they may have been imposed on the patient by his parents in an effort to discipline or to frighten him. An honest discussion of such fears, and an explanation of how baseless they are, may serve to make the patient more comfortable and help in alleviating tension and anxiety.

In many neurotic conditions the patient worries about his symptoms to a point where they become exaggerated in his mind. A reassuring attitude on the part of the physician is helpful in diverting attention from symptoms toward more basic problems that produce the neurosis. Energy may therefore be concentrated in creative efforts rather than in futile fears and self recriminations. Such reassurance is, of course, quite superficial, but it may help the patient get out of the vicious cycle of brooding about himself.

Where reassurance is used, it should not be started too early, since the patient at the start may not have sufficient faith in the physician to be convinced of his sincerity. He may believe the physician is secretly ridiculing him or does not know how serious the situation really is. Reassurance is founded on acceptance of the physician as a sincere and omniscient authority. It is for this reason that reassurance given to the patient under hypnosis will be accepted and acted upon more intensely than in the waking state.

In reassuring the patient, the physician must listen to his complaints with sincerity and respect, pointing out that they seem significant and overwhelming because they represent much more than appears on the surface. Under no circumstances should the patient be ridiculed for illogical or ridiculous fears. He, himself, usually appreciates that his worries are senseless, but he is unable to control them. Actually he may not be so much worried about the fears themselves as he is about their implications.

One of the most common fears expressed by the neurotic person is that of going insane. Panicky feelings, bizarre impulses and unreality sensations lead him to this assumption. He becomes convinced he will lose control of himself and inflict injury on himself or others. Usually he justifies his fear by revealing that he has a relative who is insane, alcoholic, or epileptic, from whom he believes he has inherited a taint. It is essential to show him that fear of insanity is a common neurotic symptom, and to acquaint him with the fact that there is scarcely a family in which one cannot find cases of mental illness. A presentation of the facts of heredity, and an explanation that insanity is not inevitable even in those with the most positive history, is most helpful. Furthermore, the patient may be reassured that his examination fails to reveal evidence of insanity.

Another fear relates to the possession of a grave physical disease or abnormality. The patient may believe that through masturbation, physical excesses, or faulty hygiene he has procured some irremediable illness. A physical examination with x-ray and laboratory tests may help convince the patient that his fear is founded on emotional factors. An explanation may be given him regarding how anxiety and worry can produce physical symptoms of a reversible nature. Where his fears are not too integral a part of his neurosis, these explanations may suffice. Even where fears are deep, as in obsessional patients, and even where he does not accept the results of the physical examination, his more rational self will toy with the idea that he may be wrong.

At any rate the absence of demonstrable physical illness will give the physician the opportunity to demonstrate to the patient that his problem is much more than a physical one, that feelings of being ill or damaged may serve an important psychologic function.

Masturbatory fears are often deep seated and operate outside the awareness of the person. The patient may, through reading and discussions with enlightened people, rationalize his fears, or he may gloss them over with an intellectual coating. Either because of actual threats on the part of early authorities, or through his own faulty deductions, he may believe that his past indulgences have injured him. He may shy away from masturbatory practices in the present or else engage in them with conscious or unconscious foreboding. Reassurance about the supposedly evil effects of masturbation, coupled with assigned reading of books which present scientific facts on the subject, usually have remarkably little effect on the patient's misinterpretations. He is unable to rid himself of childish emotions that seem invulnerable to reason. Nevertheless, the physician's point of view should be presented in a sincere and forthright manner, with the statement that the patient may not be able, for emotional reasons, to accept the explanation at the moment. Eventually as he sees how deep his masturbatory fears really are, he may be able to understand how victimized he has been all his life by the faulty ideas about masturbation which he absorbed during his childhood.

Reassurance may also be required in regard to sexual impulses and sexual relations. Many people express disappointment in their sexual life and believe there must be something basically wrong with their mate or with themselves because they are unable to experience the exquisite pleasures of sex they had imagined would come about as a result of their marriage. It is essential to reassure the person that this is not necessarily the case. Frequently an inability to experience pleasure in sex may be due to early sexual intimidations, to guilt feelings and to many other unfortunate associations.   The first sexual contact may have failed to live up to expectations.   The person must be reassured that sexual feelings have to be nurtured, especially when they have undergone a long period of repression.

In women, frigidity may be the product of years of fear and guilt.   Marriage will not automatically remove these fears.   This explanation will provide an opportunity to go into the details of the patient's sexual life and to prescribe the proper reading material.   The patient may discover that the difficulty does not lie exclusively in herself, but also in the approach of her husband who may take her for granted and spend insufficient time in love making and preparation for the sexual act.   In such cases, the husband will also require instruction and perhaps therapy.

In men, reassurance may be required for temporary impotency.   Many males are concerned about their own sexual powers, and have exorbitant expectations of themselves in a sexual sphere.   Reassurance may be given to the effect that episodes of impotency are quite natural in the lives of most men.   Temporary feelings of resentment toward a marital partner, or attempts at intercourse during a state of exhaustion, or without any real desire, interfere with erective ability.   On the basis of several such failures in performance, the individual may become panicky, and his sense of tension may then interfere with proper sexual performance thereafter.   The patient may be shown the necessity for a different attitude toward sex, less as a means of performance, and more as a pleasure pursuit.   Reassurance that his impotency is temporary and will rectify itself with the proper attitude, may suffice to restore function.

Another concern shown by patients is that of homosexuality.   Fears of homosexuality may be overwhelming. It is essential to reassure the patient regarding his homosexual

fears or impulses. An explanation that a liking for people
of the same sex may sometimes be associated with sexual
inclinations toward them, that this impulse is not a sign one
is evil or depraved, and that it need not be yielded to, may
be extremely reassuring. An effort may be made to explain
how in the development of a person he is thrown together
with children of his own sex, and how sexual curiosities and
sex play are universal and may lead to homosexual explora-
tions. Usually this interest is transfered to members of the
opposite sex, but, in some persons, for definite reasons, an
arrest in development occurs. The patient may be informed
that homosexuality represents a basic attitude toward people
as part of a neurotic problem, and that it need not be considered any more significant than any other problem which
needs psychiatric treatment.

Reassurance may be required because of infidelity of a
marital partner. Where a woman is extremely upset because
her husband has been unfaithful to her, it is probably not
only because she feels her security threatened but also because she experiences a shattering of her self esteem. She
may be reassured that infidelity on the part of the marital
partner is indeed hard to bear but that it is far from a unique
experience, occurring often in our culture. It is probably
by no means due solely to any defect or fault in herself. She
must be urged not to be stampeded into a rash divorce
simply because she feels outraged. In most cases infidelity
is a passing fancy and need not destroy the marital relationship. It is natural that knowledge of her husband's infidelity should have filled her with indignation, but she should
not act precipitously. She may find herself encouraged by
friends, family and public opinion to hate her husband, and
to cut herself from him. There are few women who can
resist acting dramatically and precipitating a divorce over an
affair that is in all probability quite insignificant. Such
reassurance may convince the woman that she really does

not desire a divorce, but that she can work out a better relationship with her husband and perhaps discover why the two had drifted apart.

LIMITATIONS OF REASSURANCE

Reassurance is apt to help the patient with everyday material problems and with fears that are based on misinterpretations. It is not so successful when applied to basic personality difficulties.

One of the most common symptoms in the neurotic person is a devaluated self esteem which fosters inhibitions in action, perfectionistic strivings or feelings of worthlessness, inadequacy and self condemnation. An attempt to inflate the patient's ego by reassurance here is usually unsuccessful.

Self devaluation may be a symptom that serves a useful purpose for the patient, protecting him from having to live up to expectations on the part of other people or his own ego ideal. Self depreciation may furthermore help him as a subversive means of pleading for love and protection on the basis of his own helplessness. He may also feel that if he prepares himself by self castigation, he will not suffer so much upon being confronted with a situation that actually brings out his shortcomings. To rebuild his self esteem by reassurance, therefore, threatens to remove an important coping mechanism. Many persons who devaluate themselves actually derive from this act masochistic gratification, insidiously doing penance for forbidden strivings and desires. Reassurance here may actually plunge the person into anxiety. Other persons secretly harbor tremendously arrogant notions of their capacities and worth. When reassured that they are all right, they become filled with rage, because they believe they will have to adjust on a normal or mediocre level. The end result may be that the patient will interrupt therapy and seek a physician who they fantasy will fulfill their grandiose expectations.

Apart from the instances mentioned, reassurance, judiciously given, is a helpful adjunct to therapy. It should, nevertheless, be used only where indicated. Where the patient has sufficient ego resources, reassurance should be minimal, and emphasis must be placed upon the fact that much of the responsibility for getting at the patient's problems has to be borne by himself. If this precaution is not taken, the patient may lose initiative in getting at the source of his difficulties, and will tend to seek more and more reassurance from the physician. Reassurance should always be coupled with efforts to bring the patient around to working more dynamically with his problems.

HYPNOSIS IN PERSUASION

PERSUASION is based upon the belief that the patient has within himself the power to modify his pathologic emotional processes by force of sheer will, or by utilization of common sense. In persuasive therapy, appeals are made to the patient's reason and intelligence, in order to convince him to abandon neurotic aims and symptoms, and to help him gain self respect. He is enlightened as to the false nature of his own concept regarding his illness, as well as the bad mental habits he has formed, and by presenting him with all the facts in his case, he is shown that there is no reason for him to be ill. He is urged to ignore his symptoms by adopting a stoical attitude, by cultivating a new philosophy of life aimed at facing his weaknesses, and by adopting an attitude of self tolerance. An attempt is made to bring the individual into harmony with his environment, and to get him to think of the welfare of others as well as himself.

Most lay psychotherapists utilize persuasion and attempt to indoctrinate their patients with their own particular philosophies of life. Results derived from this form of treatment are due to the more or less directive relationship between the patient and therapist, to a need for the therapist's approval, and to a feeling that the therapeutic authority must know what is best for the patient. The approach is a somewhat more mature one than that of guidance, since it presupposes active participation of the patient in his own cure, and aims for an expansion of the personal powers and resources. The majority of popular books on mental therapy are modified forms of persuasion.

The use of persuasion was first advocated by Paul DuBois[8,9] of Switzerland who held conversations with his patients and taught them a philosophy of life whereby they substituted in their minds thoughts of health for their customary preoccupations with disease and suffering. Much of the success that DuBois achieved by his persuasive methods was due to his own vigorous personality which exuded confidence and cheer.

DuBois recognized the importance of the interpersonal relationship and he insisted that the physician must treat the patient not merely as an interesting case, but as a friend. He declared that the doctor must be inspired by a real sense of sympathy and affection for the patient, and should show these sentiments so openly that the patient "would really be very ungrateful not to get well." The physician must be sincere in this conviction that the patient would get well because if he had any doubts, he could not help imparting them to the patient.

The aim of "mental persuasion," according to DuBois, was to build up in the patient a feeling of self confidence, to make him his own master. This was done by imbuing the patient with a belief in himself by "education of the will, or, more exactly the reason." The physician was enjoined to hammer the truth into the patient's mind with the ardor of a barrister convinced of the justice of his plea.

In order to approach the patient's problem rationally, it was first necessary to understand clearly the nature and sources of the disorder. The physician had to distinguish those symptoms of a physical nature and those of psychical origin. The analysis with the patient of his symptoms and the understanding of how these debilitated and inconvenienced him was important, for it made the person feel that the physician was interested in him and understood his suffering. The patient had to be shown how he utilized his symptoms to escape responsibilities in life. He had to be convinced that his nervousness had crushed his morale. Even though he believed his trouble to be physical, it really was mental. He was urged to chase his troubles from his mind, and he was promised that his discomforts then would all vanish. He needed no medicine, DuBois insisted, "for there is none to turn a pessimist into an optimist."

DuBois recommended prolonged discussions during which it was necessary to convince the patient of his errors in reasoning. He had to be shown that his symptoms were the product of emotional stress. Though annoying, they were not serious in themselves. The less one concentrated on symptoms, the less disturbing these would become. If the heart palpitated, let it pound; if the intestines were active, let them grumble. If one had insomnia, he had best say: "If I sleep, all the better; if I don't sleep, no matter." Undue attention aggravated the difficulty. The best way to overcome symptoms was to stop thinking about them. Fatigue, tension and fear were all exaggerated by attention. It was necessary to stop thinking of pain and suffering and to dismiss petty ailments with a smile. "The proper philosphy," he said, "easily learned, can restore the mental balance."

DuBois contended that healthy people disregarded their bodily sensations. The emotionally upset person on the other hand, concentrated on them until they became his chief preoccupation. For this reason he was upset by improper thinking habits. Notions of happiness and health must then replace ideas of disease and suffering. Happiness depended less on external circumstances than upon one's inner state of mind. One might be ill, or have some financial misfortunes, or have lost dear friends; but the intensity of his suffering depended upon the spirit with which he accepted these calamities.

The education of the "self" was the first step in securing real happiness. The patient had to cultivate the thought in his mind that he was going to get well. So long as he was convinced he would experience pain, fatigue or other symptoms, he would feel them vividly. If he obliterated these thoughts from his mind, he would overcome his problem.

Every sign of progress was to be held up to the patient and even exaggerated. Improvement was to be stressed as proof of the patient's tenacity to get well. As soon as ideas of health entered the mind, ideas of disease would vanish. The patient was to be shown that he was not alone in his trouble, that everyone had difficulties that varied only in their manifestations. While he might be concerned with his symptoms, his problem was deeper, involving attitudes which were very significant. Improvement in his attitudes toward life held forth the greatest hope for cure. Above all he must not be hopeless about the outcome, even though it required a long time to secure real improvement. The patient's nervousness existed a long time before the present difficulty. Relapses might occur as improper thinking habits returned, but these would be easier and easier to combat as one stopped thinking about himself. He had to bear his discomforts cheerfully and make it his ambition to lead a bold and active life. He had to develop confidence in his own powers of resistance.

One of the most important elements in therapy was to question the patient about his conceptions of life and his philosophy. False views were to be criticised, and those viewpoints that were logical and helpful were to be encouraged. The physician had to make an effort also to discover in the patient qualities of superiority that would elevate him in his opinion. It might even be necessary to teach him to make an optimistic inventory of his good qualities. If the patient's condition was brought about by tragic events, one had to soothe his suffering by reassuring him and sympathizing with him. If his difficulties involved irritability and emotional instability, he had to be taught the spirit of forbearance. Therapeutic efforts were not confined to the patient, but also extended to those with whom he lived.

Among the proper philosophical ideas that the patient was to imbibe were moral notions which could guide one's life and make for good relationships with others. The best way to forget oneself was to devote more thought to other people. The best road to happiness was altruism and making others happy. Tolerance, sympathy, kindness, and forbearance were the keynotes of a serene life. Religious sentiments were to be awakened and turned to good account.

DeJerine,[10] using the methods of DuBois, also emphasized the "re-education of the reason," but he stressed emotion rather than weakened will as the basis for neurosis. He speculated that the emotions under certain conditions might overwhelm the intellect and cause illness. DeJerine believed that therapy must therefore aim for a liberation of the personality from the effects of harmful emotions. The emphasis in therapy was to get the patient to talk about traumatic incidents in his life, especially fears and sorrows in the present. Unlike DuBois, DeJerine did not try to impose his philosophy on the patient, but strove to permit the patient to develop an emotional relationship with him until a state of confidence developed. When this was obtained, DeJerine practiced persuasion to encourage the patient to correct his "bad habits." He contended that to cure nervous illness, one had to fight the deceptive systems of monism, fatalism, skepticism, and determinism. Reason could overcome obsession once emotions were given a proper outlet. It was necessary to keep before the patient's mind an ideal. He had to think thoughts of the noble, the just and the beautiful. He had to learn to gain satisfactions by the fulfillment of duty, yet the brain had "always to be guided by the heart."

Modern persuasive methods draw largely for their inspiration on the work of DuBois and DeJerine. Stress is laid on cultivation of the proper mental attitude toward life, on the facing of adversity, and on the accepting of environmental difficulties and self limitations one is unable to change.

The dynamic basis of many persuasive cures lies in the enforcing of repression of symptoms by appealing to the patient's sentiments of patriotism, family pride, altruism and self respect. The therapist builds up in the patient a desire to get well in order to indulge pleasures inherent in being constructive and sociable. The patient is reminded constantly that if he regards himself as a better person, others too will have a better opinion of him. Furthermore his duties and responsibilities to get well are continuously emphasized.

Hypnosis can give force to persuasive arguments, since the hypnotic relationship facilitates the absorption and acceptance of suggestions. The patient is also capable of learning such technics as "thought control" and "emotion control" with greater ease. Under hypnosis the patient is told that all people have within themselves forces of strength, health and creativeness. Emotional illness buries these under feelings of helplessness and inadequacy. Suggestions under hypnosis can conquer neurotic feelings and liberate forces of health. Persuasive suggestions are then given the patient. If the patient is able to achieve a deep trance, posthypnotic suggestions may permit him to carry out directions with more power and determination. It is essential to remember that not even hypnosis will cause the patient to accept any philosophy that violates his basis scheme of life, or which opposes too drastically his character structure. Suggestions must accordingly be in concert with the patient's personality.

Forms of Persuasion

Persuasive suggestions have arbitrarily been subdivided nto several categories. It will be seen that they represent a point of view and a slant on life which may not always be accurate, but which, if accepted by the patient, may help alleviate his distress. In general, suggestions tend toward a redirection of goals, an overcoming of physical suffering and disease, an overcoming of the "worry habit", "thought control" and "emotion control", correcting tension and fear, and facing adversity.

1. Redirection of Goals.   If it is apparent that the patient's goals in life are distorted, he may be instructed that the most important goal in life is inner peace rather than fame, fortune or any other expedient that might be confused with real happiness.   In order to gain serenity he may have to abandon hopes of becoming rich, famous or successful.   He may be causing himself much harm by being over-ambitious. If he is content to give up certain ambitions, and to make his aim in life mental serenity and enjoyment, he should try living on a more mediocre scale.   He should give up struggling for success.   Health and freedom from suffering are well worth this sacrifice.

One can attain happiness and health by learning to live life as it should be lived, by taking the good with the bad, the moments of joy with the episodes of pain.   One must expect hard knocks from life and learn to steel himself against them.   It is always best to avoid foreboding and anticipations of what might happen in the future.   Rather one should aim for a freer, more spontaneous life in the present. He should take advantage of the experiences of the moment, and live for every bit of joy he can get out of each day.   The place to enjoy life is here; the time is now.   By being happy oneself, one can also make others happy.

It is always necessary to try to help other people with their problems.   Many persons who have suffered pain, disappointment and frustration have helped themselves by throwing their personal interests aside and living to make their family and other people happy.   Helping others always results in helping oneself.   Man is a social creature and needs to give to others, even if it is necessary to force himself to do so.   In giving he will feel a unity with other people. He can take a little time out each day to talk to his neighbors, to do little things for them.   He can seek out a person who is in misery and encourage him to face life.

The person must also avoid acting out of a sense of hopelessness. One of the pitfalls into which most nervous people fall is a hopeless feeling that paralyzes any constructive efforts. It is necessary to remember that hopelessness is merely a part of the problem. It is as much a sign of sickness as anxiety or physical symptoms. One must never permit himself to yield to feelings of hopelessness. Life is always forward-moving. Hopelessness and despair are a negation of life. If a person stops holding himself back, he will automatically go forward; for development and growth are essential parts of the life process.

2. *Overcoming Physical Suffering and Disease.* The patient, if he is suffering from ailments of a physical nature, may be told that physical symptoms are very frequently caused by emotional distress. Studies have shown that painful thoughts can affect the entire body through the autonomic nervous system. For instance, if we observe an individual's intestines by means of a fluoroscope, we can see that when the person thinks of fearful or painful thoughts, the stomach and intestines contract, interfering with digestion. On the other hand, peaceful happy thoughts produce a relaxation of the intestines and a restoration of peristaltic movements, thus facilitating digestion. The same holds true for other organs.

Understanding the powerful effect that mind has over body is important, for it lends scientific proof to the fact that physical suffering can be mastered by a change in attitudes. By directing one's thoughts along constructive lines, by keeping before the mind's eye visions of peace and health, a great many persons who have suffered physical ailments, and even incurable diseases, have conquered their suffering and even have outlived healthy people. This is because a healthy mind fosters a healthy body and can neutralize many effects of a physical malady.

Physical aches and pains, and even physical disease, may be produced by misguided thoughts and emotions. The body organs and the mind are a unity.   The one influences the other.   Physical illness can influence the mind, producing depression, confusion, and disturbed thought processes. On the other hand the psyche can also influence the body causing an assortment of ailments.   When such a condition prevails, instituting proper thought habits can dispel physical distress.

It is quite natural for a person who is suffering from physical symptoms to feel there is something organically wrong with him.   He cannot be blamed if he seeks relief.   But relief is not found in medicines or operations.   Relief is found in determining the cause of his trouble and correcting the cause.   If a person has pain resulting from a hobnail, the cure is surely not a sedative to relieve the pain.   The cure lies in removing the nail.   Worry, tension and dissatisfaction are causes for many physical complaints, and the treatment lies in abolishing destructive thoughts.

The first step in getting relief from physical suffering is to convince oneself that one's trouble is not necessarily organic. The difficulties may lie in one's environment, but usually they are due to improper thinking habits.   If there is a remediable environmental factor, this must of course be remedied.   If it cannot be altered, the person must learn to change himself so that he can live comfortably in his difficult environment.   In the latter case he has to reorganize his patterns of thinking.

Where a patient actually has an organic ailment that is not amenable to medical or surgical correction, an attempt should be made to get the patient to accept the illness, and to change his attitude toward it.   Here it is essential to discuss the problem thoroughly with the patient in an effort to reorganize his entire philosophy so he can find satisfactions in life consistent with his limited capacities.

In physical conditions of a progressive nature, such as a coronary thrombosis, cancer or malignant hypertension, the patient may be in a constant state of anxiety, anticipating death at any moment. Here it is wise to emphasize the fact that death is as much a part of living as is life, and the horrors attached to it are those that come from a misinterpretation of nature. Life must go on. Babies are born, and people pass on to a peaceful sleep that is death.

The chances are that the patient still has a long useful life ahead of him that can be prolonged by adopting a proper attitude toward his condition. If suffering and pain do not exist, this should be pointed out as a fortunate occurrence. The person should think about the present, and avoid dwelling too much on the future. No one can anticipate what the future may bring. Accidents can happen to anyone, and even a young person in the best of health does not know when he will be smitten by an illness or accident that he does not expect. The only rational philosophy is to glean whatever joy one can from the moment, to leave the future to take care of itself.

The patient is encouraged to develop hobbies and to engage himself in activities that will divert his thinking from himself. A list of activities that the patient can pursue may be prepared, and the patient should be guided into adopting new interests.

3. Overcoming the "Worry Habit." Patients who are obsessed with worrying about themselves may be urged to remember that worry is a state of tension in which energy is spent ruminating about one's problems and fears, instead of doing something positive about their solution. Worry tends to magnify the importance of petty difficulties, and usually paralyzes initiative. The worrier's thoughts are constantly preoccupied with ideas of fear, dread and morbid unpleasantness. These thoughts have a disastrous effect on the motor system, the glands and the organs.

In order to overcome the "worry habit" it is first necessary to formulate in one's mind the chief problem with which one is concerned. To do this it will be necessary to push apprehensions boldly aside in order to be able to use one's reasoning powers to best advantage. Even when worry is caused by a seemingly insurmountable problem, one should attempt to reformulate the situation to bring clearly to mind the existing difficulties. One may be worrying about an insufficient income, about a neurotic and drunken mate, about overactive and recalcitrant children, about one's seemingly hopeless situation in life. But if one takes time out to be honest with himself, he will realize that he has spent most of his energy in hopeless despair, in anxiety, or in resentful frustration, rather than in logical and unemotional thinking that can bring about a solution.

It is necessary to review all possible solutions for the problem at hand. Next, the best solution is chosen even though this may seem inadequate in coping with all aspects of the problem. A plan of action must then be decided on. It is then necessary to proceed with this plan of action immediately, and to abandon all worry until the plan is carried out as completely as possible. Above all the person must stick to his plan of action, even if he finds it distasteful.

If the person himself cannot formulate a plan, the physician may help him to do so. The patient should be told that it is better to concern himself with a constructive plan than to get tangled up in the hopelessness of an apparently insoluble problem. Until he can work out something better, it is best to adjust himself to the present situation, striving always to externalize his energy in a constructive way.

The patient must be urged to stop thinking painful thoughts. Forgetting is a process that goes on of its own accord. Worry is a process that must be learned. One can therefore help himself by controlling his thoughts and avoiding painful worrisome ideas. If action is impossible for the moment, he can crowd out worrisome thoughts by resolving to stop worrying.

Discussion of painful topics with others should also be avoided. Instead of worrisome ideas, one should direct his thoughts into unemotional channels. If he must discuss his painful feelings, he should confine himself to discussions with the doctor, not with friends or relatives. "Blowing off steam' and relating his troubles to friends often does more harm than good because the suggestions offered are usually unsound. It is better to underestimate his difficulties than to become too emotional about them. It is also necessary to get his friends and relatives to stop talking about his personal problems, if such discussions serve to stir him up. It is understandable that his loved ones will be much concerned with his illness, but they must be reminded that their concern may aggravate the condition. Often a person can forestall matters by insisting that he feels "fine," when questioned by others about his health.

4. "Thought Control" and "Emotion Control." Patients who seem to be at the mercy of painful thoughts and emotions may be enjoined never to permit their minds to wander like flotsam, yielding to every passing thought and emotion. It is necessary to choose deliberately the kind of thoughts to think, and the kinds of emotion to feel. It is necessary to eschew ruminating about resentments, hatreds, and disappointments, about aches and pains, and misery in general.

One must think those thoughts that will nourish the ego and permit it to expand to a better growth. If a person wants to be big in spirit, if he wants to be without pain, he must fill his mind with painless ideas. If he wants to be happy, he must smile. If he wants to be well, he must act as if he were well. He must straighten his shoulders, a smile on his lips, walk more resolutely, talk with energy and verve. He must face the world with confidence. He must look life in the face and not falter. He must stand up to adversity and glory in the struggle. He must never permit himself to sink into the quagmire of helplessness or give himself up to random worries, feeling sorry for himself.   He must replace thoughts of doubt and fear with those of courage and confidence.   He must think steadfastly of how he can, with whatever resources he has, accomplish the most in life. He must feel those emotions that lead to inner harmony.

He must picture himself as above petty recriminations, avoid being self centered and jealous, avoid centering his interests around himself.   Even if he suffers from pain and unhappiness, he must stop thinking about his daily discomforts.   He must give to others and learn to find comfort in the joy of giving.   He must become self reliant and creative.   Emancipation from tension and fear can come by training one's mind to think joyous and peaceful thoughts. But new thought habits do not come immediately.   One must show persistence and be steadfast in his application. One must never permit himself to be discouraged.   He must practice, more and more.   Only through persistent practice can perfection be obtained, so that the mind shuts out painful thoughts automatically.

It is not necessary to force oneself to stop worrying or to force oneself to stop feeling pain, or anxiety, or tension. Will power used this way will not crowd out the painful emotions.   One must substitute different thoughts or appropriate actions.   If he starts feeling unhappy or depressed, he should immediately raise his head and determine to rise above this emotion.   He should talk cheerfully to others, try to do someone a good turn; or he may lie down for a short while, relax his body and then practice thinking about something peaceful and pleasant.   As soon as this occurs, unhappy thoughts will be crowded out, and the entire body will respond.   A good practice is to think of a period in one's life when one was happiest. This may be in the immediate past or during childhood. One may think of people he knew, the pleasant times he had with them   This substi-

tution of pleasant for unpleasant thoughts may take several
weeks before a new thinking habit results.

   5. *Correcting Tension and Fear.* Where undifferentiated
tension and fear occurs, the patient may be told that difficulties may come from without, but that one's reactions
to these difficulties are purely personal and come from within.
By changing one's reactions, he can avoid the evil consequences of stress.   If one is confronted with tension, anxiety
or feelings of inner restlessness, it is best to start analyzing
the causes.   Is it due to a disappointment or failure?   Is
it because of a sense of hopelessness?   Once the cause is
found, it is necessary to face the facts squarely and correct
the cause by action.   It is necessary to plan a course to
follow and to execute it immediately.   If facts cannot be
altered, one must change his attitude toward them.   It is
necessary to stop thinking about the painful side of things,
and to find instead something constructive on which to
concentrate.

   One may be unable to prevent anxious thoughts from
coming into one's mind, but he can prevent them from
staying there.   He must stop saying, "I can't," and think in
terms of "I can."   So long as a person says, "I can't," he is
defeated.   Being resolute and persistent in saying "I can"
will bring results.

   The first step in overcoming tension is to stop indulging
oneself in self pity.   Tension will drag one's life down if he
lets it.   It is best to live one's life today, and let tomorrow's
problems be solved as they come up.   It may be impossible
to change the world, but it is possible to change one's attitudes toward the world.   It is necessary to learn to love
life for the living.   One must learn not to exaggerate
troubles.   He must let other people live their lives and he,
himself, should live his own.

   Many people suffering from tension and fear have helped
themselves by saying, "Go ahead and hurt all you want;

you will not get me down." Fears are best faced by courageously admitting them. It is necessary to overcome the
fear of being afraid. Fear can be conquered by stopping
to fight it or trying to master it by sheer will power. Acknowledging that one is afraid is the first step. Thereafter
he must determine to rid himself of fear by developing the
conviction that he will overcome it. A sense of humor is
without parallel. If one laughs at his fears instead of
cringing before them, he will not be helpless and at the mercy
of forces he cannot control.

Practicing relaxation may be very helpful. Each day a
person may lie on his back, on the floor, or on a hard surface
for twenty minutes, consciously loosening up every muscle
from his forehead to his feet, even his fingers and toes. He
may then start breathing deeply, with slow, deep exhalations
through pursed lips. At the same time he may think of a
peaceful scene at the mountains or seashore. Mental and
muscular relaxation are of tremendous aid in overcoming
states of tension. In spite of his fears, he should continue
his work and not yield to his irrational emotions.

6. *Facing Adversity.* In the event a patient has an irremediable environmental difficulty, he may be reminded
that there are many dire conditions in one's environment
that cannot be changed no matter how diligently one tries.
Poor financial circumstances, an unstable mate, overactive
healthy youngsters who make noise and tax one's patience,
a physical handicap, or an incurable physical illness can
create a great deal of worry, tension and anxiety. It is not
so much these difficult conditions that are important as it is
the reaction of the person to them. Life is full of hardship
and struggle; but the individual need not permit himself to
get embroiled in the turmoil and misery of the world. There
are many persons who are deformed, or deprived of sight,
hearing, and of vital parts of their body who live happily
and courageously because they have learned to accept their

limitations, and to live by the rule that it is best to get the most joy out of life as it is right now.   There are many who exist under the most miserable conditions of poverty, with no resources or education, who are not distressed by worry or nervousness because they have not yielded themselves to their emotions.

It is a human tendency to exaggerate one's plight.   If he compares himself with some other people, he will discover that he is not so badly off.   An individual may not be able to achieve all ambitions he has in life.   He may not be as intellectual as he wants to be, or as strong, or successful, or rich, or famous.   He may have to earn a living at work he detests.   As bad as he imagines his state to be, if he were to be faced with the possibility of changing places with some other people, he would probably refuse to do so.   He might be dissatisfied with his appearance and desire to possess features that would make him look more handsome and distinguished.   If this were possible, he might find that his health had become impaired, or his intellect not up to his present level.   It is better, as Shakespeare put it, to bear existing outrageous fortunes than to fly to others one knows not of.

It is necessary to make the most out of the little one has. Every person has weaknesses and should learn to live around them.   He must pattern his life so as to make his weaknesses as least manifest as possible.   He must expand all of his good qualities to the limit.   One's facial appearance may not be handsome, but the person may have nicer hair and teeth than other people.   He can emphasize these in hair style or smiling. He can appear well groomed with well-tailored clothing. If his voice is good, he can cultivate it. Thus he may take advantage of every good feature he possesses.

Instead of resigning to a sense of hopelessness it is wise to turn one's mind toward creative activities and outlets. It will take much perseverance to conquer feelings of helplessness and frustration, but it can be done.   It can be done by living honestly and courageously.   The wealthiest person is he who has not riches, but strength of spirit.   If one is dissatisfied with himself, he may imagine himself to be the kind of person he would like to be.   He may then find that he can do those things that he has hitherto felt were impossible.   He must never yield to despair or discouragement. Crippled persons have learned to walk by sheer perseverance of will.   On the other hand it is necessary not to set goals for oneself that are impossible of fulfillment.   Thwarted ambition can give rise to bitterness and greed.

The sign of character is to change those conditions that can be remedied and to accept those that cannot be changed. To accomplish this one must face the problem squarely. What is to be done about a difficult situation?   What can be done?   How will one go about accomplishing the change? This calls for a plan of action which once made must be pursued diligently without discouragement.

There are always, of course, situations one must accept. Facts must be faced.   If one cannot change things as they are, he can change his own attitude so that he will not over-react to his difficulties.   As soon as a person has decided to make the best of things, his condition will improve immediately.   Progress will be made in changing oneself. One must accept some difficulties that life imposes on him without struggling or rebelling.   He can try to rise above them by elevating his mind and spirit.   If one is handicapped by a physical illness or deformity he cannot correct, or is confronted by impossible difficulties in his environment, he must learn to tolerate his limitations.   If he is unable to possess the whole loaf, he must learn to content himself with part of a loaf.   He must disregard minor discomforts, and pay less and less attention to them.   His symptoms may be annoying, but they are not fatal.   Keeping two lists, on one side the things that have troubled him, on the other side the things that have gone in his favor, will often convince the person, after a while, that the balance is on the positive side.

It is particularly important to train oneself to overcome the effects of frustration and disappointment. These may be expressed in the form of quarreling, or holding grudges against others, or by depression or physical symptoms. There are many dangers associated with permitting oneself to become too angry. It is best here to forestall anger before it develops, by adopting the attitude that one will not be upset if things go wrong. One must force himself to regard all adversity dispassionately, with the idea of modifying the cause if possible, or changing one's attitude, if the cause cannot be removed.

Limitations of Persuasion

Most forms of persuasive therapy are, to say the least, superficial, and are often based on the acceptance by the patient of banalities uttered by the therapist who utilizes aphorisms and examples from the lives of the great to reinforce ideas that are scientifically unsound.

Persuasive therapy, nevertheless, has some justification in that it provides some people with a mental crutch where a psychological analysis of their problem is impossible. The substitution of persuasive philosophical precepts for destructive habit patterns is probably the lesser of two evils. Some obsessive-compulsive personalities do remarkably well with persuasive methods. Indeed they respond better to persuasion than to psychoanalysis.

The greatest fallacy in persuasive therapy lies in the exaggerated value attached to the reasoning powers as potentially capable of diverting inner emotional processes. There is, furthermore, an assumption that the patient is conscious of his basic defects and is therefore capable of mastering them through concentrative effort. Unconscious conflicts and emotions are the most important determinants of neurotic behavior, and this explains why reason, knowledge and will power often fail to bring about the mastery of symptoms. The same effort should, therefore, be made in persuasion as in guidance, to bring about a change in the relationship with the physician from directiveness to nondirectiveness, and to work with the dynamic sources of the patient's problems in an analytic manner to give him as much insight as he can absorb and utilize.

HYPNOSIS IN DESENSITIZATION

DESENSITIZATION is a process which enables the individual gradually to face and to accept painful aspects of his personality. Freed of the necessity of defending himself, the hope is that he will then become capable of living a more productive life.

Elements most painful to the person, and hence subject to suppression and repression, are damaging memories, particularly of experiences which threaten the individual's security or self esteem, traumatic sexual incidents in childhood, hostile and sexual impulses of various types, and material which points to the fact that he is an inferior, evil or contemptible person. The extent to which such elements are acknowledged will depend on the degree of repression. This, in turn, is conditioned by the intensity of the associated anxiety, and the capacity of the person to cope with this anxiety through his available ego resources. There are thus elements which are conscious and fully known to the person. There are others, so frightening, that they have been totally shunted out of awareness by the mechanism of repression.

The pathologic consequences of suppression and repression are legion. The individual over-reacts to incidents that threaten to bring the hidden material to his attention. He may elaborate symptoms such as phobias, compulsions, paralysis, amnesia and other hysterical manifestations in an effort to give vicarious expression to the repressed material as well as to shield it from awareness. Only by facing the forbidden experiences, impulses or conflicts, by dissociating them from past misinterpretations, and by re-evaluating them in the light of present day reality, is it possible for the person to gain any real relief. Only then will the person become desensitized to their effect.

The method by which desensitization is implemented during therapy varies with the extent of repression. The more conscious material may be handled through discussion, confession and ventilation. The less conscious material will require interpretation from the physician of repressed memories, conflicts and motivations through observation of the patient's free associations, dreams and transference phenomena.

Hypnosis is extremely helpful in desensitization, since it produces a relationship with the physician of such confidence and intimacy that the patient is enabled to talk about matters he would be incapable of facing in waking life. In deeper trance states, repressed memories can be recaptured by direct recall, or by regression and revivification, with associated catharsis and desensitization. Desensitization may also be achieved through hypnotic drawing, dramatics, play therapy, and the production of experimental conflicts. These technics will be discussed in a later chapter since they involve analytic methods.

In utilizing confession and ventilation, the patient is encouraged to talk about those things which bother him most in his past life or in his present day relationships. His responsiveness will depend on the confidence and trust he has in the physician.

The patient may be told that most people have bottled up within themselves memories and experiences which have a disturbing effect on them. The attempt to obliterate emotional experiences by banishing them from the mind is not usually successful. Disturbing ideas keep obtruding themselves into the stream of thought. Even when will power triumphs and suppression succeeds, casual everyday happenings may remind the person of his conflict. In addition to memories, there are also impulses and desires of which the person is thoroughly ashamed, and which he dares not permit himself to think about. Among these may be desires for extramarital sexual gratification, homosexual interests, hostile strivings and impulses of a fantastic and infantile nature.

The uncovering process must never be forced upon the patient. To force him to reveal inner fears of a traumatic nature prematurely, may cause him such panic that his resistance to further revelations will be raised. Actually the patient, himself, has built up so hard a crust of repression that it keeps him from admitting his deepest fears even to himself. It is essential to let him feel his own way and choose his own pace with casual encouragement.

In continued discussions with the patient, it may be emphasized that every individual alive has difficulties and problems of which he is ashamed, that the patient probably is no exception and may have impulses or may have had experiences which make him feel he is wicked. Discussing the patient's problem in this roundabout way may make it possible for him to face his difficulties more openly. For instance, where it is obvious that the patient has a suppressed homosexual wish, the physician may weave into the discussions the fact that every person alive, at certain times in life, develops friendships with and crushes on people of the same sex. This is by no means abnormal, but merely a developmental phase in the life of the individual. Some people, for certain reasons, continue to have ideas which were normal at an earlier phase. As a matter of fact, most people have fears of homosexuality. The patient may then be told that it would be unusual if he did not have such ideas. He may then casually be asked whether he has.

As the patient realizes that he will not be ridiculed or condemned for his impulses, he will become more and more able to face his problem openly. The feeling that the physician is his friend will inspire him to elaborate more completely on his inner fears. The frank acknowledgment by him of his difficulty, and its repeated discussion will serve to clarify his position, and permit him to elaborate a new point of view. For in the clear light of logical discussion most painful impulses are robbed of their horror.

Ventilation by the patient of his fears, hopes, ambitions

and demands often gives him relief particularly when they are subjected to the uncritical and sympathetic appraisal of the physician.   Hitherto the patient has retained memories, conflicts and impulses that he has dared not admit to himself, let alone others.   A growing confidence in the physician makes him feel that he has an ally who will help him bear fearful inner secrets.   Being able to share his secrets with an understanding person robs the experiences of much of their frightening quality.   In addition, the patient finds that his judgment as to the viciousness of his experiences may have been distorted.   The very act of translating his fears into words lessens their terrifying hold on him.   The fact that he has not been rejected by the physician, even though he has revealed his shortcomings, encourages him to re-evaluate the sinister nature of his experiences or desires.

Many of the patient's disturbing fears and ideas have their origin in fantasies or in mistaken notions he has obtained from others.   By talking about his ideas he gives the physician the opportunity to correct misconceptions that he has hitherto accepted.   He may need clarification on phases of life relating to his physical functions or interpersonal relationships.   The patient believes many of his fears and impulses to be unique to himself.   When he receives the assurance that his fears are more or less universal, he may become convinced that it is his attitude toward his fears that has been abnormal.

In the event the patient confesses to a truly reprehensible incident in his life, the assurance that this incident does not necessarily pollute him, that many persons are compelled for neurotic reasons to do things which they regret later, that their subsequent actions can fully neutralize what has been done before, can be very reassuring.   The patient may be urged to spend his energy doing something positive in the present, rather than to wear himself out regretting the past.   He may, if he desires, make some restitution to the person who has been injured by his act or to society in general.

Discussion of the patient's problem is continued until he no longer reacts emotionally to it. The repeated analysis of unpleasant and disagreeable attitudes and experiences permits him to face his past fears and conflicts with diminished inner turmoil. For example, if the person has had a very traumatic experience in his past, its constant review and discussion will permit him to dissociate it from irrational fears. He will develop a capacity to tolerate disturbing emotions. This process is associated with an increase of insight and the ability to deal with his problem on a reality level.

Much of the value that comes from confession and ventilation is based upon the fact that the patient becomes desensitized to those situations and conflicts that disturb him, but which reality demands that he endure. The tolerance of pain, disappointment and frustration are inordinately low in neurotic persons, and it is necessary to build up the ability to deal with difficulties and painful experiences without collapsing.

The method of confession and ventilation has certain serious limitations inasmuch as the most important sources of conflict are usually unconscious. It is often impossible to verbalize the basic causes of anxiety. Nevertheless there are many conscious conflicts that plague the person, ventilation of which has a beneficial effect.

The more unconscious memories and conflicts will require an analytic approach. Hypnosis is invaluable here. The mere induction of the trance serves to dissolve many resistances to recall. Important traumatic experiences, fears, and impulses of which the patient is ashamed may be divulged by the patient while under hypnosis. These must never be presented to the patient in the waking state, and it is best to wait until the patient feels sufficiently strong to talk about them himself.   The fact that he has expressed himself freely during hypnosis will enable him to do so much more easily in waking life.   Dramatics, drawing, play therapy and regression are important technics which aid the recall of repressed material.

In cases where the individual has irrational attitudes that develop from his relationships with people, or where he has phobias, he may be repeatedly urged for purposes of desensitization, to expose himself to those situations that incite painful emotions.   The experience is then subjected to discussion, and the patient is trained to face gradually those situations without quaking.   For instance, if the patient has a fear of closed spaces, he may be instructed to lock the door of his room for a brief instant for the first day; to increase the interval to the count of ten the next day; then to one-half minute, extending the time period each day, until he discovers through actual experience that he can tolerate the phobic situation.   Other phobias may be treated in a similar way varying the suggestion.   The physician must appreciate, of course, that the patient's fears may be rooted in deep unconscious conflicts and may not yield to such densensitization therapy until the sources of fear are uprooted through analytic understanding.

Feelings of hostility are powerful in many patients and will require desensitization therapy.   Hostility is an almost inevitable component of the neurotic adjustment, arising from defects in interpersonal relationships.   Often a fusion of love and hatred such as existed in early childhood has never been resolved.   Because of existing character defects, the patient is constantly frustrated in the expression of his basic needs, and his neurotic impulses frequently get him into difficulties with others, creating incessant hostility. Unfortunately most people in our culture have a great fear of expressing rage because of the rejection or retaliatory punishment that this entails.   As a result of the repression of aggression, drainage through autonomic channels may be the only release.   Psychosomatic illness is thus a frequent consequence.

During hypnosis, the problem of hostility may be discussed with the patient by demonstrating to him how and under what situations his hostility is aroused.   He must also be shown why he feels he must repress the expression of his anger.   Substitutive reactions may be suggested.

In deep hypnosis an artificial situation can be created that would justify the patient's open expression of aggression. A scene may be re-enacted in which he is unfairly exposed to criticism by another person, or his rights jeopardized, and the patient is encouraged to express his resentment verbally and by appropriate motor acts.   Although the patient may realize the artificiality of the situation, the fact that he has expressed himself even in play may facilitate the expression of aggression in the waking state.

For instance, a man applied for therapy for a gastrointestinal disorder for which no organic origin could be found. Significantly his illness was exacerbated whenever he was in the presence of people whom he admired or respected. His interpersonal relationships were oriented around a need to submit himself to the opinion of others, to comply and to act submissive, principally because of uncertainty regarding the validity of his own ideas and convictions.   He was aware of the fact that he resented having to comply with all demands made on him, but he felt powerless to resist.   On the occasions when he had attempted to assert himself, he had become overwhelmed with so much panic that he was unable to persist in his effort.   He was also certain that he was disliked by people.

It became increasingly apparent that his fear of self expressiveness was associated with the notion that he would be rejected or punished.   His idea that others disliked him was the product of his own hostility that he projected toward the world.

Discussion of the need to be assertive and to defend one's

rights and convictions brought forth many examples from his own experience of how disaster had followed such a course of action.   The rise of dictatorship, he insisted, was based upon the powerlessness people felt in coping with authority who could punish one for nonconformity.   He was aware of his rage, but he was certain that he had best never show his resentment toward people.   This was uncivilized and merely made it more possible for people to despise or hurt him.

Under hypnosis the patient was regressed to the age of five, and in the guise of first his mother and then his father, I encouraged him to play with other children, to stand up for his rights if others imposed on him.   I also urged him to forget that he had been taught to be obedient at all times. At progressively more mature age levels, the same process was repeated with the enactment of fictitious incidents in which the patient was able to assert and to defend himself. Finally, the posthypnotic suggestions were given to the patient to the effect that he would want to be able to talk back to people and to ask for things when he desired them. When this wish became strong enough, it would overcome any resistances he had hitherto felt to self expressiveness. He would want to be more and more assertive in his behavior. The patient accepted these suggestions and tried them out cautiously at first, then more boldly.   The gradual realization that he could ask for things and not be rejected, that he could even get angry and show others that he was resentful without being hurt, produced a remarkable change in the patient's patterns of adjustment.   He became more self confident and was soon able to make demands and to refuse to conform with injunctions he felt to be unfair or against his best interests.

Many of the beneficial results of desensitization are a result of a reintegration of the individual in his attitudes toward himself when he finds he no longer must be a victim of inner fears.   The ability to express fearful memories, strivings, and emotions rebuilds his self respect and removes the damaging effects of hostility, tension and anxiety.

HYPNOSIS IN RE-EDUCATION

UNLIKE persuasive therapy which is founded on unscientific and frequently irrational premises, re-education attempts to teach the patient the nature of his difficulties with the object of giving him insight into some mechanisms of his neurosis. The re-educational method that the physician applies will depend upon his training and theoretical orientation. In all cases the aim is to assist the patient toward a more harmonious adaptation to his environment by inculcating in him new adaptive goals and attitudes i line with biologic and social needs. An alteration is a. tempted in the character structure itself.

The character structure of the person is the machinery by which he regulates his relationships with the world and with other people. It issues to a large degree out of experiences and conditionings in childhood in relation to parents and early authorities. Secure and loved children develop patterns of interpersonal reactivity that are conducive to a healthful adaptation. On the other hand, insecure children, as a result of a disturbed home, neurotic parents, rejection or overprotection which produces unhealthful identifications and a devaluated self esteem, develop a character structure that militates against a healthful adjustment.

Reaction patterns are always elaborated to preserve the integrity of the individual, to insure his security and self esteem. As a result of disturbing early experiences and conditionings, the person may become excessively dependent, perfectionistic, or power-driven, or he may develop the notion that he cannot depend upon anyone except himself. He may harbor bloated ambitions, and expectations of himself may become inordinate and out of proportion to his intelligence, capacities, or available opportunities. He may believe that others must fulfill his demands and consequently show little spontaneity and initiative. He may detach himself from people and attempt to function without ties to others. He may be resentful and fail to establish any form of satisfying relationship with another person. Countless other attitudes and impulses may develop on the bedrock of unfortunate early experiences, and these are incorporated in the adult character structure.

The consequence of disturbed attitudes and strivings is maladjustment to life and to people. Difficulties in interpersonal relationships inevitably produce anxiety and hostility. These emotions have a damaging effect on the individual and cause assorted neurotic manifestations and symptoms.

Character drives have such profound security values for the individual that even insight into their irrational nature fails to prevent their operation. The patient may see how in an interpersonal situation he feels victimized or exploited without real provocation. Yet he is unable to prevent feeling the way he does. He may find himself competing blindly, or imposing his will or views on others at all times. Knowledge of how irrationally he is acting has little effect on the compulsive nature of his strivings.

Under these circumstances one may inquire whether it is possible to change character drives by bringing them to the attention of the patient. The answer to this query cannot be dogmatic. The ability to change will depend on a certain "will" to develop to a more complete fulfillment of the self. It will depend upon the ability of the person to tolerate insecurity and anxiety which are inevitable in the abandoning of customary behavior patterns and defenses. It will depend upon what pleasures and secondary gains are associated with retention of maladaptive reactions. Unhealthy as they are, many character traits possess subversive values of an exorbitant nature. To abandon them may mean to the person that he will have to face a life which will have neither meaning nor glamor. For instance, the power-driven individual may base his self evaluation completely on how strong a front he presents to the world. His sole pleasure consists of making himself invincible. The only other alternative he knows is accepting his weaknesses, which is equivalent to being destroyed.

The process of changing character responses is difficult and prolonged. It consists of bringing to the conscious attention of the person his maladaptive attitudes, demonstrating to him what difficulties are consequent to their exploitation. The person is shown the reasons for their development in his past life and for their persistence in the present. Finally, he is helped to adjust with new, healthful, adaptive patterns.

In psychobiologic therapy there is less emphasis on exploring the origins of character drives, and more emphasis on the retraining of habit patterns, regardless of their sources in constitution or in specific inimical experiences. During the process of retraining, early difficulties that originally produced the disturbing character patterns may spontaneously be remembered by the patient. As part of the training, the patient must be taught to face his early childhood experiences, and, if necessary, to change his attitudes toward them.

Among the best known of re-educational systems is that of Riggs.[11, 12] Riggs advocated treatment of psychoneurosis in a new environment such as in a sanitarium. Here the patient received daily treatments from the physician in the form of personal discussions. In addition he obtained group therapy which involved lectures in psychology and in human adjustment The patient followed a routine schedule daily which included rest, exercise, relaxation, occupational therapy, entertainment and social activities. Emphasis was placed on social living and upon re-education of ideals and goals.

Success in re-educational therapy will depend in part upon

how accurately the physician is able to diagnose the patient's
character drives and to understand the ways they interfere
with his adjustment.   It will depend also upon the ability
of the patient to grasp the significance of his trends and to
gain insight into how they operate in his everyday experiences.

In some forms of re-educational therapy, particularly
where too short a time is available to go deeply into specific
character trends, it may be necessary to give the patient a
general description of emotional problems and mechanisms
in the hope that he will be able to apply this knowledge to
himself.   Explanations are made as simple as possible and
may be supplemented by prescribed reading.

Among popular books on the general subject of emotional
difficulties are those by Osler,[13] Riggs,[14] and Strecker and
Appel.[15]   Problems relating to childhood are discussed in
such books as Sayles,[16] Thom,[17] and Williams.[18]   The book
by Levy and Munroe[19] is splendid for family problems.
Books by Horney,[20] Robinson,[21] and Edman[22] may also be
prescribed.   An excellent bibliography of selected reading
may be found in Twyeffort,[23] Bradley and Bosquet,[24] Mudd
and Whitehill,[25] and Appel.[26]

Discussions with the patient take up the reading material
and involve how the patient has applied what he has read to
his own difficulties.   The physician leads the discussion
and asks pertinent questions to see whether the patient has
been able to gain any intellectual insights.

This approach is, of course, very diffuse and usually
touches only upon conscious problems.   Nevertheless the
patient may derive much from the reading and from the
discussions which can allay baseless fears and lay down a
foundation for personality change.

Another method of re-education involves analyzing and
interpreting for the patient his specific character drives,
once the physician has obtained a clear understanding of

them. The aim here is to get the patient to adopt a new philosophy of life based on an understanding of his personality in operation. This method is not so hit and miss a procedure as the previous one, and is somewhat less directive although the relationship with the physician is still an authoritarian one.

The physician teaches the patient to regard his symptoms as the product of emotions and distorted goals in life. He outlines for the patient the disturbed attitudes and strivings which get him into difficulties with people. Next he helps the patient apply the knowledge about himself to immediate life situations. An evaluation is made of the patient's assets and these are compared with his liabilities. From this the patient often learns that he has concentrated upon his liabilities more than on his assets. He may come to the realization that he has been so provoked by his failures that he has minimized any good qualities that he possesses. Indeed when his assets are brought to his attention, he may be surprised that he has accepted them without realizing their proper value. He may gradually become cognizant of how exclusively he has focused his attention on his bad features, blotting from his mind his good points. Redirecting his attention on the latter gives him new goals toward which to strive. This may break up a vicious chain of frustration and despair. An investigation of the patient's objectives may disclose ambitions that he is unqualified to fulfill which have contributed to his sense of defeat. An attempt is made to modify these ambitions within the range of the patient's capacities, energies and environmental opportunities.

There is much in this type of approach that resembles guidance. However it is more nondirective, the patient being actively encouraged to solve his own problems, and to recognize how his compulsive drives initiate and maintain his unhappiness.

A re-educational approach strives to give the patient insight into the neurotic ways he involves himself with people, into his disturbed patterns of adjustment. Conversational discussions may reveal only the more superficial character drives, and an analysis of the patient's free associations, dreams and transference manifestations may be required to get to the core of the patient's problem. Hypnoanalytic technics may be invaluable as an aid to diagnosis and to the understanding of the genesis, function and consequences of the patient's impulses and strivings.

Of utmost importance is the relationship with the physician, for the learning process, which is the vehicle of the re-educational method, is facillitated through a positive, cooperative relationship. Insights cannot be smuggled into a patient's mind. Even where the physician has a sound idea as to the dynamics of the patient's disorder, explanations to the patient will have no lasting effect unless the patient has confidence in the doctor. There are, of course, some persons who have progressed far in working out their own problems, who have developed to a point where a mere pointing out of the meaning of a character drive can have a profound therapeutic effect. Unfortunately this is rare, and considerable time may have to be spent in establishing a good relationship before the patient develops the motivation to change.

Re-education may take the form of teaching the patient to think unemotionally, to face facts bravely, to adjust to painful memories and impulses without panic, to meet stresses of life with courage, and to forsake fantasy in thinking. Each trait that the patient exhibits may be taken up in detail, discussing its origin, purpose, value to the individual, and the ways it interferes with his happiness and adjustment. More adaptive substitutive patterns may then be instituted.

A discussion of the life history for instance, may reveal to the physician an inordinate attachment to a domineering

parent who continues to infantalize the patient. The latter's dependency is brought to his attention, and he may be
shown how certain of his symptoms are based on the need
to cling to people, and to repress his resentment. He may
be shown the wisdom of visiting his family at increasingly
infrequent intervals, and the need to make his own decisions
and to find outlets for his energy and interests. It is to be
expected, because neurotic reaction patterns are so deeply
imbedded that this advice will not be heeded at first; but as
the patient constantly experiences emotions associated with
the giving up of his independence, he may agree with the
physician's observations and gradually experiment with new
methods of adjustment.

Where a patient is too compliant, it may be pointed out to
him that he has always felt the need to be over-respectful
toward authority. His security is bound up with this reaction. However, as a human being he has a right to his own
opinion, and he need not accept the wishes or orders of
other people unless he wants to. He can review in his mind
the pros and cons of any advice given him, and then can
accept it or reject it as he sees fit. If he does not want to
follow the orders or judgments of other people, and they
expect him to, he can explain to them why his own plans
seem best. Should he decide to conform with the wishes of
others, he must be sure this is what he really wants, and is
not what he feels forced to want. Above all he must be
logical rather than emotional in his choice of action. Specific
suggestions on how to function independently may be given
to him. The help of other people with whom the patient
lives may be enlisted in this training process. Frequently it
will be discovered that the patient's problem is exaggerated
by members of his family who refuse to permit the person to
emancipate himself. The extent to which the patient accepts these re-educational suggestions will, of course, depend
on how much he really desires to be independent.

An individual who has a power drive may be shown how

this is a dominating motif of his life, permeating every thought and activity. He may be partly aware of how he strives for power and strength in all of his interpersonal relationships. What he may not be aware of is how mercilessly his drive rules him, and how it results in his forfeiting normal goals. The person must be shown that this trend brings him into conflict with others and brings out retaliatory hostilities. It is necessary to get the patient to see the need to adopt a more mature attitude, readjusting his standards in line with the reality situation. Other outlets than power may then be substituted to satisfy the patient's drive for self assertiveness and self esteem.

The same technic is used in dealing with other compulsive neurotic patterns, as detachment, aggression and perfectionism. They are brought to the patient's attention and he is shown why they stir up difficulties for him. He is challenged in his assumption that they are the only way of life, and substitutive responses are suggested.

The patient may be acquainted with the ways in which his character drives are insatiable and operate insidiously. He may be shown that unknown to himself he lashes out at others, or vanquishes them in actual deeds or in fantasy, or renders himself invulnerable and strong, or retreats from competition, or engages in any number of facades that become for him basic goals in life and make the ordinary pursuits of life meaningless.

Such unhealthy attitudes perhaps might be understandable were we to concede what is probably not true, that the patient really was a contemptible and inferior person, and that he had to eliminate adult and realistic methods of dealing with problems. The patient must be shown the need to stop taking refuge in childhood defenses and to face his difficulties with decision and courage. However, because he has utilized his defense for so many years, he must understand that they may not vanish immediately. They will keep cropping up from time to time. If they do, there is nothing of which to be ashamed. When he becomes sufficiently strong, he will not need these defenses. Yet he must not abandon his patterns out of a sole conviction that they are wrong, or out of a desire to please the physician. Rather, as he realizes the implications of his neurotic drives, he will want to substitute creative goals and patterns for those that have resulted in his present unhappiness.

The physician should actively encourage a conscious analysis by the patient of his customary trends, as well as stimulate him to substitute new ways of thinking and acting. In the event the old patterns start emancipating themselves, it may be necessary to bring them to as complete a halt as possible by deliberate effort. This involves an elaborate inquiry into the patient's daily routines, in order to get him to inject his new attitudes into every phase of his activity. The patient should be reassured and encouraged that he has the capacity to change, that others sicker than himself have done so successfully.

Usually the patient will be surprised to find that his character patterns are regarded as problems, because he has accepted them as natural and normal. As soon as he realizes that they involve him in difficulties with people, and are in themselves responsible for much of his turmoil, he is supplied with a valid motivation to alter his scheme of life. This, in itself, is insufficient to produce change, because his customary character strivings are for him the only way he knows to gain security and to bolster self esteem. Furthermore, normal attitudes and patterns are so enigmatic to him that he may display for them feelings of contempt or indifference. Nevertheless, the conviction that he must tolerate suffering or abandon certain character drives brings his conflict to a more constructive level. He is confronted with a choice for which he, himself, will have to assume a measure of responsibility.

Many persons faced with this choice are unwilling or unable to give up their destructive drives. The knowledge that frustration or pain will follow their pursuit is not enough to make them relinquish the gratifications that accrue from the propitiation of neurotic goals. An extreme example of this is the alcoholic who appreciates the physical, social and moral hardships that inevitably follow his bouts of drinking. Even in cases where the patient refuses to abandon his immature objectives, the knowledge that he is responsible for his own plight is healthier from a therapeutic viewpoint that the conviction that may have existed previously to the effect that the sources of his misery lay outside of himself.

In cases where the person is convinced that his adjustment is eminently unsatisfactory, where he realizes that his suffering does not compensate for the gratification that comes from indulgence of his immature drives, where he is convinced his reaction patterns interfere with biologic and social goals, he will be motivated toward experimenting with new attitudes and reactions toward people.

Once reaction patterns that are inimical to adjustment are clearly defined, and a more adaptive substitutive reaction suggested, a long period of experiment and training is necessary before unhealthful attitudes are replaced by those of a more mature nature. Success is never immediate and relapses occur frequently; but with each relapse the patient usually gains new insight. As a general rule, the patient will fail at first to integrate new reactions. He should be forewarned not to be disappointed, and reminded that time is a factor in the re-educational process. Habit patterns that have persisted over a lifetime do not vanish within a few weeks or a few months.

Even where the patient has the motivation to change, a struggle will be necessary to achieve a reorganization of the character structure. In spite of all good resolutions, the patient, at first, will find himself responding automatically in line with his customary habits.   He will, however, become more and more conscious of his reactions, and, as they occur, he will be better able to subject them to intellectual analysis and logic.   Even though this may fail to stop him from following his usual patterns, he will become more and more aware of their irrational nature, and he will have a greater determination to substitute constructive behavior tendencies.

For instance, a perfectionistic person may becomes conscious of the fact that his impulse to do everything meticulously extends itself into every aspect of his life and poisons his relationships with people.   He will see, as the physician brings it to his attention, that the slightest failure to perform flawlessly suffices to create tension and panic.   He may learn that the reason for his disturbance lies in the fact that when he is not perfect, his image of himself is shattered, and he feels unloved and unlovable.   Life then becomes a constant series of frustrations, since it is obviously impossible to be human and to do things perfectly every minute of the day.   The patient will, as he becomes aware of his inordinate expectations, find himself toying with the philosophy of self tolerance, which, at first, he will not wish to accept, probably because being mediocre is equivalent to being no good at all, and because he is not yet convinced that perfectionism is not really the keynote of life.   As he tests the truth of the physician's exhortations, and as he realizes the extent to which his perfectionistic strivings dominate him, he may attempt to catch himself before yielding to perfectionistic impulses. He will review in his mind the reasons why he must be perfect on every occasion.   He may eventually even try to substitute for this impulse the attitude that he can do things in an average manner.

In dealing with specific character traits, an attempt may be made to trace their source in early experiences and conditionings.   If the origin of neurotic character trends becomes apparent, the patient may be shown how they arose in response to unfortunate environmental circumstances or because of childhood misinterpretations. Automatically he is reacting to his present day situation as if he were still a vulnerable child who must defend himself against hurt or must comply with authoritarian expectations. This will reinforce his motivation to change.

Hypnosis may be used to produce experimental conflicts in order to create situations reminiscent of the original sources of trauma. This will help demonstrate to the patient how he reacts automatically to a situation symbolic of an early difficulty, and will eventually result in desensitization as well as the creation of insight into existing reaction patterns. Experimental conflicts can also demonstrate to the patient in a dramatic manner how his various drives operate in his daily functioning.

For example, a patient who complained of depression and loneliness, and who was manifestly detached from people, insisted that he was a sociable person who enjoyed the company of women, but that he did not want to get too involved until the right woman came along. He resisted accepting the interpretation that an intimate relationship was probably distasteful or dangerous to him and that he defended himself by detachment. Under hypnosis a fictitious situation was suggested to the effect that he had met a young woman who appealed to him so much that he wished to marry her. It was suggested that he would have all the emotions and feelings associated with such a situation when he awoke, although he would not remember my suggestions. Upon awakening the patient had an intense anxiety attack, and it was possible to demonstrate to him from this incident, and from the dream that occurred that evening, the function his detachment from women served in allaying a fear of being injured in a close relationship. Hypnosis thus can aid the patient in accepting the need for new, more mature reaction patterns.

In appraising what attitudes and reaction patterns are normal or abnormal, the physician must scrutinize his own standards carefully.[27]   He should regard with suspicion those character drives and actions which though culturally condoned are actually opposed to the patient's best interest. Even though the culture praises such ideals as ambitiousness, perfectionism and rugged individualism, the perpetuation of these traits may breed such hostile attitudes that they interfere with the best interests of the patient.   The physician himself may cherish certain attitudes that constitute for him the proper goals in life.   It is always necessary to subject his attitudes to an honest appraisal to see if he puts too much value in ambitiousness, perfectionism, detachment, dependency, narcissism or power devices.   Unless he does so he is apt to consider these traits as perfectly normal, and to re-educate his patients along improper lines.

HYPNOSIS IN RECONDITIONING

THE FACT that neurotic patterns of behavior are the product of faulty conditionings suggests that normal behavior patterns may be substituted by a process of reconditioning.

Among the earliest work along this line is that of Jones[28] who experimented with a child who had been bitten by a rabbit, and had developed great fear of the animal and of rabbits in general. Jones believed that if he could get the child to associate the rabbit with a pleasant emotion, fear of the creature might be lost. He decided to feed the child appetizing foods when the latter became hungry, at the same time exposing the child to the sight of the rabbit held at a distance; then gradually diminishing the distance. The experiment was successful and the child no longer experienced fear of the rabbit.

Other reconditioning experiments have been performed by Yates,[29] Max[30] and Mowrer and Mowrer.[31] Yates, treating a girl who was upset emotionally by the presence of men, had her repeat the word "calm," associating to it ideas of security, well-being, and peace. She gradually learned that constant repetition of the word in the presence of men sufficed to maintain her emotional composure. Max treated a homosexual patient who was obsessed with homosexual thoughts whenever he came in contact with a certain inanimate object. Presenting this object to the patient at the same time he has given an electric shock sufficed to terminate the power of the object to excite homosexual thoughts. Mowrer and Mowrer treated enuresis by constructing an apparatus that was placed in the bed of the enuritic child, which when wet caused a circuit to close and to ring a bell, awakening the child. They discovered that after three or four such experiences, the impulse alone to urinate aroused the child.

All of these experiments are dependent upon reconditioning

the individual to painful or pleasurable stimuli. Because hypnosis is capable of intensifying emotional stimuli, and because it renders the patient more susceptible to the establishing of conditioned reflexes,[32,33] it would seem to lend itself admirably to this therapeutic technic.

An example of how reconditioning is effected under hypnosis may be illustrated by the case of a woman who had, since childhood, experienced an intense dislike for orange juice which gradually had extended itself to other citrus fruits. Even the sight of an orange nauseated her, and on several occasions she had to leave the dinner table when this fruit was served. Her reaction caused her great social embarrassment. She associated her dislike with the fact that her mother had forced her, during childhood, to drink castor oil which had been mixed with orange juice. Indeed, whenever she tasted a citrus juice, she imagined she was imbibing castor oil.

Treatment consisted of discussing with her the mechanism of conditioning in relation to her own experience. Under hypnosis she was asked to dream about the happiest and most enjoyable episodes in her life. She was enjoined to fantasy the most pleasurable experiences that might happen to a person. Then a suggestion was given her that she would feel unbounded happiness and pleasure in the trance, as if the experiences were happening all over again or as if she were fulfilling her fantasies. As soon as she responded to these suggestions, she was asked to imagine herself in an orange grove while enjoying the same emotional state. Suggestions were then made that she would lose her dislike for fruit juice because the dislike would be replaced by pleasure. Indeed she would, to her surprize, find herself wanting to drink orange juice because she realized she did not dislike it as much as she had imagined. A sip of diluted orange juice was given her and she admitted that it produced no nausea.

During later sessions, these suggestions were repeated, and she was given stronger and stronger concentrations of citrus juices.   When she was capable of drinking undiluted orange juice, a posthypnotic suggestion was made to the effect that she would be able in the waking state to drink fruit juices of all types, and to look at fruits with enjoyment instead of disgust.   Those suggestions were successful and the patient overcame her phobia.

Phobias that have been established on the basis of for-tuitous conditionings are most easily influenced by this technic.   Habits which the patient finds difficult to break, such as excessive smoking, nail-biting, eating, and alcoholic indulgence, and some forms of drug addiction respond very well to this method.   The aim is to replace the pleasure feelings associated with these habits with disagreeable emotions, in the effort to get the patient to abandon his habit.

In the trance state the patient is told that he will exper-ience less and less of a desire to indulge his habit, and its control will contribute to his self respect and feelings of happiness.   Painful or disgusting experiences in the life of the individual, and fantasies of a disagreeable nature which he brings up in the trance, are linked to his craving.   When an association is established in the patient's mind, the con-ditioning process is tested by permitting him to indulge his habit in hypnosis.   For instance, in an alcoholic patient, nausea and vomiting may be associated to the drinking of alcohol, and success in the conditioning process is achieved when the patient disgorges a drink he is encouraged to imbibe.   Following the successful establishing of the con-ditioned reflex, posthypnotic suggestions are made along the same line.   The patient will require regular reinforcement of these suggestions for a considerable period thereafter.

In some instances, it may be possible to condition an individual to react comfortably to interpersonal situations to which he customarily responds with tension and discomfort. For example, a patient, who lived out of town and could spend only a few weeks in therapy, complained that when he was in the presence of other people, he was intensely disturbed and uncomfortable. In the trance it was determined that he felt competitive with others and anticipated criticism and attack. Feelings of relaxation were induced by suggesting a peaceful isolated scene on the seashore. Then in fantasy a person was introduced. The patient was urged to maintain his tranquillity by thinking and talking about those subjects with which he was most conversant, avoiding controversial topics. The pleasurable emotional tone persisted until the patient found himself engaging in a fantasied argument with his companion. By shifting the conversation, he again relaxed. Gradually, more and more people were introduced in the scene, and the patient was able to appreciate quite vividly how his tranquillity was upset by his own attitudes. He was able to transfer to the waking state what he had learned in the trance. In a group he experienced the same feelings of comfort and relaxation, and he was able to maintain his tranquillity by choosing and concentrating on the more pleasurable aspects of the situation.

Success in reconditioning is possible only where the symptom or habit does not serve a vitally dynamic purpose in the life adjustment of the individual. Where a symptom has a deep symbolic value, particularly as a defense against anxiety, reconditioning suggestions will usually be unsuccessful until the patient has achieved emotional insight.

In phobias of anxiety hysteria, for instance, exposing the patient to the phobic situation while undergoing an artificially imposed state of happiness or ecstasy, may awaken the patient or cause him to condition in an opposite direction, that is, to associate fear with conditions which hitherto had been associated with happiness or ecstasy.

In some instances the patient may seem to respond favorably to an imaginary situation in which he exposes himself to his phobia.   An agoraphobic patient in a state of induced ecstasy may, if given a suggestion that he imagines himself outdoors walking around, execute these directions, creating the impression that he has overcome his phobia.   However, the patient is quite conscious that he is playing a role, and will willingly go through the motions suggested to him provided he is not actually exposed to his phobia.   In the waking state he will still respond with undiminished terror when faced with a real situation.   It is important to remember that symptoms usually have an important symbolic significance and that reconditioning may be unsuccessful until the symptom no longer serves a vital function.

A patient with claustrophobia, revealed, through his associations and dreams, that the situation that made him most happy was one in which he was in close contact with his fiancee.   He was extremely dependent upon this woman, and when separated from her felt an abysmal loneliness.   He was constantly preoccupied with thoughts concerning her whereabouts, and whenever they were apart, he could scarcely wait until they were reunited.   His fantasies were concerned with his being embraced or fondled by a maternal woman.

As a child he had been overprotected by a solicitous, domineering mother who had babied and mothered him to excess.   He apparently wanted to perpetuate the mother-child relationship in his later contacts with women.   Even consciously the thing he wanted most was a love relationship with a woman older than himself.   In deep hypnosis this desire was fulfilled in fantasy by suggested dramatized situations in which he was close to an older woman.   The patient fairly exuded happiness on suggestions that he was being petted by his fiancee.   At the same time a suggestion was given him that he was together with her in an elevator, in the attempt to get him to associate being in a closed place with being embraced by his fiancee.   He responded favorably to this while in a trance.

However, in real life his claustrophobia did not vanish. With an analytic technic it was found that this symptom was in part the result of a feeling that he was trapped and might suffer mutilation in a close contact with a woman. Only after his relationship with women straightened out to a point where he felt he did not have to violate his independence or freedom in closeness, was it possible to recondition him successfully.

ILLUSTRATIVE CASE

THE FOLLOWING case illustrates the use of hypnosis with a directive, persuasive and re-educational approach. The symptom for which the patient sought help was premature ejaculation which was so severe that intercourse was impossible. A transcription of the entire treatment (which consisted of eight sessions over a period of a little more than one month) follows.

FIRST SESSION (April 1)

The patient presents his problem which is premature ejaculation, so severe that complete penetration is impossible. His motivation for therapy is a desire for a normal sex life. Responses to the Rorschach cards and Goodenough test indicate severe neurotic problems. However, he sees no difficulty in any other area of psychobiologic functioning than the sexual one. There is no desire on his part to inquire into his interpersonal relationships and for this reason a directive approach is decided on at the start.

Pt. I have been suffering for many years, Doctor, of what I believe is premature ejaculation. It is an outgrowth, I imagine, from a period of masturbation in childhood. And I put off marriage because that fear was constantly present in my mind. In going to some sources of books, I happened across Dr. Robinson's book, who cited cases similar to mine, and whereby he had done very good work along those lines that were cured. Well, I then went to see a medical doctor who examined me and said there was nothing wrong organically, but that as a result of the masturbation, he thought that a certain conditioning was set up which will be, has to be overcome. He wasn't very specific as to what channels I might use, but it was evident that he, as a medical man, found nothing wrong organically, that he could do nothing for me.

Dr. I see. How old are you?

Pt.   Thirty-six.

Dr.   And you are married.

Pt.   Married only a short time.

Dr.   How long?

Pt.   Six weeks.

Dr.   And you felt for a long time your condition was hopeless?

Pt.   My conviction that it wasn't hopeless dates back about eight months ago, and when I broached the subject of marriage, to my doctor, and told him frankly that the fear of being unsuccessful has kept me from marrying, and truthfully by nature I don't want to live alone, he said he thought it would be perfectly all right for me to venture into marriage, feeling certain that I wouldn't encounter too much difficulty and it would wear off in time.   And I married, as I said, six weeks back.

Dr.   Yes.

Pt.   Of course I'm trying to regulate myself as much as possible.   I've had a better attitude than when I was single, but not sufficient improvement in performance to be at all successful.

Dr.   I see.

Pt.   Now I was thinking if as the doctor had mentioned that there was nothing organically wrong, I thought perhaps hypnosis would help.   If it is not too extreme conditioning of that habit.

Dr.   As you get into the thing and get an idea as to what's behind this premature ejaculation, we can then discuss whether hypnosis is the method of choice.   At first I want to ask you just a few more questions.   When you married your wife, how long did you know her?

Pt.   Oh, about three months.

Dr.   How old a woman is she?

Pt.   Thirty-four.

Dr.   She's never been married?

Pt. No.

Dr. And had she had any relations before?

Pt. No, she hasn't.

Dr. Were you able to penetrate?

Pt. Not fully. Her hymen has not been dilated.

Dr. Are you in love with her?

Pt. Very much.

Dr. Is she understanding?

Pt. Very.

Dr. And patient?

Pt. That's right, very much so.

Dr. What about her own sexual feelings? Is she responsive or cold?

Pt. Yes, she's quite responsive.

Dr. Does she have an orgasm?

Pt. On occasion, she doesn't permit herself to go too far, but on occasion she does when I play with her. See, that's the peculiar thing, I might add that might be helpful, that I could play with her until she does reach an orgasm. But the minute I insert, I mean, it happens. I mean the ejaculation comes.

Dr. Yes.

Pt. But it has always been a source of surprise to me that I could hold back indefinitely and have it arise until I try to insert. She is so stimulated sometimes that she has an orgasm and she likes it.

Dr. When she has an orgasm, is it easier for you to control yourself? Or the ejaculation, does it come, none-the-less?

Pt. It comes immediately when I try to insert it.

Dr. I see. Ah, now let us go back a little bit farther. Supposing you tell me about your first relationships with women. How far back do they go?

Pt. Well they go considerably far back. Going up to a prostitute's home on occasion.

Dr. And do you remember the first time?

Pt. Yes.

Dr. What was the occasion? Can you describe it to me?

Pt. Well, if I remember, I think there were three of us, two friends and myself, and we went up to a place in mid-town New York. There were three rather attractive girls. I think the experience was the same even at the first time, if I remember correctly. I think the ejaculation came very fast there, too. The girl was nice; there wasn't anything repulsive about it as I remember her. But the experience has been in that way, and it's been that way ever since more or less.

Dr. Now, supposing we go back now into your early childhood. Start in with your parents. Are your parents alive?

Pt. My mother is, my dad passed away a short time ago.

Dr. What sort of person is she?

Pt. Well, very fine, very homelike. The family spirit has been very fine all through the years. The feeling of devotion and loyalty between members and between parent and children, it's been a high type.

Dr. And what about your relationship with your mother. What sort of a relationship was it?

Pt. Well. . . .

Dr. Were you attached to her, were you very fond of her, or were you detached?

Pt. No, normally fond. We always had a high regard not only for mother, but for father and mother I mean.

Dr. Did she domineer you?

Pt. No.

Dr. You could do pretty much as you wanted?

Pt. That's right.

Dr. And what sort of a person was your father?

Pt. Very much the same. He was of a religious nature.

Dr. Was he a domineering person?

Pt. No.

Dr. Restrictive, repressive?

Pt. Not restrictive, no. He was liberal minded.

Dr. And you loved him?

Pt. That's right.

Dr. Did you prefer your mother or your father?

Pt. No, it was about equal there. There was no preference for either of them.

Dr. And what about your brothers and sisters?

Pt. I have no brothers; I have three sisters, older than myself.

Dr. And their personalities are what?

Pt. They're very much like my own.

Dr. How do you get along with them?

Pt. Very well indeed.

Dr. How would you describe your own personality?

Pt. Well, it's difficult to define.

Dr. For instance, how do you get along with people?

Pt. Very well, very well.

Dr. Do you get along on submissive or domineering lines?

Pt. No, just the middle type.

Dr. You can hold your own with people.

Pt. Definitely, socially and in business. I am in charge of several people.

Dr. Are you able to adopt a leadership role?

Pt. Definitely I am; I have no difficulty along those lines.

Dr. Do you get at all hostile towards people?

Pt. No.

Dr. Now what about symptoms? Do you get any depressive symptoms of any kind?

Pt. No.

Dr. Any anxiety?

Pt. No.

Dr. Do you have any phobias of any kind?

Pt. No.

Dr. Any fears, any obsessions of any kind?

Pt. No.

Dr. Do you feel compelled to do certain things?

Pt. No, no.

Dr. Any headaches or stomach trouble or other physical complaints?

Pt. No.

Dr. Do you feel tense? Emotionally tense?

Pt. Occasionally, yes; emotionally, no.

Dr. Any insomnia?

Pt. No.

Dr. Any nightmares?

Pt. No.

Dr. Alcoholism?

Pt. No.

Dr. Sedatives?

Pt. No.

Dr. How about dreams? Do you dream?

Pt. Well I have not for the longest time; I never did, ah, often. It's a rarity with me.

Dr. You weren't a nervous child?

Pt. No.

Dr. Do you remember any dreams you have had at all?

Pt. No, I really couldn't say. I really couldn't say.

Dr. Do you recall any repetitive dreams as a child?

Pt. No.

(Up to this point in the interview it would seem that the patient has no problems other than the symptom of premature ejaculation. He is not aware of any difficulties in interpersonal relations.)

Dr. All right, I'm going to show you some cards of ink blots, and I'd like to have you look at these and tell me what comes to your mind. It's not really a test, merely impressions as to what may be going on in your deeper emotional life.

Pt. I see.

Dr. You've probably heard of the Rorschach test.

Pt. Yes, I have.

Dr. I'd like to know what you see. This is the first card.

Pt. Butterflies.

Dr. Anything else you see?

Pt. That's about all.

Dr. This is the second card.

Pt. Two animal figures, nothing else.

Dr. Do you have any ideas about them?

Pt. No, not really.

Dr. Perhaps if you turned them upside down you might see something else.

Pt. (*Long pause.*)   No, I'm afraid not.

Dr. This is the third card.

Pt. There seem to be two animal figures. That's all.

Dr. That's the fourth one.

Pt. Something in the insect family. (*Pause*)

Dr. This is the fifth card.

Pt. Represents a sea gull.

Dr. What makes it a sea gull?

Pt. The shape.

Dr. This is the sixth one.

Pt. I notice one characteristic of all of them, though. You do want me to state what I think?

Dr. Yes.

Pt. It's the fact of the similarity to the biological diagrams of a woman's vagina.

Dr. For instance, where?

Pt. Right along the edge.

Dr. Do you see that in any of the others?

Pt. Yes, I noticed a characteristic in most of them.

Dr. I see, but you didn't mention that.

Pt. No.

Dr.   What else do you see?

Pt.   Nothing.

Dr.   This is the seventh.

Pt.   Represents a statue or something.   (*Pause*) Looks like two animals perched on top of something or other, that's about all I can get out of it.

Dr.   You see anything else there?

Pt.   No.

Dr.   This is the eighth.

Pt.   Two lions standing.

Dr.   This is the ninth.

Pt.   (*Long pause.*)   I can't see anything (*Hands card back.*)

Dr.   All right, this is the tenth one.

Pt.   Squirrels feeding.   Tree branches here, and that's all I can get out of it.

Dr.   All right, fine.   Now I'm going to come back and ask you a few questions.   In this one, (*second card*) you saw two animals there.   What are the animals doing?

Pt.   They're holding up their paws.

Dr.   Do the red spots have any significance?

Pt.   No.

Dr.   How about this?

Pt.   Ah, a butterfly.

Dr.   Where would you say that the female genitals were?

Pt.   Well, they're covered.

Dr.   Where?

Pt.   That's the way they're turned in like.

Dr.   Would the thigh be somewheres?

Pt.   Yes, right along here.

Dr.   What could this red part be?

Pt.   It could be blood from an intercourse.

Dr.   Blood from an intercourse?   I'm going to show you the next card, that's the third one.   You mentioned there were two animals, what are they doing?

Pt. Well it's just like a pose.

Dr. Just like a pose. Now what about the red spots there, what could those be?

Pt. Well I couldn't say.

Dr. I'm going to show you this card, the ninth card that you couldn't see anything in. Now look closely and tell me the first thought that comes to you.

Pt. Well that too, might be the walls of the woman's vagina.

Dr. Anything else?

Pt. No.

Dr. Now I'm going to give you a paper and I'd like to have you draw me a picture of a person.

Pt. I don't suppose I'm very good at drawing.

Dr. I see you've got the head of a man there. Supposing you draw me the picture of a woman. (*Patient draws a crude picture of a woman's head.*)

> (*It is quite apparent from the tests that the patient is severely neurotic, that he has problems in relationships with people, that he conceives of intercourse as a bloody act. He masters his anxiety by minimizing his productivity, by detachment, and by an intellectual attitude toward life. Self esteem is markedly inhibited and assertiveness very low. One defense that the patient has is avoiding the fact that he has any real problems. It would obviously be futile to do any therapeutic work on his basic problems until he becomes aware of them and is motivated to correct them. His present motivation is to eliminate his sexual defect, and he does not wish to go any deeper.*)

Dr. From your history, from the way things have been going with you, you feel everything has been perfectly normal except this one symptom, premature ejaculation. You would be happy to have everything remain at its present level if your sexual relations could be better?

Pt. Yes.

Dr. There is no other problem that you would want corrected?

Pt. No.

Dr. There seem to be some indications from the Rorschach that there are other problems that involve your relationships with people. For instance, there are indications that you detach yourself a little bit more than is good for you, in the attempt to avoid stimulating situations. Almost as if in keeping apart from them nothing bad will happen. Of course, these tests could be wrong, they are merely indications.

Pt. I see.

Dr. There are indications also of an overevaluation of the intellectual aspects of life to a minimization of the more emotional aspects.

Pt. Yes.

Dr. This could include the sexual element too. Now what we have to decide on is what our objective will be in treatment. Are we just going to shoot at the sexual symptom, or are we going to shoot at the broader issue of your relationships with people, which would be a much more ambitious procedure, and involve a much longer period of time?

Pt. Well that's the difficulty, doctor. You see, I don't have much time to devote now. And I'm in a terrible state right now as far as time is concerned to have this thing checked before it goes too long. That's what I'm up against.

Dr. What do you mean time?

Pt. Well for one thing, it's hard getting away from my business, of course, and then evenings it would be difficult to get away.

Dr. I see.

Pt. And I want to get over this before it gets worse. Of course the period of time enters into it, something I should have done a long time ago I mean; instead I waited.

Dr. Well I can tell you that there are other problems that you have besides sexual ones, but that if you'd like to work hypnotically with only the sexual thing we can do so.

Pt. Yes.

Dr.   Tackle this one thing and leave the others alone.

Pt.   Yes, I think for the time being at any rate.

Dr.   Always with the idea that I may be able to present you with more data about what I think about yourself, the significance of which you can evaluate.

Pt.   Yes.

Dr.   I think we will need a period of ten sessions to see if we are going to be successful, or if other things have to be worked through before we can be successful. In other words, if it's not bound up with other problems it will be corrected. But if it's intermeshed with many other problems which involve your relationships with people, it may take a longer time.

Second Session (April 2)

In this session the patient brings up masturbatory misconceptions. These are clarified and an attempt made to correct them. The ideas about masturbation are presented in an authoritarian manner since the motivations of the patient will allow of no other approach at this time. Hypnosis is induced and a medium trance achieved. The patient appears to be quite responsive to suggestions. The nature of his hypnotically induced dreams indicates what the Rorschach brought out: passivity and impaired biologic drives.

Dr.   Have you been thinking about our last talk?

Pt.   Yes.

Dr.   Did you have any other ideas after I had talked to you?

Pt.   No.

Dr.   Or any thoughts?

Pt.   I thought that masturbation could have been the cause.

Dr.   Could you tell me something about your masturbation, when it started, what fantasies were associated with it and so forth.

Pt. Well, it started in early childhood, about ten or eleven years. I might have been about ten or twelve.

Dr. Do you remember the circumstances under which it started?

Pt. No, no.

Dr. And what happened?

Pt. Well it was just the imagination of, oh, sexual intercourse.

Dr. Do you still have sexual intercourse fantasies with masturbation?

Pt. That's right.

Dr. Any erection trouble with masturbation?

Pt. No.

Dr. Any fears associated with it?

Pt. No.

Dr. Do you have any conscious fears about sexual intercourse?

Pt. No.

Dr. Any thoughts or fantasies occur when you want to engage in intercourse?

Pt. No. Well, the same as any other men feel, the desire is there, it's frequent.

Dr. Is there a desire to penetrate?

Pr. That's right.

Dr. I see. Now why do you think that masturbation was the cause?

Pt. Well years back, I mean, in earliest periodicals and literature, I found things that hinted at masturbation being the cause of physical harm. At that time and in earlier youth I felt as though there's nothing that could be done about it. It was only later on after I read further and found that there could be, that something could be done about it. That's when I started investigating.

Dr. In other words, you had read material to the effect that masturbation can cause premature ejaculation?

Pt. That's right. Of course maybe I was under the impression that it was the, the fundamental cause of impotency in man. That's why I feared and shied away from any serious thought of marriage.

Dr. I see.

Pt. Until one day when I read otherwise.

Dr. How about the frequency of masturbation?

Pt. Well, that's hard to say.

Dr. How frequently did you used to masturbate when you were a boy?

Pt. As often, I should say, at the rate of about three times a week.

Dr. Three times a week, and that continued through when?

Pt. Yes, it's continued through to a later period in the twenties.

Dr. How about now?

Pt. No.

Dr. When did you stop masturbating?

Pt. About five years ago.

Dr. Do you think that masturbation is a normal or abnormal thing?

Pt. I've always considered it abnormal until I consulted this physician who told me that there was nothing abnormal about it.

Dr. Did that surprise you?

Pt. Yes, it did. It did.

Dr. Did you know that practically all children masturbate? Boys and girls?

Pt. No, I didn't know that; it's only at a recent date that I discovered that a good percentage of them do. I always thought it was the exception.

Dr. Masturbation is the yielding to the sexual impulse that is normally present in all children. Almost universally children are led to feel that it is evil.

Pt. That's right.

Dr. It is extremely important that your misconceptions about masturbation be clarified and corrected. We will have the best chance to overcome your symptom when we do this.

Pt. I see. I might add this, which might be helpful. As I say, all through the period of years I felt that due to a long period of masturbation I thought that the difficulty was purely organic and that it could not be cured, and I was so amazed when I found that it was nothing organic at all, that it was something that was built up in the mind. Especially in my particular case and that it might have caused a barrier.

Dr. The effects of this misconception probably did. But even though we correct the misconceptions, it may take time for you to overcome years of fear. Not long ago there was a tradition of guilt about sex so profound that all text books and all literature decried the evils of masturbation. There were times when books were written to that effect which were completely fantastic, utterly opposed to science, utterly opposed to biology, and utterly opposed to facts.

Pt. I see.

Dr. Now, I am going to give you certain scientific facts for what they may be worth on masturbation. But whether you utilize them and whether they can immediately disperse your old misconceptions is an entirely different story. A child, when he's very little, is entirely dependent upon the parents. When he's little he has no other way of life. In the course of his development and growth, the normal child eventually will give up much of his dependency and become independent and assertive. He does this by exploring his environment and finding pleasures within himself, and his own capacities to do things through his own efforts rather than to get things from the parent. That's part of the normal growth of the individual.

Pt. Yes.

Dr. Now, what occurs is that as his brain develops, the child becomes more and more cognizant of his own body. He gradually explores himself, his feet, his eyes, and even his genitals which are, after all, part of him.

Pt. Yes.

Dr. The genitals are very delicate and sensitive.

Pt. Sensitive.

Dr. And he gets a certain pleasure sensation from the handling that is perfectly normal. Biologically it is important because it serves to teach the child that he can find pleasures within himself, that he doesn't need all pleasures from the parent. So that it serves as one way of beginning to break his dependency on the parent, the mother in particular, for all kinds of gratifications. In the course of genital manipulation, the child finds that the pleasures he gets serve as a means of alleviating tension.

Pt. That's right.

Dr. That adds to the growth of the self, ego growth we call it. It's perfectly normal. Mind you the child does not make a career out of masturbating. He merely manipulates his genitals occasionally; at first out of curiosity, then for pleasure. When he finds other pleasure outlets, genital manipulation does not become too important. But if the parent restrains the child, if the parent punishes the child— which many sexually repressed parents do—it teaches the child that there's something evil and bad, not only about his sex organs, but more importantly about doing things for himself and finding pleasures within himself and through his own resources. He is apt then to feel that being independent is bad or dangerous, and he may cling to his dependency strivings.

Pt. I see.

Dr. Now, as the child develops, the sexual feeling continues to be strong. Tension builds up. This is particularly the case during puberty when the sex organs mature. Mas turbation is the usual outlet for these tensions due to the fact that sexual intercourse is, for social and economic reasons, taboo. Where the child has no great guilt feelings about masturbation, he will relieve his tension without fear. Where such guilt feelings exist, tension may drive him to masturbation, but the aftermath is disastrous. He hates himself and his parents and the world. He believes himself doomed to eternal suffering, and feels that he has, through masturbation, injured himself physically.

Pt. What you say, doctor, I know is right, because when I have been tense I have had the urge.

Dr. The release of tension through masturbation, if not hampered becomes no problem at all. But if the child feels restricted and evil for this impulse, masturbation and sex become a problem. They are overvalued. The greater the restriction, the more important sex becomes for him, and the more evil he feels.

Pt. Right.

Dr. Sex and masturbation may dominate his thinking.

Pt. That's right.

Dr. The same could be said for any frustrated biologic drive. If a hungry person satisfies his appetite, he doesn't think much about his stomach. But if he is unable to satisfy his appetite, if he remains hungry, his thoughts will be constantly on food.

Pt. The child feels it's wrong and bad to masturbate, but he does anyway.

Dr. Most authorities feel that the only hurt that can come through masturbation are the thoughts of evil that are associated with it.

Pt. Exactly. Well, I did feel all the way through childhood, I had a terrible sense of guilt and perhaps that's what was built up in me.

Dr. It was built up, and nurtured, and gradually gave rise to many misconceptions about your sex organs.

Pt. That I do remember vividly, having that terrific

sense of guilt and shame for myself, I mean, all the way through.

Dr. This guilt and shame reflects itself in other ways. The Rorschach cards I showed you last time indicate that there is an association, perhaps unconscious, between sexual intercourse, blood, and hurt of some kind. There may be misconceptions about the female sex organs too. There's a link somewhere, and through hypnosis we may be able to get the answer, to correct that misconception, too. Once we correct the misconceptions of masturbation, sexual relations, and misconceptions in reference to a woman's sexual organs, you will have the best chance to enter into a normal sexual relationship. But sometimes it takes a little time to break a habit.

Pt. I expect so.

Dr. But once we have the road cleared we should make progress.

Pt. I hope so.

Dr. Now I want to talk about hypnosis. Have you ever been hypnotized?

Pt. No, I haven't, but students in the classroom, I've seen it, students being hypnotized.

Dr. I see, you've seen hypnotic process.

Pt. Yes.

Dr. What do you think about hypnosis?

Pt. Well, I, from what I've seen of it and studied of it, I think it's a very valuable science.

Dr. Hypnosis is suggestion.

Pt. That's right.

Dr. And the ability to incorporate suggestion. Practically all people can be hypnotized. It's a matter of concentration.

Pt. Yes.

Dr. Supposing I give you an example of what the hypnotic process is all about. I'd like to have you clasp your hands this way, keep your feet down. Clasp your hands and then, for a moment, close your eyes and imagine that you are looking at a vise. One of those heavy metal vises with jaws that clamp together with a screw. Imagine that your hands are like the jaws of a vise, and that they gradually begin to press together, harder and harder and harder. I'm going to start counting from one to five. When I reach the count of five, your hands will be pressed together so firmly that it will be difficult or impossible to open them up. It will be just like the jaws of that vise. Imagine that you're looking at the vise now, and I begin to count. One, tight; two, tighter; tighter; three, tighter and tighter still; four, as tight as a vise; five, so tight, so firm that they get cemented together. You notice that even when you try to separate them, they're so firmly clasped together that the harder you try, the more firmly they're clasped. And even though you try to pull them apart, they become very closely clasped together, just like that. Now, slowly, they begin to open up, and then you'll be able to open them up. Slowly, they open up. And now you're able to separate them slowly, just like that. Good. Now pull them apart. That is one of the phenomena of hypnosis, the ability to visualize something and feel it is so.

Now another phenomenon is this. Supposing you bring the palms of your hands down on your thighs and you watch your hands. Watch either hand, say the right hand. I want you to begin experiencing all the sensations and feelings in your hand no matter what they may be. Perhaps you'll feel the sensation of roughness of the trousers on the your hand. Perhaps you'll experience sensations; perhaps you'll get little tingling sensations in your fingers. No matter what sensation you feel, I want you to concentrate more and more and more on the feelings in your hands. Just watch your hands.

Now you'll begin to notice an interesting thing. As you

watch your hand, you'll notice that one of the fingers will move. You don't know which one of the fingers will move first, whether it will be on the right hand or the left hand. But one of the fingers will move ever so little. It may be the middle finger or the thumb, or the little finger, or the ring finger. Whichever finger it is, it will move soon. You don't know exactly when. It will move and jerk as you watch it. Perhaps you'll notice that the space between the fingers will gradually widen, the fingers spreading apart, the space becoming wider and wider, just like that. And as you notice the space increasing, you'll become aware of the feeling of lightness in your fingers. Your hand and fingers will begin to feel light.

Slowly your hand will begin to lift and rise, slowly rise and lift, lift, pulling up, up higher, and higher so that the hand and fingers lift and rise, slowly rise, up in the air as if they're like a feather. Rising and lifting just like that. Higher and higher and higher; slowly, imperceptibly and even perhaps without your knowledge, the hand will lift up toward your face. It will begin to rise, and you'll begin to feel the sensation of heaviness and sleepiness in your whole body except the right hand.

You'll begin to feel tired, very tired. You'll begin to get drowsy. Your eyes will get heavy, very heavy. They'll get so heavy and tired and sleepy they blink. They blink and you get tired and drowsy.

Your breathing now becomes deeper. The hand continues to rise up, and your breathing gets deep, and your eyes get heavy, and your body gets heavy, and you get sleepier, and sleepier, and sleepier. And as the hand rises, you'll notice that you'll get sleepier all over until when the hand touches your face, you'll be asleep, firmly asleep, deeply asleep. And you'll get drowsier and drowsier and drowsier, and finally when the hand touches your face, lean the cheek against the palm of your hand to support the head and go to sleep, go to sleep. You are tired, very drowsy. Your eyes are blinking. Now your breathing gets deep and automatic. Slowly your hand begins to lift up, up, up, higher, higher, lifting straight to your face, and as it lifts your eyes get so heavy that it's difficult to keep them open. You'll be going into a deep restful sleep. Your hand is moving towards your face, and you're getting drowsier and drowsier and drowsier. You're going to sleep; you're going to sleep; you're going to get sleepier, and sleepier, just like that.

I want you to rest this way for a few minutes, and at the end of that time I'm going to talk to you again, and you're going to be asleep, deeply asleep. And when I talk to you next you'll be much more deeply asleep than you were before. (*Pause*)

As you sit there, I want you to continue to feel the sensation of deep restful sleep. This time I'm going to ask you to open your eyes when I count five and look at a shiny object. When I show it to you, you're going to notice that as you gaze at it, it will be impossible to keep your eyes open, and that the harder you stare at it, the more tired your eyes will get. And finally they'll get so tired that they'll close and again you'll go to sleep, deeply asleep. One, two, three, four, five. Slowly open your eyes and stare at the object, and as you stare at it, your eyes will get heavy. They blink, they burn, they feel like lead, and then, when they feel so tired that it's impossible to keep them open, they'll close and you'll go into a deep restful, relaxed comfortable sleep. Your eyes get tired, they're tired and you get drowsier and drowsier and drowsier. Stare at the object as long as you possibly can. And then your eyes will begin to close and you'll go to sleep. Very tired, tired and drowsy. Get sleepier, very sleepy. Go to sleep, go to sleep, go to sleep. And as you sleep, your whole body will relax, from your head right down to your feet. I want you to sit this way in a deep sleep, drowsy sleep, until I talk to you next.

When I talk to you next, you'll be still more asleep than you were before, and I'll give you more suggestions that you'll find it easy to follow. Go to sleep and I'll talk to you soon. (*Pause*)

Now, I'm going to ask you slowly to wake up, and after you wake up, I'm going to count from one to five. As I count from one to five, at the count of five, you'll notice that your eyes will again have become so heavy that it will be difficult or impossible to keep them open. Slowly open your eyes, and then I'll count. One, they blink, two, they get heavy; three, get drowsy; four, get sleepier and sleepier. They start closing. You get tired. Five, they close. Your breathing gets deep, very deep and automatic.

Now I'm going to start stroking your left hand. You'll notice something very interesting; the left hand will start getting extremely heavy, very heavy, as I stroke it. It will get heavier and heavier and heavier so that it will feel as if a hundred pound weight is pressing down on the arm. It will feel as if two bands strap your arm down, at your elbow and at your wrist. It will feel as if a suction pad pulls your arm down against your body. It will feel as if it's made of lead, heavy and stiff, so that when I reach the count of five, it will feel so heavy that even when I try to budge it, it will feel heavy and stiff, and it will be impossible for you to lift it. It will be impossible for you to lift it. I may, by pulling it, possibly get it up a little bit. It will come down, but it won't lift up. One, heavy; two, heavier and heavier; three, as heavy as lead. Visualize a heavy stiff lead bar. Four, heavier and heavier; five, heavy and stiff. The muscles become rigid and stiff so that when I try to pull it up, it stiffens up just like that. And the harder I pull, the stiffer it gets. You'll notice now that even though you try to move it, the harder you try to move your arm, the heavier it will feel. The harder you try to move your arm, the heavier it will feel.

I'm going, now, to count from one to five. At the count of five, you'll find that you are able to move your arm. It will lose its stiffness, and you will be able to move it. One, two, three, four, five. Good. And now you're going to notice an extremely interesting thing. You're going to notice that as you sit there, you'll feel your arm so heavy and stiff that it will be impossible for you to move it. But this time you, yourself, will count from one to five, and when you reach the count of five, you'll notice that suddenly the arm will loosen up and get limp and you will be able to move it. At the same time your eyes will continue to be closed, and you go into an even deeper state of sleep. So count from one to five. At the count of five, you notice suddenly the arm will be able to move.

(The purpose of this technic is to start giving the patient a feeling of capacity of controlling muscular function as a means of building up a feeling of self confidence, to show him he is not entirely helpless about influencing his physical self.)

Pt. One, two, three, four, five.

Dr. You can move your arm now, good. Now I want you to go to sleep even deeper, and in a few minutes, I'm going to talk to you again. *(Pause)* Now, as you sit there, I'm going to give you a suggestion. Visualize yourself walking along a street with me. We go along together, we walk toward a church yard. We enter the church yard. We notice a tall church in front of us, the spire and steeple. As you visualize that, indicate the fact that you see it by your hand rising up about two inches. As soon as you visualize ourselves walking along the street to the church yard, indicate it by your hand rising up. Your hand rises up.

As you observe the church, the spire and the steeple, notice a bell. The bell begins to move. You get a sensation as if you hear the bell clanging. As soon as you get that sensation indicate it by your hand rising up. Your hand rises up.

Now I'm going to ask you to wake up slowly, as I count from one to five. At the count of five, you still will be drowsy, but your eyes will be awake, open. And then, after that, I'm going to say "Sleep, sleep, sleep, sleep," and as I say "Sleep," your eyes again will become very heavy and tired, so heavy that it will be impossible to keep them open. And then they'll close very tightly. One, slowly start opening your eyes; two; three; four; five. Sleep, sleep, sleep, sleep; your eyes are tired and heavy, and you're going into a deeper and deeper and more restful, more relaxed, more comfortable sleep.

As you sit there this time, you'll notice that your entire body becomes heavy, very heavy and stiff; it's almost as if it's frozen. I'm going to count from one to five; at the count of five, your body will be so heavy and stiff and cramped that when you try to get out of the chair, it will be impossible for you to move out of the chair no matter how hard you try. It will be impossible for you to get out of the chair. One, heavy; two, stiff; three, heavier and heavier; four, as heavy as lead, as heavy as lead, as heavy as lead; five, it's heavy and stiff. No matter how hard you try to move or to budge or to wiggle in your chair, the harder you try the more solidly implanted you are in your chair. Try it and you'll see that the harder you try the more stiff you get. Your whole body begins to stiffen up.

And now, I'm going to ask you again to count from one to five. As you, yourself, count from one to five, at the count of five, even though you're deeply asleep, it will be possible for you to move a little in the chair. Count.

Pt. One, two, three, four, five.

Dr· You can move, good. Now I'm going to ask you to visualize something again. This time I approach you and I have a bottle in my hand. You notice that there is a label on the bottle with a flower printed on it. Imagine that there is perfume in the bottle. As soon as you visualize the bottle and label and flower, indicate it by your hand rising. Your hand rises. Now I'm going to unscrew the cork on the bottle and bring it close to your nose. You'll actually be able to smell the odor of perfume. As soon as you do indicate it by your hand moving up. Your hand rises.

Imagine now that you are in a surgeon's office, because of a finger that has become very, very painful. Your finger has a boil on it, and the doctor says it's necessary to open it. It's necessary to make an incision in the finger, in order to relieve the pressure, in order to take out the pus. And, in order to do that, he injects novocaine around the wrist, like this, to create a wrist block, anesthesia of the hand. So the feeling in the hand will get numb. There will be no feeling of pain.

As you sit there, imagine that your hand has been injected and that you feel as if you're wearing a thick, heavy leather glove. I'm going to count from one to five, and as I reach the count of five, you'll notice that you get a sensation of wearing a thick heavy leather glove. The feeling will be so real that it will be as if you're actually wearing a thick heavy leather glove. As I count to five, you get the sensation that your hand is different from the other hand, that it's wearing a glove. As soon as you get the impression or feeling that your hand is wearing a thick, heavy leather glove, indicate it by your hand rising up in the air—like that.

You'll notice that whereas the right hand is sensitive, this hand begins to feel numb even when I prick it deeply. (*The hand is pricked with a needle.*) You notice that? Even when I prick it deeply there's a numbness here. Any pain?

Pt. No.

Dr. As you sit there, I'm going to suggest to you that you imagine yourself in a theater observing a play. You're sitting in the audience, and you notice the stage in front of you. The curtain is drawn. Now I'm going to count from one to five, and at the count of five suddenly the curtains will be drawn apart, and you'll see action on the stage. You'll visualize a play. No matter what you visualize, tell me about it without waking up. As soon as I reach the count of five, you'll see a flash of action. One, two, three, four, five.

Pt. It's in a green sitting room.
Dr. Yes?
Pt. Somebody's sitting at the piano, playing.
Dr. What?
Pt. Two other people reading.

(*As in his response to the Rorschach cards, movement in this fantasy is minimal. A restriction of creativeness, activity and biologic drive is suggested.*)

Dr. A scene, a quiet living room scene. What you have visualized is a fantasy. Fantasies and dreams are of the same caliber, except dreams are more vivid, but they're essentially the same. Now tonight when you go to sleep you'll notice that you probably will dream. You probably will dream, and if you do remember the dream, I want you to bring it in to me. Tonight when you go to bed you will dream, and if you do remember the dream, bring it in with you when you come to see me next.

Now, next time we try this I'm going to repeat "Sleep, sleep, sleep, sleep", and as I do, you'll notice that your eyes will get heavier and heavier and heavier, and finally they'll close, and you'll go into a sleep which will get progressively deeper and deeper.

As you sit there, now, I'm going to give you the suggestion that you have a dream or a image that is like a dream. As soon as you've had that, indicate it by your hand rising, lifting. As soon as you've had a dream or fantasy that's like a dream, indicate it by your hand rising, no matter how long it takes. (*Pause*) Now your hand rises.

Listen carefully to me. When you wake up, you may or

may not remember the fantasy or dream that you've had. It makes no difference. If you remember it, tell it to me. You may not remember other things that happened; it's immaterial. But this is important, when you wake up, you'll notice that when you look at me, your eyes will begin blinking, that it will be impossible to look at me without your eyes jerking and blinking. I'm going to count from one to five, and when I reach the count of five, your eyes will open up, and you'll blink. No matter how hard you try to control it, the spasms will continue. You'll not be able to stop yourself from blinking. Then I'm going to say, "Close your eyes," following which I'll say, "Slowly open them." And this time your eyes will not blink when you look at me. This time you'll notice that your eyes will not blink when you look at me. The first time they will, and then I'll ask you to close them, and the second time they will not blink. One; at the count of five open your eyes. They will blink spastically as you look at me; two, three, four, five. Notice how your eyes are blinking? Now close them. Slowly, as you open them now, it will be possible for you to look at me without your eyes blinking. Good. Good. How do you feel?

Pt. Sleepy.

Dr. Fine, what do you remember?

Pt. Meeting my wife, taking her out walking to the theater, a dream.

Dr. Fine, now tomorrow we meet again at four-fifteen.

Pt. Four-fifteen.

THIRD SESSON (April 3)

Patient has a dream, in response to my suggestion, which indicates he is putting me in a paternal role. In hypnosis an attempt is made to analyze what may be behind his lack of penial sensations in intercourse. He exhibits resistance to this probing, and obviously does not wish to analyze. Suggestive and persuasive commands are given him to adopt a different attitude toward sexual relations.

Pt. It is amazing. I did have somewhat of a dream last night. I don't really remember it well. It is very short, too vague. It is a peculiar thing, I dreamt of my father, and it is the first time I have. It didn't consist of very much.

Dr. Can you tell me what it was?

Pt. Yes. I was walking into a church, and he was sitting there and sort of made room for me to sit next to him. I don't remember very much—there wasn't very much beyond that.

Dr. I see.

Pt. But I saw him sitting there, and naturally I walked over to sit down along side of him.

Dr. Do you have any association to walking into church?

Pt. Well, I have been going to church more. In my youth I did attend services with my Dad. He was religious and I always managed to attend with him.

Dr. And with your Dad do you recall a certain feeling of closeness?

Pt. Closeness? Yes.

Dr. Now, did your Dad demand that you go to church?

Pt. No, he didn't have to. I mean I knew that he desired it that way and I went. And I rather liked it—I mean —it was nice—the associations with home.

Dr. You were quite fond of your Dad?

Pt. Yes.

Dr. Your fantasies about your Dad, are they always of a pleasant variety?

Pt. Yes. Very.

Dr. Did you have any other feelings or ideas in relation to him?

Pt. No. After I left you I thought of him.

(In response to my suggestion the patient had a dream which turns out to be a transference dream. Apparently the patient desires and expects me to play a paternal role. If his feelings toward his father are not too ambivalent, he may be very responsive to prestige suggestion.)

Dr. What happened when you left?

Pt. I went home. I didn't tell my wife I came to see you. We tried sex.

Dr. What happened?

Pt. Well, the same thing.

Dr. Can you describe that more in detail?

Pt. Well, yes. After about 10 or 15 minutes of preliminaries I tried to insert it.

Dr. You had an erection?

Pt. That's right. And upon insertion it was the same thing—I—it lasted for I should say a little over a half minute —between a half minute and a minute.

Dr. Between a half minute and a minute. You inserted your penis?

Pt. That's right.

Dr. Did you get any sensation when you inserted it?

Pt. No, no.

Dr. Did you get any feeling of pleasure, or did you get any feeling of pressure; was it anesthetic or what?

Pt. It was almost anesthetic.

Dr. Almost anesthetic.

Pt. Yes. The feeling of pleasure is somewhat, I imagine secondary, because of the tension that I'm under at that particular moment. You see, that fear is always there with me. Will I succeed or will I not succeed?

Dr. The fear that you will or will not succeed is there.

Pt. Fear that I won't succeed.

Dr. I see. Then the insertion isn't so much the desire for pleasure as it is wondering about the success.

Pt. That's right. That is the thing.

Dr. So that you never have actually permitted yourself to feel any sensations in intercourse.

Pt. That's right. That's exactly what it is.

Dr. Now yesterday, briefly, before we started hypnosis, we emphasized several things. First, the masturbatory misconceptions, and, second, the fact that there may be other elements operating of which you may not be aware. Now we're not going to work in too great detail because you don't want to change everything. We want to accomplish as much as we can in as little time as possible. I'm going to give you strong suggestions that will enable you to function sexually. If your difficulty is not too deep, these will enable you to function. If it is on a more complicated basis, it may be necessary to go into more material.

Pt. I see.

Dr. One thing that may be essential is to capture fantasies or associations th t occur in the process of inserting your penis.

Pt. Yes.

Dr. We may possibly do that under hypnosis. What I'm going to have you do is work out a plan, an ordered plan of establishing a better contact with your wife in order that you overcome whatever fears there may be.

Pt. Yes.

Dr. Has she read any medical books on sex?

Pt. Yes, she has.

Dr. How about yourself, have you read anything?

Pt. Some things, not much.

Dr. I'm going to give you a list of books. Perhaps you and your wife can read to remove as many misconceptions as possible about the sexual function and the sexual act.

Pt. I see.

Dr. Now, we will use hypnosis again. Did you feel relaxed yesterday?

Pt. Yes. I was wondering, doctor, is there any way of knowing, am I susceptible to suggestion, or is it just my willingness to cooperate? I mean I have no way of telling.

Dr. Whether you are complying voluntarily or automatically in a trance is not material. It is not necessary for you to comply. Actually every person who is hypnotized asks these questions about hypnosis. It is not necessary that you concern yourself too much with them. The way we're utilizing hypnosis here is not so much in a sense of creating a sense of passivity, a sense of compliance, but rather of you participating with me to achieve certain effects and a certain mastery of functions. As you proceed you will get the idea.

Pt. Yes.

Dr. It will be possible for you to control your own functions, and, through the medium of hypnosis, you, yourself, will begin to be able to master certain sensations and functions. You will be able to translate that over into the sexual area, eventually.

Pt. I see.

Dr. All right, now supposing you lean back in your chair and again bring your hands down and watch your fingers; watch your fingers, and as you watch your fingers, this time rapidly, you'll begin to notice that your hand will get light, that the fingers will slowly lift up in the air, and that you will begin to sleep, sleep, sleep, sleep. Your eyes will get heavy and then close and your hand will lift up toward your face, straight up. Just like that. And when it touches your face, lean your head up against the palm of your hand and go to sleep. It is moving up, you are getting drowsier and drowsier and drowsier. Sleep, sleep, sleep, sleep, sleep. You're very tired. Very tired. Drowsy, drowsy, very drowsy. From your head right down to your feet. You're going to get so tired and drowsy and sleepy. You are going into a deep restful sleep. Your hand is moving up, up, up, straight up to your face. Your whole body is heavy except for your arm. You get drowsier and drowsier and drowsier. As soon as your hand touches your face, just relax and sleep. Now you are asleep. Sleep for a few minutes and then I'll talk to you again. You'll be more deeply asleep. (*Pause*)

As you sit there, I'm going to stroke your arm, your other

arm, and as I do you'll begin to notice that it gets heavy, very heavy, and that the heaviness sweeps down, right down, from your shoulder to your finger tips, so that the arm gets just as heavy as lead and stiff, stiff, just like a board. Heavy and stiff. Heavy and stiff. As I stroke it, it gets heavier and heavier and heavier. I'm going to count from one to five, and at the count of five, it will feel so stiff and rigid that even when I try to budge it, it will not move. One, heavy; two, heavier and heavier; three, as heavy and stiff as a board; four, stiffer and stiffer and heavier; five, just as heavy as a board. When I try to budge it, it remains heavy and stiff, and you yourself will notice that even though you try to budge it, the harder you try, the heavier it will feel, until the muscles become so achy and so heavy that it is impossible to lift it.

At the same time, your entire body begins to feel heavy and stiff and rigid, almost as if you're made of iron. I'm going to count from one to five, and at the count of five, you'll notice that your entire body will have become so heavy and so stiff that even though you try to budge out of the chair, you cannot. You'll notice that the harder you try the heavier you feel. One, heavy; two, stiff; three, heavier and heavier; four, as heavy as lead; five, heavy and stiff, and when you try to move out of your chair, the harder you try, the heavier and stiffer you get, so that it is impossible to budge even though you try. It is impossible to budge. Try and you'll see that the harder you try to get up, the heavier you feel.

Now as you sit there, I'm going to ask you, yourself, to count from one to five, and you'll notice that now that you count from one to five, at the count of four it will be impossible for you to move your body or arm, but at the count of five, your body will relax, so that it will be possible for you to move your body and to move your arm. Go ahead.

Pt. One, two, three, four. . . . five.

Dr. Now you can move your arm and body. You noticed that, didn't you?

Pt. Yes.

Dr. Good. Now I'm going to ask you, as you sit there, to visualize yourself again walking with me toward the church, and as we walk you go into the churchyard, you see the tall spires and steeples and the bell. As soon as you hear the ringing of the bell, your hand will rise to indicate that to me. (*Hand rises.*) Now it comes down again, and you begin to feel more tired and more sleepy, drowsier and drowsier and drowsier.

In a moment I'm going to count from one to five, and at the count of five, this time, your eyes will open up, but you will still feel drowsy. You'll still feel sleepy, and the moment I say, "Sleep, sleep, sleep," your eyelids will feel just like lead, and even though you try to keep them open, you'll notice that your eyes shut firmly. One, two, three, four, five—sleep, sleep, sleep—your eyes shut.

Now listen carefully to me. I'm going to stroke your hand again, and I want you to go to sleep and to dream. It may take a little time or it may come shortly. You'll have a dream, and this time your dream will indicate your feelings, your deep feelings about your father, no matter what they may be. The dream will be about your deep feelings about your father. As soon as you have that dream, your hand will rise to indicate that to me. Continue to sleep, continue to sleep, continue to sleep. I want you to sleep. Perhaps you'll visualize the scene on the stage, by looking at the stage and noticing the curtain opening up. I want you to report to me exactly what you see. No matter what it is that you see. It will appear just like a dream, because a dream is nothing more than thoughts that occur in a state of sleep. I want you to tell me about it as soon as you see that, indicating that you've seen it by your hand rising. (*Hand rises.*)

Like that.   Go ahead now.   I want you to tell me just what you dreamed.   What did you see?

Pt.   Father sitting on a chair, reading the paper.   People sitting around the table playing cards.

(*The passive content of the dream will be noted.*)

Dr.   Good.   Now as you sit there, I'm going to give you some suggestions.   It is essential for you at this point to begin to have certain feelings restored to you.   You have a desire to function, to function well sexually.   Your left hand will move, will rise about two inches, if you have that desire.   It will be able to rise if you have the desire to function well sexually.   (*Hand rises.*)   You have that desire, your hand moves and now you bring it down.

If you have the desire to function sexually as you indicate, then it will be possible to remove the causes that prevent you from functioning sexually.   It will be possible to do that in two ways; understanding what is blocking you from functioning sexually, and retraining yourself, so that you can function well sexually.   Now if you have a real desire to overcome this, and I believe you have—you've indicated it to me—then you will have the desire to go into whatever feelings and whatever fantasies are important.   You'll have a desire to tackle this thing.

I want you to visualize yourself in this theater, watching yourself on the stage.   This time you will be performing sexually with your wife.   You're on the stage, you play with her, you have an erection, and then you insert your penis.   You then suddenly get a flash through your mind, thoughts that come to you in a flash about what goes on underneath the surface—fear, disgust or whatever it is as you insert your penis.   As soon as you see this, indicate it to me by your hand rising.   (*Hand rises.*)   Your hand rises.   Tell me about it.

Pt.   It was just an ordinary flash.

Dr. What was it?

Pt. Light.

Dr. A flash of light. A flash of light. What emotion was there with that flash?

Pt. None.

(Patient is so severely repressed that he is unable to acknowledge his deeper feelings. I decide at this point to use a more persuasive than analytic approach.)

Dr. None. All right. Now listen to me. If there is no emotion of fear, if there is no emotion of disgust, if there is no emotion of a sort that would inhibit you, then it will be possible for you to put into action what I am going to suggest to you. From now on, I want you, when you go to bed with your wife, to go to bed, not with the idea of performing, not with the fear that you may fail, not with the intense desire and expectation that you are going to succeed, but rather not caring anything about your performance. I want you, instead of feeling you've got to satisfy your wife, merely to insert your penis with the idea of seeing what sensations you can get out of the insertion. It will make no difference whether you have an orgasm immediately, no difference whether you can last any length of time. Merely experience whatever feelings, whatever sensations there may be in your penis. In other words, I'm going to give you a very strong suggestion, and that is that it will be possible for you to begin to demonstrate to yourself that you can have feelings. Up to this time you functioned with an anesthetized penis. I want you to begin to have certain feelings in your penis, no matter what they may be. I want you to feel less that you are performing, and more that you have sex for whatever pleasure there is. I would like to have you take your wife into confidence and tell her that you are going to work at this thing, not from a feeling that you've got to perform—because the very challenge of performing may block you and cause you to fail—rather you are going to do it from now on with the idea of feeling what pleasure you can get out of it.   On that basis, it will not be a challenge to you.   It makes no difference who the man is, if he feels challenged, if he feels that he is going to fail, it will interfere with his performance.   And I want you to enter into this new relationship with her with the idea of not caring whether you perform well or whether you do not perform well.   Do you understand me?

Pt.   Yes.

Dr.   You understand me thoroughly and are you desirous of working at this from this point of view?

Pt.   Yes.

Dr.   You believe you will be able to do this?

Pt.   Yes.

Dr.   Good.   I want you to try to do it and to work at it without the idea of succeeding at all, without the idea of a challenge, but merely with the idea of engaging in an activity that may have pleasure values for you.   I'm going to make that a strong suggestion.   At the same time I want you to observe yourself, to observe what ideas accompany the sexual act, to observe whether any fear appears, to observe whatever ideas occur so that you can tell me about them. When you go home, it will be possible for you to feel that you are experiencing something important.   As you sit there, I'm going to suggest that you will feel a sense of strength developing in you.   You will feel more self confident.   You will feel better and stronger, better and stronger.

I want you to be more deeply asleep.   Feel yourself dozing off and getting very sleepy.   When you wake up, when I wake you up, you'll notice that your left arm is stiff, very stiff, very, very stiff.   When I yank on it, it will become stiffer and stiffer and stiffer and more rigid.   When you wake up, your arm will become so stiff and rigid, that it will be impossible to budge it.   It will be impossible to budge it

until I say, "Count." When I say, "Count," you'll count
from one to five, and you'll notice that at the count of five,
it will then be possible to move your arm. When I wake you
up, you will notice that the arm is heavy and stiff, hugs your
body and that the harder you try to move it, the heavier
it feels. But when I say, "Count," you will count from one
to five, and at the count of five, the arm will loosen up and
then it will be possible to move it. One—start waking up—
two, three, four, five. (*Patient awakens and tries to move
his arm unsuccessfully*.) Count.

Pt. One, two, three, four, five.

Dr. Now you can move your arm. Good. How do you
feel?

Pt. Relaxed.

Dr. Good. I'm going to repeat what I said to you because some of this may possibly be obscure now. It is
very, very essential to work at this systematically. We
are going to try in a very short time, to correct a tendency
that you've had all your life. You must enter into sexual
relations with your wife on the basis that you're not
damaged, that you are functioning all right, that whatever
is causing your premature ejaculations are the product of
misconceptions and fears that go way back in your life that
have no bearing on the situation today. You must look
upon sex as a pleasure function, and not think of satisfying your wife for the time being. Your not thinking of
her will in the long run be beneficial to her. You must stop
regarding sexuality as a means of proving yourself because
it cannot do that for anyone. The more a person feels he
has to perform in sex, the more he feels he's got to succeed,
the quicker he's licked. I'd like to have you, until I see
you next, experiment and see what feelings you can develop.
Look upon it as a pleasure experience. Don't even think
about how long it is going to last. Just see what pleasures
you can get out of it. Just experience whatever feelings

come up.   If you want to take your wife into your confidence, so much the better.   If you don't want to, all right.

Fourth Session (April 9)

*Patient expresses discouragement.   He is reassured and an
attempt is made to convince him that there is a connection between
his symptom and his attitudes toward women.   He refuses to
admit this.   In hypnosis an attempt is made to condition him to a
firmer control over his physical functions including the sexual
function.   Authoritarian, forceful suggestions are used to get
him to divorce his early misconceptions from his present day life.
His passivity and fear of aggression are brought up and a hobby is
suggested to permit him to express aggression.*

Dr.   Well, how are things?

Pt.   Not much good.

Dr.   Why not?

Pt.   I'm afraid I haven't responded to the suggestions you
made.   Somehow I acted the same way I always did.

Dr.   After all, a pattern of this type that goes so deep has
to be worked at before a change occurs.   It never comes
immediately.   Have patience, it will come if you have a
strong enough desire.

Pt.   I have that.

Dr.   You just can't take a lifetime and throw it out the
window in a few days.   How long have you been coming here
now?

Pt.   A little over a week.

Dr.   Knowing the path along which to move and not being
so concerned about immediate results is important.

Pt.   Yes.

Dr.   When did you have relations?

Pt.   Last night.

Dr.   Well what thoughts came to you during this?   Did
you have any ideas or thoughts about it?

Pt.   No, no, there's only one thought at all times that's
utmost in my mind, and it's the eagerness to succeed, to

prove, to bring home to myself that I'm perfectly normal.
That was the thought that was always in my mind. I can't
seem to grasp any other thoughts.

Dr. The thought has been to prove yourself.

Pt. That's right exactly.

Dr. What sort of person is your wife? Can you describe
to me the feelings you have for her, the kind of relationship
you have with her?

Pt. Well, I don't know if I can put it into words very well.
I mean it's a closeness, the intimacy is there naturally, and
there's a great fondness and admiration we have for each
other. If I might add the mere fact that she is so lovely.
I'm just, of course—I know it must mean an awful lot to
her. She pretends it doesn't, and she's perfectly willing to
be patient and all that stuff. Which makes me that much
more eager. I mean, had she probably, ah, well let's see
now, how will I put it? Well, had she seemed more disappointed, more disillusioned, perhaps I would feel differ-
ently.

Dr. How would you feel then?

Pt. Well, oh, I feel as though if that's the way it is, I
wouldn't care so much. It would just have to right itself,
yes or no, I would have to gamble on the outcome of it.

Dr. In other words you wouldn't be so eager.

Pt. Eager, exactly. The mere fact that she's so lovely
about it, so fine, so patient.

Dr. Supposing you never succeeded in having relations
with her. What do you fantasy?

Pt. I don't know. At first, well for the first two or three
weeks of our married life, I thought it would end up in an
annulment. You hear about these things and it's logical
to assume that your case will not be different from anybody
else's. Of course that was a terrible thought, and I succeeded in dismissing that mostly, I think, because in her
attitude, I mean, whereby she feels that the sex angle is that

while it's of great importance, it's not of paramount importance. And, she's very much in love with me, and she ad-
mires me and all that sort of thing. Of course, I, as a man,
know the other thing plays a very important part, and
marriage based without that simply can't succeed. Well
I'm not as I was the first two or three weeks.

Dr. You did talk to her then? And are you convinced
that even though you are never able to have complete relations, she won't leave you?

Pt. Yes, I really am.

Dr. You're sure?

Pt. So far, yes.

Dr. All right, now we have to go on because you do want
to break this thing up.

Pt. Um hum.

Dr. First, it's good that you feel that she's not going to
leave you under any circumstances. That will prevent you
from getting too anxious.

Pt. That's right.

Dr. Second, it will be good for you to feel that you
mustn't perform, that there's no challenge. It has nothing
to do with your masculinity. It's a problem. You're not
impotent, because you do have erections.

Pt. That's right.

Dr. And it's merely the fact that just as soon as you insert, you have an ejaculation.

Pt. That's right.

Dr. We're working on a basis of giving you a certain sense
of mastery over your impulses, but at the same time it's
necessary to divest you of fears, misconceptions about your
own functioning. You are not damaged. Look, if it were
true that masturbation produced this in you, then you
wouldn't be able to have an erection when you kissed her,
hugged her and made love to her.

Pt. I see.

Dr. So that the masturbation thing has nothing to do with this picture.   There seems to be a peculiar association to the female genital organ.

Pt. Um hum.

Dr. And the contact with the female genital organ, whatever that happens to mean to you.

Pt. Yes.

Dr. And it may have a content and a meaning to you of a particular kind that is different than for other people.

Pt. I see.

Dr. What about your attitudes towards female sex organs?

Pt. Well, I've never given it much thought.   My passion is the same as everybody else's, I suppose.

Dr. By that you mean what?

Pt. The same as any man's thought on these things.

Dr. Well what do feel about it?   I mean on a conscious level.

Pt. Well, I, I don't know how to put it.   What do you mean when you say, how do I feel about it?

Dr. Does it repulse you, do you get frightened by it?

Pt. No, no.

Dr. Do you feel excited by it?

Pt. No.

Dr. Do you feel it's nasty?

Pt. No, no, no.

Dr. You don't have any feelings.

Pt. No. None.

Dr. Neither positive nor negative.

Pt. No, neither positive or negative.

Dr. Just an indifference?

Pt. That's right.

Dr. Behind that indifference there may lie certain fears.

Pt. Um hum.

Dr. Because things like this don't happen by magic.

The fact that it's disassociated and disconnected from what's going on in your conscious life doesn't mean that it's not there.

Pt. Yes.

Dr. Here you have an erection, and just as soon as it comes in contact with the female sex organ it disappears.

Pt. That's right.

Dr. Yes, so that it's the contact with the female organ; and what I'm trying to do is to establish a connection and a continuity between the act and the symptom.

Pt. Um hum.

Dr. So that if there is any fear, we can bring it up into consciousness and you can get rid of it.

Pt. That's right.

Dr. But actually you have, you feel, no associations to the female sex organs that are either repulsive or exciting.

Pt. I've never felt, not consciously at any rate, I've never felt any repulsion or fear.

Dr. Well it may not be there, or it may. And what about your relationships with women in the past? Have you been attracted to any particular type of woman?

Pt. No.

Dr. Say a passive type of woman or an active type of woman, what kind of woman has appealed to you?

Pt. The passive type, more or less.

Dr. And your wife is a passive type?

Pt. That's right.

Dr. Now supposing you just relax yourself and breathe in deeply and then go to sleep. Sleep, sleep, sleep. As you sit there you're going to feel tired and drowsy, and slowly, automatically, even perhaps without your knowledge, your hand, your right hand will lift up. It will rise towards your face, begin to lift and rise, slowly rise and lift as you get sleepier, and sleepier, and sleepier. Very tired and drowsy and sleepy, from your head right down to your feet. Your hand will begin to rise and lift straight up towards your face, and you'll go into a deep restful, relaxed, comfortable sleep. Slowly the hand will rise, and lift. Your eyes get heavy, you get tired and sleepy. The hand is moving up now, moving up, rising straight up towards the face, and when it touches your face, you'll be asleep, in a deep sleep. Very tired, very sleepy. (*Pause*). Now as you sit there, I'm going to ask you to begin counting slowly from one to five. This time, as you count slowly, from one to five, your arm, your left arm, will begin to stiffen up, and to get heavy, so that at the count of five, no matter how hard you try, the arm will have gotten so stiff and so heavy that it will be rigid and will not move. It will not move. It will not relax even though you may try hard to make it relax. It will stay glued up against your thigh. Count slowly, and as you count, your arm will begin to get heavier and heavier and heavier, and it will get so heavy and so stiff that it will not move.

Pt. One, two, three, four, five.

Dr. Notice how heavy and stiff and rigid it is. I'm going to pull at it now, and try to budge it, and it will become stiffer and stiffer and stiffer. And as you sit there, you begin to notice more and more that the arm stiffness continues almost apart from you. Without any participation on your part it continues to be stiff and rigid until you, yourself, give yourself the command to move it by counting from one to five. Now start counting, from one to five, and as you count from one to five, the rigidity will gradually leave. As you count from one to five, the rigidity will gradually leave.

Pt. One, two, three, four, five.

Dr. The arm can move. Now, the arm will stiffen again through your own suggestion. Count from one to five. As you count from one to five, the arm will stiffen and remain in a fixed position, it will stiffen and remain in that position. Even though you try to move it in either direction, it will remain exactly as it is, stiff and rigid and firm. Count from one to five.

Pt. One, two, three, four, five.

Dr. You notice how stiff it is? And when you try to budge it, it remains exactly as it is, and it will get stiffer and stiffer and stiffer, and it's impossible for it to go down. It remains stiff, it remains stiff, and it remains rigid just as it is now. And the harder you try to bring it down, the stiffer and heavier it becomes. Now it's possible for you to control that, the stiffness, and the rigidity; it's possible for it to remain stiff and rigid. And you're going to notice this, that it will be possible for you to control all your body functions better and better, even the function of your penis, which too, eventually, will become stiff and rigid when you insert it in the vagina. So that when you insert it in the vagina, you will be able to feel that it remains stiff and rigid, that it continues to be stiff and rigid, just like your arm remains stiff and rigid, and that no matter what happens, it continues to remain stiff and rigid and firm. And I'm going to ask you now to count from one to five, and at the count of five, you will be able to move your arm down to the body.

Pt. One, two, three, four, five.

Dr. Now, your arm moves down to your thigh. I want you to sit back in the chair, breathe in deeply and go to sleep deeper. In a few minutes I'll talk to you, and you'll be still more deeply asleep. (*Pause*)

As you sleep, listen to me. Eventually you will liberate yourself from whatever fears, whatever anxieties there exist in your relationship to women, and in your contact with the female sex organs. It makes no difference about the origin of the anxieties. It makes no difference how strong the anxieties are. It will be possible for you to dissociate your own feelings from your fears, if there are fears. Let us assume that there is something that is operating within you, say a childhood misunderstanding or fear of the female sex organs. We do not know that there is a connection, but the probabilities are that there is some difficulty. It may be the result of experiences with your own mother, or the result of early experiences with women, it may be that even your father enters into the picture in some way. Regardless of how this thing started, regardless of what anxieties, what fears, what distrust, what hostilities may exist in your relationships with women, they have absolutely nothing to do with present day facts. They have absolutely nothing to do with your wife. Eventually you will deal with life less on the basis of early associations, early conditionings, early fears, no matter what they may have been, and more on the basis of present day reality. It's not really necessary to unearth or to examine everything about your early life to produce results. It is not essential to our task right at this moment. We're going to work on the assumption that there is some sort of anxiety, some sort of fear in relationship to women, but that it is not important to bring it out at this time. No matter what your associations were before, no matter what difficulties you had with your mother, or other women, no matter what fantasies you may have had when you were little, or what fears there were, they did happen in the past. They are not a part of your present life. You must dissociate them from your present life.

Let us assume now that you do go to bed with your wife with the idea of getting whatever pleasure you can out of it. I'm going to suggest that you gradually throw away the other motivations, that is performing and pleasing her. Assume that it makes no difference how long it takes, really assume that, and go into sexual relations as a means of pleasing yourself, of seeing what pleasure you can get out of it. The suggestions that I'm giving you now about fitness, and your own ability to control stiffness and rigidity, will continue to operate in other areas. And I'm going to extend that suggestion so that it will lend strength and capacity for erectiveness in your sexual functions.

You can, if you wish, try to isolate yourself from the fears no matter what they may have been, no matter what they are. At the same time let yourself assume that it makes no difference how long your penis remains erect. It may go down immediately, and if it does, you must get yourself to a state where you don't care. It may go down shortly after you insert it, and if it does, you must not care. It may continue in there for a minute, and then go down; it may continue for two minutes or three minutes or even more in a fully erect position. The important thing is you must insert it with the idea of seeing if there is any pleasure associated with intercourse. See if there is any pleasure associated with inserting it. Insert it with the idea that it makes no difference to your wife; it only makes a difference in how *you* feel. Finally, you must separate whatever anxieties or fears that exist in relationship to women, and in relationship to their sexual organs from yourself. Just go ahead with the idea of getting as much fun out of sex as possible.

If you do all these things, you will notice that it will be possible to feel stiffness and rigidity in your penis that will enable you to function well. I'm going to give you another strong suggestion to that effect. You must now begin to dissociate, remove, whatever fears there may be. Don't concern yourself with them so much. It may not be necessary to look into them or to investigate them. If they're there, it will be increasingly possible to dissociate yourself from them, to remove them, to feel that they need not matter to you, that you can function and do well without them. I'm going to repeat the suggestion that the ability to control the stiffness in your penis will become more and more and more pronounced.

As you sit there, I'm going to ask you now to continue to sleep, continue to sleep, and again count slowly from one to five. At the count of five, you'll notice that your whole body will stiffen up and become rigid, firm, rigid, firm. As you sit there the rigidity will increase until I give you the command to loosen up. Count from one to five, and the whole body will stiffen up. It will be impossible for you to get out of the chair, and you continue to sleep until I give you the command to loosen up again.

Pt. One, two, three, four, five.

Dr. Even though you try to get up out of the chair, the harder you try, the stiffer you feel. In a moment, I'm going to talk to you again. In the meantime continue to sleep. (*Pause*) Now I'm going to count slowly from one to five, and at the count of five, the stiffness will be gone and you'll slowly awaken, slowly awaken. Then we'll talk some more. One, two, three, four, five. Open your eyes and wake up. How do you feel?

Pt. Drowsy.

Dr. I'm going to work with you in other areas besides the sexual one, because I think from your associations, that you have other problems like the ability to express aggressiveness and action. Do you have an opportunity in your work to express aggressiveness?

Pt. It doesn't call for a great deal of aggressiveness.

Dr. How about your relationships with your employees?

Pt. They're very good. They've always been good.

Dr. Good in a sense that they're congenial?

Pt. Yes.

Dr. It would be very, very helpful to you if you would be able to have an opportunity to express certain forceful feelings. It is important for you to practice being firm and holding your ground, being assertive and demonstrative. But this won't develop right away. It will take time. Do you have any athletic outlets?

Pt. Physical? No.

Dr. Physical exercises would be helpful, as an outlet for forceful actions.

Pt. Yes.

Dr. Are you interested in any hobby? It would be good

if you could get interested in something that would give you a chance at motor expression. Do you have any ideas you would like to talk about, any impressions or feelings?

Pt. No, but I have led a restrictive life.

Dr. The ability to express yourself forcefully in some sphere would be helpful to you.

Pt. Yes, I can see that.

Dr. Because you have led too restricted an existence.

Pt. That's right.

Dr. A passive kind of life.

Pt. True.

Dr. It's a little difficult to know exactly in what area your interests may lie. For instance, I knew a man who wasn't at all aware of the fact that he was inhibiting his aggression. He believed he was being civilized in hardly moving a muscle.

Pt. Yes?

Dr. And so I asked him why he didn't take up a hobby. He replied, "Well, what hobby?" We worked and we worked on this, and finally he took up fencing. He was terrified the first few times that he might hurt somebody. Well it took effort and courage to go ahead. He began seeing that he didn't kill anybody in fencing, and he got rid of a lot of pent-up aggression within him. I don't know what hobby you might find interesting, but something like that would be extremely helpful.

Pt. I was thinking about golf.

Dr. Even golf, you could just take a good lusty swing at the ball, even get mad at it.

Pt. (*Laughs*) Well, that's true, I don't get mad often enough.

Dr. Try it, even if it's only a ball you get mad at. Wallop it as hard as you can.

Pt. I will.

Dr. Get the aggression out of your system. Do you play golf now?

Pt. No, but I will. I can see what you mean.

FIFTH SESSION (April 10)

The patient has been able to recognize his lack of aggression as a problem. He has made an important gain, feeling for the first time sensations in his penis during intercourse. He apparently has accepted the suggestion given him to regard sex relations as a source of pleasure rather than as an arena in which he proves himself. We discuss the flowing rather than the spurting character of his ejaculations and connect it to the use of the penis as a urinary rather than sexual organ. In hypnosis strong persuasive arguments are given him, and an attempt is made to remove misconceptions about masturbation.

Pt. I couldn't help but feel last time I left the office riding on the subway that we're on the right track. I mean what you had said seemed just right home.

Dr. Particularly in what respect.

Pt. About the aggressiveness in me not being there.

Dr. Do you have any ideas about that?

Pt. No, I haven't.

Dr. Have you been aware of this lack all along?

Pt. Yes, I have been aware of that.

Dr. How far back does it go?

Pt. Well, about ten years is all I can remember. I've reproached myself more or less for it during that time.

Dr. How?

Pt. To me it was symbolic of a certain weakness.

Dr. All right, we can work on that along with the other if you wish. Has anything else happened since I saw you last?

Pt. Yes, but there wasn't much difference in my sex relations.

Dr. There was no difference at all?

Pt. I think, though, I detected a difference in feeling

there. In other words I wasn't as anxious to perform and do good. The tension was less.

Dr. Good.

Pt. Yes, the desire to succeed wasn't as strong as it generally is. Another interesting thing is that for the first time when I inserted my penis, I think I really detected a difference.

Dr. Are you sure of that?

Pt. Yes.

Dr. You didn't concentrate your attention on the performance.

Pt. Yes. Somehow the ultimate outcome wasn't as important as it generally is.

Dr. Did you have an ejaculation last night?

Pt. Yes.

Dr. Were you able to observe if the ejaculation was a spurting ejaculation or a flowing one.

Pt. Well, I don't recall.

Dr. Did you note any muscular spasms as you ejaculated?

Pt. No, no.

Dr. It was just sort of like urinating?

Pt. That's right.

Dr. Well, it will be interesting to follow this along. When you masturbate is it a flowing or spurting ejaculation?

Pt. No, that's a spurt.

Dr. There's a difference, then. Now, do you recall any urinary fantasies or urinary activities as a child?

Pt. No, none of that kind, none at all.

Dr. There was never any such thing as bed wetting?

Pt. No, no.

Dr. Any such thing as noticing a little girl urinate?

Pt. No, no, nothing like that.

Dr. There is a difference in the two types of ejaculation.

Pt. I noticed that.

Dr. The flowing off may remind you of the urinary function.

Pt. It does.

Dr. And the absence of sensation in inserting the penis may be referable to the fact that the penis is not used as a sexual organ, but rather as a urinary organ.

Pt. I see.

Dr. I want you to concentrate on your feelings in your penis, on the ideas that came to you in intercourse. I want you to get as much pleasure out of the feeling of intercourse as possible.

Pt. That's right.

Dr. It is necessary to retrain your entire attitude toward sex and the sex act.

Pt. Yes.

Dr. This can be done. You must recast your attitudes so sex comes to have pleasure values for you. Now I want you to go to sleep. I'd like to have you lean back now and watch your hands   Just keep gazing at your hand, breathe deeply and then slowly begin to feel yourself getting drowsy, and then your hand will begin to get light. It must begin to move a little bit, the space between the fingers will widen and you'll begin to notice that the hand will start lifting up slowly, rising, and lifting, right up towards your face. As it rises and lifts up towards your face, you get sleepier and sleepier until finally you go to sleep. Your hand will continue to rise and lift. You get sleepier and sleepier and sleepier, and the hand will rise toward your face, until it touches your face. When it touches your face, you will be asleep, deeply asleep. You will get drowsy, you'll breathe deeply, you'll go to sleep. Your hand touches your face now. Breathe in deeply. Sleep; lean back and go to sleep. In a moment I'll talk to you, and you will be still more deeply asleep. (*Pause*)

I'm going to suggest to you that as you sit there, you, your-

self, count from one to five, and at the count of five, you'll
be cognizant of a stiffness and rigidity in your fingers, in
your hand, in your arm, that makes the hand stretch itself
out, and the arm will stretch itself out, this way. Go ahead,
start counting now. Count from one to five.

(*An attempt is made here to get the patient to participate as
much as possible in the therapeutic process in order that he begin
to express more aggressiveness.*)

Pt. One, two, three, four, five.

Dr. So that the arm becomes stiff, and even though you
try to relax it, even though you try with all your might to
move it, the harder you try the stiffer and heavier it becomes.
Do you notice that?

Pt. Yes.

Dr. Do you notice that even when you try to make it
relax and to become soft, that it's stiff and outstretched, hard
and rigid?

Pt. Yes.

Dr. Now as you sit there, I'm going to stroke this arm
again and only as I count from one to five will it become soft
and come down. One, two, three, four, five. Now it
comes down. Good. Sleep deeply. (*Pause*)

As you sit there, I'm going to ask you to visualize that
scene in the theater where you noticed action. The last time
you saw that scene the movement on the stage was extremely
passive, people were sitting or standing. There was very
little movement. All that is indicative of the lack of aggressiveness, the lack of assertiveness, the lack of movement
in your life, the lack of push, the lack of masculine forcefulness. I would like to have you look upon the stage in your
imagination now, and notice before you a picture of real
forcefulness, of activity, of movement. I want you to
notice that and as soon as you see that tell me about it. See
if you can visualize and feel a scene of movement and forcefulness.

Pt. Someone dancing, a man and woman.

Dr. Now as you sit there, I want to see if you can visualize yourself in an aggressive role. Visualize yourself in the most aggressive role that you can possibly bring to your mind. As soon as you get a fantasy of that kind, tell me about it without waking up.

Pt. Swimming in a championship contest.

Dr. Did you visualize yourself swimming in a championship contest?

Pt. Yes.

Dr. Good. Now a problem that we have to tackle that's bound up with and associated with premature ejaculation is the idea of masculine forcefulness. It's necessary for you to bring out this material and see the significance of how far back it goes, and then take certain active steps with my help toward an entirely new orientation in regard to people, life, yourself and your own impulses, aggressive and sexual. As a child were you an aggressive child?

Pt. No.

Dr. Did you get into fights with the other boys?

Pt. Rarely.

Dr. How did you make out in those fights you got in?

Pt. Same as average, winning, sometimes losing. I tried to avoid any kind of trouble. I was afraid.

Dr. What happened to you that made you become so passive? Something occurred that put the floodgates on your aggressiveness, forcefulness and strength. What did happen to you is possibly not known to you now. But perhaps you may be able to recapture it through the medium of dreams, either now or later in the future. Of course, it is not absolutely essential to get the cause, but it's very essential to correct the effect. But getting the origin may make it possible to correct the effect more rapidly. Even though you may not possibly have the desire to get to the origin of your problem, because of time or any other reason, you still will be able to correct the effect of lack of aggression and lack of forcefulness that has permeated your whole life. Now, as you sit there, do you know of any incident or any series of incidents that frightened you?

Pt. No.

Dr. Did anything happen to you that made you feel that being hostile, being assertive, being forceful, having push, was not the proper or desirable way to be?

Pt. No.

Dr. Nothing like that. You will become increasingly aware of how important this problem is to you. You will become more and more aware of the fact that there is something lacking in your life, which will make you want to cooperate with me in a plan I shall outline for you. The first part of the plan involves your relationships with your wife. There is nothing more disastrous to effective sexual functioning than to look upon it as an arena in which you must demonstrate your virility and masculinity. Sex is no place of display. It has a different purpose. It is a procreative function that has pleasure values. You must regard sex in terms of pleasure not performance. For that reason again I'm going to give you a forceful suggestion that when you go to bed with your wife and want to have sex with her, that you do it on a basis of your wanting to see how much fun you can get out of it. There may, perhaps, be the feeling that you don't know whether you can have fun, but in spite of that a part of you will desire to have pleasure out of sexuality. And that part of you will grow and will undermine the other part.

If you have any anxiety at all about this, if you have any tension, if you have any fear, or if you have any reluctance about coming here, I will expect you to tell me about it because it's very important. Also I want you to tell me about all the sensations you feel when you insert your penis in the vagina, no matter what those sensations may be—constriction, tingling, feeling of oppression, pain, pleasure or whatever sensations you may have. Observe them and see what feelings come to you, pleasure feelings or other feelings. Again I'm going to suggest that less and less you will look upon sex as an arena of performance, and more and more you must regard it as a means of finding important values and pleasures for yourself. You must begin to regard sexuality as a source of pleasure and not as a means of displaying or proving yourself.

Let us now discuss the matter of your self confidence. As a result of the work that you do with me here, you are going to find that you can become more assertive, more self confident, and more active than you've ever been.

Before we go on further I should like to explore an area with you that may be important. I'm going to give you a suggestion that you begin to feel yourself getting small as you sit here, that you feel yourself going back in time, getting little, very little. Your head is getting little, your arms are getting little, your legs are getting tiny. Feel yourself getting tinier and tinier, and going back, back, back in time to a point, let us say, when you were six years of age. Let us say that you visualize yourself as a little boy of six. Listen to the clock ticking, so that as the clock ticks back, ticks the time far back, you get little, very little. And when you talk to me next, you will be a little boy, you will be six years of age. As soon as you feel yourself six, as soon as you feel yourself small, you will indicate it by your hand, your left hand, rising up about two inches. Feel yourself getting small, little, six years of age. As soon as you do, your hand will rise up and indicate that you feel like six. Everything will be as it was when you were six years of age. Your hand rises now. How old are you?

Pt. Six.

Dr. What grade are you in?

Pt. Two-B.

Dr. You must have skipped, how old were you when you started school?

Pt. Five.

Dr. Now as you sit there, do you know your teacher's name?

Pt. No.

Dr. How do you get along with the other kids?

Pt. All right.

Dr. Do they fight with you?

Pt. No.

Dr. Do you get mad at them?

Pt. No.

Dr. Do they ever get on your nerves?

Pt. No.

Dr. How do you get along with your mother?

Pt. Well.

Dr. And your father?

Pt. Well.

Dr. And with the other people in the family?

Pt. Well.

Dr. Has anybody ever picked on you or wanted to hit you?

Pt. No.

Dr. They didn't? You're not afraid to fight, are you?

Pt. No.

Dr. Good. Now you begin to get a little bit older, older. You're thirteen years of age. You're exactly thirteen years of age. You're thirteen. The next time I talk to you you'll be thirteen years of age. How old are you now?

Pt. Thirteen.

Dr. What grade are you in?

Pt. Junior High.

Dr. Do you like school?

Pt. Yes.

Dr. How do you get along with the kids?

Pt. Well.

Dr. Do you get into fights with them?

Pt. Occasionally.

Dr. Does anybody in particular pick on you?

Pt. No.

Dr. Who do you fight with?

Pt. Boys.

Dr. Why?

Pt. Get in little arguments.

Dr. How do you get along with your mother?

Pt. Fine.

Dr. And father?

Pt. Fine.

Dr. Do they ever pick on you?

Pt. No.

Dr. How about masturbation? When did you start masturbating?

Pt. About ten.

Dr. Did anybody teach you masturbation?

Pt. No.

Dr. How did you learn about it?

Pt. I don't know.

Dr. Can you see yourself masturbating now?

Pt. Yes.

Dr. Do you feel that any harm can come to you if you masturbate? What do you think about it?

Pt. I do.

Dr. Do you think it's wrong?

Pt. Yes.

Dr. What may happen to you?

Pt. I don't know, it's just that it's wrong.

Dr. Did anybody ever tell you it's bad?

Pt. No.

Dr. Well, how do you know it's wrong?

Pt. It just doesn't seem right.

Dr. As you sit there, I'm going to tell you that all youngsters masturbate. No physical harm will come to you. But if your own feeling about masturbation is that it can do you harm, your own fear of masturbation can create guilt feelings which may cause anxiety. As you sit there I'm going to tell you that whatever fears, whatever destructive feelings you have had about masturbation, you will eventually get over them. Nothing will happen to you.

Now I want you to go back, or forward, whichever it may be, to the first time you put your penis in a woman. And I want you to describe to me in great detail how it happened, all your feelings, all your fears, if there were any, all your ideas, everything, just as if you were living through it again. As soon as you feel yourself there, tell me all about it as if you were living through that experience again.

Pt. I remember going into the room with a girl undressed.

Dr. Who was the girl?

Pt. I don't know, she was a prostitute the first time.

Dr. Did you go with the other fellows?

Pt. Just one other fellow.

Dr. What sort of a girl is she?

Pt. She was an attractive girl.

Dr. Younger, older than you?

Pt. Older.

Dr. What happens now?

Pt. Well, we got into bed. Of course I was very nervous.

Dr. Did you have all your clothes off?

Pt. Ah, yes.

Dr. Did she?

Pt. Yes.

Dr. And then what did she do, what did you do?

Pt. Well, then we had intercourse.

Dr. What happened?

Pt. Well, I don't remember exactly the length of time before I ejaculated. I can't remember that. But I think it was very shortly.

Dr. Were you excited?

Pt. Yes.

Dr. And what happened directly afterwards? I'm interested in your thoughts, your ideas about that.

Pt. Well, I got dressed and left.   I repeated it several times after.

Dr. That first time, how did you feel about it?   Did you feel that it was or wasn't all right?

Pt. No, I felt it was all right.   Being there I just felt that the act itself wasn't right.   That is, I wasn't successful with it.   Because I remember that I was with a friend of mine, and we occupied two separate rooms.   I had gotten out so much sooner than he, and I was sitting and waiting for him in the ante room, and I felt that it was wrong to be through so much faster than he.

Dr. Were you ashamed of yourself?

Pt. Well, yes.

Dr. Did you feel that you weren't as good as he was?

Pt. That's right.

Dr. Do you feel that ejaculating prematurely makes you less of a man than other men?

Pt. Yes.

Dr. What happened after that?   Did you go back to the same girl?

Pt. Once or twice after that.

Dr. And what happened?

Pt. The same thing.

Dr. Was there any fear of this girl at all?   Or disgust with her?

Pt. No, no.

Dr. I see.   As you sit there return to your present age. (*Pause*)   It seems to me that we have a clue to what may be the basic problem here.   There are doubts about your masculinity, some doubts about your aggressiveness, some doubts about yourself in comparison to other men.   You have, for some reason, unfavorably compared yourself to other men, and that unfortunate comparison has influenced you and caused you to use a symbol wrongly.   That is, you believe that you are less of a man than other men because you ejaculate prematurely.   That is a wrong concept because basically

you are a masculine person.   It's only a misinterpretation
of facts that has caused you to perform in this way.   You
are not impotent, and you are not unmasculine.   You are a
masculine person, and you must begin to exercise aggressiveness and build up a concept of your own aggressive activity.
Your own feeling of masculinity in your relationship to others
will finally spread to the sexual sphere also.   I'm going to
give you a strong suggestion to that effect.   From the
moment you leave here, you must begin to plan little actions
that are aggressive in nature, no matter what they may be.
It may be certain things that you do in your work.   It
may be certain things that you do in relationship to other
people.   It may be in the field of hobbies or activities.
Whatever they are, before you come back next time, I want
you to have done something that demonstrates a display of
aggressiveness. Not destructive, but active and assertive aggressiveness. You understand me?

Pt.   Yes.

Dr.   It's extremely necessary that we build this thing up
to a point where you can exercise your aggressiveness, because that's completely bound up with your whole concept
of yourself and also your sexual functioning.   Do you see
that?

Pt.   Yes.

Dr.   Good.   Continue to sleep now.   In a moment I will
wake you up and talk to you again.   (*Pause*)   And now
slowly your eyes will open as I count to five.   It makes no
difference whether you remember or do not remember what
is said here, you still will feel a compulsion to abide by the
suggestions that I've given you.   One, two, three, four,
five.   Wake up. . . . How do you feel?

Pt.   All right.

Dr.   Feel relaxed?   How have you been sleeping?

Pt.   Well, I was always a good sleeper, but I think I have
been sleeping better in the past week.

Dr.   You have relaxed better?

Pt.   Yes.

Dr.   Good.   The things I have suggested to you are apt to create some tension and anxiety.   There are reasons why you have inhibited yourself.   The reason our efforts should be successful is that as a kid you were aggressive.   You were forceful and expressive and then something happened to you that blocked you.   I have an idea that it is bound up with masturbation and with fears that through masturbatory activities you had done yourself some irreparable harm.

Pt.   Yes.

Dr.   And there may have been an idea about masturbation that you should be more retiring than others because you might not be able to hold your own.

Pt.   That's right.   There was something very secretive about it to begin with.   As a result of that I was perhaps a little more retiring.

Dr.   Yes, and it is important to exercise aggressiveness. Whatever you do to express your own aggressiveness isn't so important as long as you do it.   If you experience a little tension or anxiety about it, we'll discuss it.   We'll try to overcome it so that eventually you'll be able to feel more and more expressive, aggressive, assertive, and more self confident.   You will be able to express yourself in all fields of action better, including your sexual activity.   But there again the urgency of performing must be put down.   The pleasure values are the important things here.

SIXTH SESSION (April 17)

The patient has noticed that even though he ejaculated prematurely, pleasure sensations continue to be present in his penis, and the character of the ejaculation has become spasmodic instead of flowing.   Further persuasive and re-educational suggestions are given him under hypnosis in the attempt to restore his sexual functioning.   He evidences no desire to probe more deeply into his lack of aggressiveness and other character defects.

Pt. I'm sorry I had to miss the last session, but something bad has been happening to the entire business world. Our firm is feeling the slump and I had to stay in the office. The bottom has fallen out of the market.

Dr. How about your personal problems.

Pt. In spite of myself, I feel I'm just racing against time. I mean this is something I should have undertaken a long time ago.

Dr. Well, but now look, the urgency is part of your problem.

Pt. I see.

Dr. And what have you done about it? What has occurred?

Pt. Not much of a change other than I don't feel as keenly about it as I did another time. In other words, the idea of performance and disappointment of failure, I mean, it doesn't play as big a part.

Dr. It's important not to let the challenge element of it get you.

Pt. I see.

Dr. Now, in your own observance of your sexual feelings, what has happened there?

Pt. Well, there too, I found a slight change insofar as the sex act itself is concerned. Several weeks back my primary interest was being successful in the act. Now I seem to be getting more pleasure out of it.

Dr. But still the thing that disturbs you is a sense of frustration.

Pt. Exactly.

Dr. And perhaps a hectic anxiety that this next time it's going to be successful.

Pt. I can't seem to overcome that. I try to fight it but I can't.

Dr. I will just keep bringing it to your attention over and over again, because understanding is the thing that will help you. You just can't look upon it as a challenge. Sex is not meant as a challenge.

Pt. Yes, I understand.

Dr. All right, so that you began to notice that you could get certain more pleasure out of sex?

Pt. That's right.

Dr. What precisely happens as you begin sex play now? How long after you start sex play do you insert?

Pt. I should say about ten to fifteen minutes.

Dr. Now does your wife have an orgasm?

Pt. No, but if I continue playing with her she does, as I did on one or two occasions.

Dr. Does that make you feel better?

Pt. Somewhat.

Dr. When you insert, what sensations have you noticed?

Pt. Well, the sensation is the feeling of having inserted. Prior to coming here I mean, my mind wasn't . . . I mean it was just that one thing, and I actually didn't feel any-thing, but now I get more feeling.

Dr. You get more feelings in your penis?

Pt. That's right.

Dr. Good, that's what I've been wanting you to see. That you can concentrate your attention on sensations and feel it's a pleasurable experience.

Pt. That's right.

Dr. Do you feel the orgasm when it comes?

Pt. That's right and last time for the first time it was spasmodic.

Dr. Spasmodic?

Pt. Yes, yes.

Dr. I see, it isn't a flowing?

Pt. No, no.

Dr. That's a great deal of progress.

Pt. Yes.

Dr. Now again we're going to work on the element of

considering sex a source of pleasure and less a challenge. In addition we must work on the business of expressing your assertiveness, your aggressiveness, your forcefulness in other areas. Have you had a chance, the opportunity, to work at this forcefulness of expression?

Pt. Yes, in one or two instances I found that I had been more forceful. In business I found that I'm a little more assertive, a little more forceful in some of the enterprises and dealings with problems that come up. But I don't know, it may be due to the conditions of business today. I mean this rapid change. But in general I think, due to our meetings, there is appearing a little more forcefulness. I do feel a little more that way.

Dr. Very good, and you've got to continue that because that's terribly essential, very vital. Supposing you lean back in your chair now. Would you be more comfortable if you'd lie down?

Pt. No.

Dr. Just lean back in your chair, put your hands down and this time I want to have you very rapidly begin to feel yourself sinking into a deep, restful, relaxed, comfortable sleep. And as you do your hand, your right hand, will rise and lift, lift, slowly rise, just like that, right up to your face. And when it touches your face, you'll feel drowsy and tired, and sleepy, very sleepy, and drowsy and tired. The hand keeps rising and lifting, and you get sleepier and sleepier, from your head right down to your feet. Tired and drowsy and sleepy; you go into a deep sleep. Begin to sleep now, go into a sleep.

Now, as you sit there, I'm going to stroke your arm and the arm is going to start feeling heavy, heavy just like lead. Good . . . now go to sleep deeper and I'll soon talk to you. (*Pause*)

You have developed certain habit patterns and fears that are affecting your functioning. Your functioning has been impaired in several areas, mostly in the area of aggressive action and forcefulness, and in the area of your feelings of masculinity. Very fortunately you happen to be a masculine person and your aggressiveness has not been squashed. It has merely been snowed under. It's a matter of removing the restraints and the inhibitions. Then you will go forward. If it were true that your masculinity was crushed completely, you would not be able to have an erection as frequently as you do. Therefore your problem is not like the problem of a person with impotency, because you do have erections when you make love to your wife. Something happens to you as you insert that makes you feel as if you are not masculine.

We are going to work on the two areas. We're going to work on the area of your assertiveness, your forcefulness, your ability to express activity in your relationships with people and in your attitudes toward life. And then we're going to work more specifically on your sexual impulse. We're going to work at it until you overcome it.

I am going to suggest to you that you will overcome it in spite of any doubts, in spite of any fears that may come up. You are going to overcome this problem of premature ejaculation, and you're going to be able to function in a perfectly normal manner. You may doubt it, you may have fears about it; but the doubt and fears are merely products of your own emotional chaos. They will not deter you; you will, you must overcome the problem. You can, and you will.

I'm going to ask you to visualize certain things for me, and to tell them to me as you sit there with your eyes closed and in a drowsy state. I'm going to give you certain suggestions. I want you to start dreaming. The immediate feeling may be that you can't dream. That again is merely a block, an inhibition. You can dream, and if there is nothing more than just visualizing something, visualize it and tell it to me.   As a last resort you may actually picture yourself in a theater looking up at a stage noticing actions in front of you just as if you were looking at a play.   But whatever method you utilize, it's necessary for you to dream or fantasy things so we can make progress faster.

I am going to ask you now to dream about or to visualize something that arouses you sexually, something that is intensely stimulating to you sexually.   No matter what it may be, I want you to have a sexual fantasy or a dream about something that is intensely exciting sexually for you.   No matter what it may be, have that dream or fantasy and then tell me about it without waking up. (*Pause*)

Pt.   A man and a woman walking into a hotel room, both undressing and lying on the bed.   The man starts making love to the woman.   They are both nude.   He starts with kissing her, fondling her, holding her breasts.   That excites him when he holds her breasts.

Dr.   All right, now I'm going to ask you to have another dream or fantasy, and this time it has to do with something very fearful, something frightening.   No matter whatever connection there may be, even though it's a remote one, tell me about it without waking up.

Pt.   I had a dream of walking into a room, noticing a man or woman about to leap from a window.

Dr.   Now I'm going to give you another suggestion and that has something to do with the thing that you had previously been dreaming about.   I'm going to give you the suggestion to repeat that fantasy, to visualize a man making love to a woman, fondling her breasts, becoming intensely stimulated.   Visualize the man having an erection and then going through the process of having intercourse.   Now I want you to imagine that it takes place and as you visualize or fantasy or dream it, this arm over here will slowly lift up and become stiff and rigid; and it will remain that way so long as the man in the dream has an erection.   The moment you see him losing his erection this arm will begin to loosen up, lose its rigidity and come down. I want you to fantasy that scene and be stimulated sexually. As you do notice his penis become erect, automatically and without any effort your arm will stiffen up, straight out in front of you, and will remain that way so long as the man has an erect penis. Go ahead. As soon as the penis no longer is erect the arm will drop down. (*Patient's arm stiffens and then relaxes*) Now I notice by actual time that this took a minute and five seconds. Can you describe what happened in your fantasy?

Pt. Well there was an erection, the man inserted and remained that way for that length of time.

Dr. Yes, a minute and five seconds. Now have you ever timed how long your penis remains erect in the vagina?

Pt. No, maybe a few seconds.

Dr. Gradually that period will increase, gradually it will increase and the time that you have a full erection will become longer and longer and longer. It will increase to a point where it eventually will become normal. Now the normal period is as you know between three minutes and ten minutes. I'm going to give you a suggestion that gradually you are going to feel in control because you will be able to control the erectivity of your penis. Whatever sensitivity exists will not force you to have a premature ejaculation. You will be more concerned with the pleasure you get out of sex than with the performance.

As you have sexual relations, I want you to keep in mind a picture of yourself as a forceful person engaged in some forceful act. I'm going to give you a suggestion now in which you visualize yourself as a forceful person doing something forceful no matter what that may be. I want you to visualize yourself doing something forceful no matter what that may be. I want you to visualize yourself as a forceful person doing something forceful.   As soon as you do that or dream it, tell me about it without waking up.   (*Pause*)

Pt.   I had a dream about addressing a jury on the behalf of the defendant.

Dr.   And doing a good job?

Pt.   Yes.

Dr.   Good.   I'm going to give you two suggestions. First, I want you to practice being forceful and assertive in your business, in your relations with people, because you realize this is important for you.   And, second, exercise force and assertiveness in your relationships with your wife. When you have sex next, I should like to have you observe the length of time that elapses from the time of insertion of the penis to the time that you withdraw.   This may be a little difficult at first because you will feel challenged.   The very time element is the thing that concerns you so much. So that looking at a clock may have certain panicky connotations for you.   But you will overcome those panicky feelings; perhaps you may not even think of them.   Observe the time from when you insert the penis to when you remove it.

Again I want you to feel that the pleasure function in sex is the primary concern.   As you insert your penis, observe your feelings and sensations and do not be concerned with how long it lasts.   Enjoy the act and orgasm.   As you have sex, you can then visualize yourself as a forceful person; visualize yourself in a capacity of doing something forceful even though you may have to utilize a fantasy of being a forceful person.   I want you to tell me what that fantasy is. Do not be concerned with the time even though you do want to know how long it lasts.   Again I repeat, even though you feel obligated to regard sex as a challenge, you will be less and less concerned with it as a challenge and more as a pleasure function.   Have you told your wife that you're coming to see me?

Pt.   No.

Dr. How do you feel about telling her that you're doing something about yourself?

Pt. I'd rather not.

Dr. If you would rather not, it isn't necessary to tell her unless you, yourself, decide to do so. I'm going to ask you now slowly to start waking up as I count. At the count of five begin waking up slowly, open your eyes and wake up. When you wake up, you'll have a sense of relaxation. You must follow the suggestions that I've given you. You will even though you do not think about them or force yourself to do them. They will come about more and more automatically. I'm going to count from one to five, and at the count of five open your eyes and wake up. One, two, three, four, five. (*Patient opens his eyes.*) How do you feel?

Pt. All right.

Dr. Good. Let us discuss the business of telling your wife about your treatments. Do you feel that if you told her, she might not respect you?

Pt. Well I guess that's it. Yes, I feel that if I did, I would have to more or less elaborate on the entire thing and my background and all. I don't care to do that.

Dr. You feel perhaps ashamed of it?

Pt. Somewhat, yes.

Dr. What parts of it?

Pt. Well, if I had to go into detail about the masturbatory period and the whole thing it might not look right. I mean in that case the question might arise why hadn't I told her about this sooner?

Dr. Actually it's your worry and guilt that makes it seem so terrible a situation. Because there's nothing that you've gone through that is so unusual. All people go through early experiences of which they are fearful or ashamed. Our culture makes people feel guilty about sex. If you talk to your wife, you probably would find that she also felt guilt feelings about sex when she was little. It is not necessary to tell your wife unless you feel you want to. Now how has she reacted to you in the past few times you had sex?

Pt. Same way, very lovely, very understanding.

Dr. Yes?

Pt. Optimistic and all.

Dr. Well, you must not regard her optimism as tolerance, as if she's standing by and waiting for great things to happen.

Pt. That's right.

Seventh Session (April 23)

The symptom of premature ejaculation is beginning to clear up. In addition the patient finds that he is more active and assertive in his interpersonal relationships. Another attempt is made to motivate him toward going more deeply into his personality difficulties and to swing him into a nondirective or analytic type of therapy. He continues to show resistance to this effort.

Dr. Well how have things been with you?

Pt. Well I noticed a slight improvement, a real improvement. One thing I saw was I was a little, I'm not as tense and excitable as I was, and I also found a little improvement in the time element. I think it's increased somewhat.

Dr. Have you actually timed it?

Pt. Well not that far, but mentally I've tried to recall the time, and I find there's an increase of almost half a minute to a minute.

Dr. Well that's fine.

Pt. Yes, I thought so.

Dr. That's very, very fine, but we're not satisfied with that only. It has to continue. Now altogether how much time would you say elapses in intercourse?

Pt. Well, now it's close on, I should say, it's close on to a minute and a half.

Dr. Well, that's more like it now. Now have you noticed anything about your ideas or thoughts during the process of intercourse?

Pt.   No, my thoughts are pretty much alike, the original form, that is the anxiety to be successful, but with less degree of tenseness.

Dr.   Without any great degree of urgency?

Pt.   Yes.

Dr.   Has your wife noticed any change?

Pt.   Yes she has, yes.

Dr.   What is the relationship between the two of you now.   Does she know about your coming here?

Pt.   No, she doesn't, no.

Dr.   And you're not anxious to let her know?

Pt.   No, I'd rather not unless it was absolutely urgent.

Dr.   It is not urgent.   If it is part of a problem that has to do with deep feelings toward her, we should understand it.   For instance, I treated a man who had a problem of this sort and who was afraid to let his wife know that he came here for definite psychological reasons that were more important than the premature ejaculations.   Until we clarified these reasons, his symptoms persisted.

Pt.   I see.   Well the actual reason, I suppose, is that it would presuppose that I was aware of this thing long, lon₁ before.   Perhaps I should have consulted her about it prior to asking her to marry me.   And, insofar as I did not, an impression of my neglect might arise, and I would feel at a loss for an answer.   Other than to say that I did consult a physician who said it was perfectly all right to marry, other than that, I mean, I couldn't very well explain it.

Dr.   How much does she know about how long this thing has been going on?

Pt.   Only from the day of our marriage.

Dr.   Well it's all right for her not to know anything more about it if you do not want to tell her.   It isn't a really spectacular or permanent problem; believe me when I tell you that.   The sexual difficulty is not the most significant thing compared to the overall picture.   As a matter of fact you will notice that your sexual life will improve as you get confidence in your ability to go ahead and not look upon sex as a performance, but as a source of enjoyment. If you are not too urgent about it, you'll find this thing will straighten out. Perhaps then you will want to work more on your deeper personality problems.

Pt. Well I see the change from day to day. Of course I'm still eager to have it one hundred per cent normal, because almost normal is not enough, I mean.

Dr. That eagerness is understandable, but if you can just get yourself into a frame of mind where it's not too urgent or important, it will continue to improve. There is nothing more that blocks a person's effectiveness than to feel challenged and incapable of meeting the challenge. It's like a man I knew, who illustrates how feeling challenged and comparing himself unfavorably with others destroyed his sexual capacities. He was functioning well sexually until he met a woman he believed was his ideal. He married her and after that found himself to be a little frightened and couldn't have an erection. He got very panicky and the next time he tried it, success was so important to him that he couldn't have an erection. He was in a state of terror. It turned out that his wife's approach to him was one of making demands, and instead of reassuring him she began to compare him unfavorably with her previous husband. Thereafter he couldn't function, and the more upset he became, the less the possibilities of success. His sexual problem was, like others, the result of a difficulty in relationships and self evaluation. I told him exactly the same thing that I told you: "Look, just don't get panicky, don't look upon sex as a challenge. If you can straighten out your relations with your wife, and realize that because you feel you are not as good as her first husband sexually, and if you can stop feeling challenged and have sex for pleasure, you will overcome your impotency." He, too, was able to correct his sex problem, but it was necessary later to work on why he permitted himself to be thrown by a statement of his wife. That took a longer time.   The sexual function is one of the first affected by a relationship problem.

Pt.   I see.   A friend of mine told me recently that he knew of one fellow who had suffered from the same thing and took a series of injections and said it seemed to help him.

Dr.   Some types of impotency are glandular and the treatment is injection with testosterone.

Pt.   I see.

Dr.   But your type of problem is psychological, not physical.   Testosterone would contribute little.   If I thought it would be helpful, you'd get it.

Pt.   Yes.

Dr.   What is necessary is building up your own confidence in yourself, of not being too much concerned with whether you succeed or fail.   What about your activity in other areas —your aggressiveness, your outspokenness, your forcefulness?

Pt.   Well, too, I found that it improved since last week, since the several times we spoke about it.   There, too, as I think I said before, I don't know whether it's the condition that brings it about, or because the business picture has changed so completely that out of necessity I may find that I'm a little more aggressive.

Dr.   Whatever the cause, it doesn't matter so long as you go ahead.

Pt.   Well, I do find I'm a little more assertive.   There's no question about it.

Dr.   Fine.   Did you have any dreams since I saw you last?

Pt.   Yes, I did some, but they've been so vague that the next day I tried to recall them and couldn't very well.

Dr.   You can't remember any of them?

Pt.   No, but there have been some.

Dr. The important thing now is to go along in the same direction of putting yourself in a position where you are outspoken and effective in what you do.

Pt. Yes.

Dr. If anything happens to your business in the impending recession, how do you believe you will react?

Pt. Well that's not affecting me as far as my condition is concerned. This is so much more important to me. I mean we've been through good times and bad times. It's a cycle and I'm accustomed to it. It's not having too great an effect on me. This thing is really paramount.

Dr. It is paramount, but you're beginning to see your way clear. You're improving because you actually have gotten hold of some of the causes now. You can see that it's on the basis of your own undervaluation of yourself, the challenge to your masculinity. Once you overcome this, there isn't any real reason why you just can't barge ahead, go forward. We have spoken about the origins of this thing and how far back it goes. A person carries over with him in his present day functioning, attitudes and feelings that started when he was very little. And unconsciously without even knowing it, these become a pattern that dominates the person's life. It's necessary to challenge that pattern. Ask yourself if you still are functioning like a little boy functioning under the aegis of a mother who is directing you, and a father who is supervising or condemning you. It's necessary to take stock of yourself.

Pt. That's right.

Dr. You're grown up now and life is an entirely different proposition than when you were little. It may be important to inquire psychologically into yourself, to see the disparity between what you were and what you are. You're not living in the past now. I think that if your relations with your wife become perfectly all right to you, you may be happier than you've ever been in all your life. But you'll continue to be happier if you get to the source of your trouble.   That will require more treatment and a different approach, more or less analytic.

Pt.   Certainly I'm very much happier now than I was a month ago, not through any difference or attitude on my wife's part.   It's just that I have more confidence now that this thing will work out, where a month ago I was very scared, very panicky.   Today I am not.   Of course a great deal of that is due to her very lovingness and considerateness.   I mean, she seems to make very light of it.   She has all the patience in the world, and she is very confident that in time this will wear off and everything will be fine.   She's very happy under the conditions as they are today, so naturally if everything gets well, so much the better.

Dr.   You feel she's happy with you now?

Pt.   Well that gets me to thinking sometimes.   Is it so, or is she trying to ease my mind and just trying to be nice? Because after all a woman does have to be satisfied, she gets aroused from time to time, and that's all there is to it.

Dr.   It is true that woman needs sexual gratification, but the very fact that you love her and she feels loved, and makes a physical contact in being in your arms, can be gratifying, appeasing and satisfying.

Pt.   That's what she says.

Dr.   To repeat, the sexual act to you should not be associated with running a hundred yard dash in nine seconds flat.   It should rather be an experience that is an act of pleasure.   And you find that you can do that right now?

Pt.   Yes, I do.

Dr.   You notice a change in your sexual responses?

Pt.   That's right.

Dr.   All right, supposing you lean back and go to sleep. Watch your hand, keep gazing at it; you'll notice that it will slowly get light, will rise and lift straight up in the air. As it approaches your face, you'll get drowsier and drowsier, and your eyes will get heavier and heavier until they go to sleep, until they shut. And as the hand rises, a sense of sleepiness will creep over you from your head down to your feet, and you will go into a deep, restful, relaxed, comfortable sleep. Your hand rises, goes up, up, straight up, up towards your face, and you get drowsier and drowsier. Now lean your head against your hand and rest and sleep for about a few minutes, and at the end of that time I'm going to talk to you again, and you'll be still more deeply asleep. (*Pause*)

Both in your work here with me while you are asleep, and in your actions outside, you will develop a certain sense of mastery, of confidence and assertiveness such as you probably have never known before. This will lead to an entirely different attitude towards yourself and towards your functions, including your sexual functions.

You have gone through experiences with me that have demonstrated to you the power of your own will and the effect that thinking and conceptualizing through suggestion has upon your physical functions. I'm going to ask you now to visualize that same scene where you feel sexually aroused, where you visualize something that stimulates you sexually. As you do, your left arm will gradually rise and become stiff, so stiff that it will be impossible for you to move it. It will become so stiff and rigid, it will be impossible for you to budge it. Now visualize a scene that is sexually arousing, stimulating, and as soon as you do, your arm will become so stiff and rigid that it will be impossible for you to budge it. Your arm is outstretched in front of you now; it's rigid and it's firm and stiff and it's going to remain that way until I give you the command to bring it down. . . .

Now slowly the arm comes down, right down to the th'gh, and you're going to be able to feel in better control of your own functions including your sexual functions. You'll notice that your assertiveness will increase within yourself, but in addition you will have a desire to inquire more deeply into your problems, so that you can improve most successfully.   You will find that the sexual act is not one in which you feel challenged, but one in which you can get pleasure. Your erection will get more vigorous and will remain with you, and the length of time it persists will continue to improve.

You will notice that the sex act will last longer and longer as you get confidence in yourself.   This does not necessarily mean that you have to be consistent in the upswing. Perhaps you will be, but there may be times when, for certain emotional reasons, there may be a temporary slipback. That means nothing, and I want you to be in a position where you pay no attention to having an ejaculation prematurely. Do not get panicky about it because next time it will probably be better.   Look upon sex less and less as a challenge, and more and more as a source of pleasure, and you will find that you do well, and will be able to have normal, good, sexual relations.

Even more important is that you reorient yourself in your attitudes towards people, towards yourself and towards life and that you feel that you can be capable of an aggressive, demonstrative stand in the world.   The latter will probably require deeper therapy.

Now I'm going to ask you to repeat for me that scene in which you go into a theater, sit down, look up at the stage and notice that the curtain opens and you see action on the stage.   You see something on the stage.   Whatever it is, I want you to visualize it vividly, and as soon as you do, raise your left hand which will indicate to me that you've seen the scene on the stage.   (*Patient raises his hand.*)   Now bring your hand down and tell me what you saw on the stage.

Pt.   There's a courtroom scene with a judge and an attorney addressing a jury.

Dr.   On any particular issue?   Or is he just addressing the jury?

Pt.   Well he's addressing the jury in defense of a murder defendant.

Dr. I see. Continue to sleep, continue to sleep, continue to sleep. Breathe in deeply now, very deeply. I'm going to ask you to visualize another thing with me. Visualize yourself walking along the street with me. We enter a church yard and we notice, right in front of us, a tall church steeple. You look at the church steeple, and you notice that there is a bell, and you notice the bell moving. As soon as you get the impression of the bell moving, you hear the bell clanging or get an impression of it clanging. Indicate this by your hand rising up just about an inch. (*Patient's hand rises.*) Good, now bring your hand down.

As you sit there again, I'm going to reinforce the suggestions that I've given you. Basically you are a fairly well integrated person, you can function fairly effectively as you are, but you must not be satisfied with the way you're functioning because you have the potentiality and the capacity to do better, to do more for yourself. You are not taking advantage of your own abilities and capacities, you are not doing what you're capable of doing yet, but you're getting there. You're seeing more and more clearly that you've been stymied, that as a result of what has happened to you before, you have restricted yourself and your capacities. You are going to be able, as you sit there, to envisage a life for yourself of far greater possibilities.

One of the most important steps that you took was to get married. It showed that you were not satisfied to live a celibate life, a life in which you would operate as if you were damaged. I don't know how you got the misconception about masturbation, but it really did not injure you physically. You have done nothing, absolutely nothing, of which you need be ashamed. Some children get the idea that when they do something that's pleasurable, of which the parents perhaps do not approve, that it's tantamount to being a murderer. You are not an evil person and never were. But you yielded too much to the forces of conscience, you yielded too much to the demands you imagined society imposed on you. Those were misconceptions. Fortunately you were able to correct those misconceptions before you got too old, before you could not enjoy yourself. It's up to you now to go forward further, to live a much more happy and integrated life than you've ever lived before. You're making steps in that direction and you must continue to make steps. You're going to be happier and happier as days go by, and you will improve in every area including the sexual area.

I want you to sit there for a few minutes and then I'll wake you up. (*Pause*) Now as you sit there, I'm slowly going to ask you to begin awakening. First, I'm going to count from one to five, and at the count of five, you'll slowly open your eyes and then wake up. One, two, three, four, five. Slowly open your eyes. (*Patient opens his eyes.*) We've gone through what I think is the fundamental basis of this symptom of yours, what caused it and how it affects you now, don't you think so?

Pt. Yes, I do.

Dr. So that now it's a matter of going deeper to understand how your personality problems started and how they affect you now. You'll notice that there may be tendencies for you to feel discouraged, for you to feel that you are going backward. But this will be temporary and you'll be able to snap out of it.

Pt. I did feel hopeless about it, but I don't now.

Dr. Good.

Eighth Session (May 6)

The patient missed several sessions ostensibly because of business emergencies. Actually as he began to function well sexually, he saw no further reason for continuing, since his motivation for therapy was merely the desire to have successful sexual relations. Resistance apparently was created by suggestions to probe deeper into his problems, which probing he undoubtedly regarded as a threat to his character defenses. He reports a definite improvement in his sexual life, his premature ejaculations no longer interfering with successful intercourse.

Dr. It's been a long time since I saw you.

Pt. Yes.

Dr. How are things?

Pt. Very nice.

Dr. I see.

Pt. Progressing very nicely. It's just been about a week that improvement is really marked. There's been a complete change in the time element.

Dr. How long do you go in intercourse?

Pt. Well last time I went very long. About a week ago, for the first time in intercourse, I found that the time element was extended to a considerable degree. By that I mean, it was at least three minutes. But as elated as I was over that experience, it turned out to be an unfortunate one in this respect. I imagine prior to that my wife probably wasn't sufficiently aroused to make any particular difference as to the length of time, but in this case, having lasted that length of time, she naturally was aroused to a pitch where she was almost ready for an orgasm, and I couldn't stay with her and she was quite upset about it. Of course the next day everything had been forgotten and it was all over. But it had somewhat of an effect on me. As I say, ordinarily I would have been very elated over the fact that the time was extended to what it was, but having let her down that way had an effect on me. So much so that the next night I just wasn't good for anything. I got an erection and I lost it, and I got it back again. It was a question of a minute and it was all gone. And then after that it came back again better than before, and has been going that way for over a week now. Say about five days I have had a normal erection and a normal insertion. I find that without any difficulty it will last a good number of minutes. And that idea is just naturally leaving me as I go along, the idea that it's just a performance. The confidence is instilled, I mean I feel in other words today that now there is no reason that I

have to prove myself. I do not see how I can improve
further.

Dr. It's just a matter of deciding how far you want to
go. You have shown a symptomatic improvement.

Pt. Great thing, to me a tremendous thing.

Dr. You're not taking too seriously your wife's being
disconcerted last week?

Pt. Fortunately I married the type of girl she is. She's
very sweet, she's very lovely. As I say it was just mo-
mentary, not that she said anything, but that feeling natu-
ally had to be there. Of course the next day it was as
though nothing had happened, which in itself made it a
little easier for me. Yes, she's had orgasms since then. Of
course, she, too, feels the same way. I mean at that first
experience, she probably didn't realize at the moment that
the fact that I did improve to such an extent—all she could
feel at that time was the feeling that . . . but I suppose today
she realizes that step by step she's going to lead a normal
life.

Dr. It's just a matter of time.

Pt. That's right.

Dr. You are functioning fairly well now?

Pt. That's right. Well, I feel today that if I can possibly
extend that another minute or two at the most, it will be
fine, nothing to worry about.

Dr. Well, there's no reason why you can't. But again
you must be warned about the business that there may be
setbacks. Have courage to go forward. It's discouraging
to be set back for a little while, but it's nothing permanent.

Pt. Well, I'm very happy over the results I've enjoyed
so far.

Dr. How about your own personal life?

Pt. Well, I don't know that it has been changing just as
you stated. I mean I think I am a little more assertive, but
I don't, ah, by that I mean, I really feel so good over this

prospect, that I know at least that there's a chance that I will be all right. It's been proven that I have improved. I feel it. I know it's there. It's not my imagination, so naturally that in itself has given me a different feeling.

Dr. I see, how do you feel about coming back here? Do you feel that you have the understanding, and that you've got the drop on this thing so that you can proceed on your own? How do you feel?

Pt. I don't know.

Dr. Well you can continue coming here and we can work more intensively at personality problems toward more assertiveness.

Pt. I suppose so.

Dr. But you have overcome one hurdle.

Pt. I see.

Dr. Just the feeling of self confidence about this thing. . . .

Pt. That's sufficient.

Dr. That's sufficient?

Pt. In time you feel that it will improve as I go along?

Dr. It should.

Pt. Say, I think it's almost, I would say almost normal today. Now if I can only extend that a little then it would be normal.

Dr. We can continue until you feel that you've gone as far as you like in the sexual or any other area.

Pt. Yes.

Dr. And you seem to feel that you've gotten as much out of coming here as you can. Now in your contacts with people have you noticed any change?

Pt. Yes, I am a little more assertive, a little more forceful in small ways perhaps, but nevertheless it's sufficient so that I can detect a little change. With that, too, I am sure that it's due to the realization, I mean I think it is the, ah, due to our talks that I'm beginning to see that and act accordingly.

(At this point I decide to show the patient the Rorschach cards to see if any structural changes have occurred.)

Dr.   I'm going to show you these cards again and I want you to tell me what you see again.   This is the first card.

Pt.   I see an eagle, the shape of an eagle.

Dr.   The whole thing?

Pt.   Yes.

Dr.   This is the second.

Pt.   I see a pair of little dogs.   Their paws meeting. That's all.

Dr.   This is the third.

Pt.   Poodle dogs with their paws meeting.   I can't seem to determine the position though.

Dr.   Turn it any way you wish.

Pt.   They seem to be standing on their hind legs.

Dr.   Who?

Pt.   These, the dogs.   No more.

Dr.   Dogs standing on their hind legs.   Where do you see the dogs?   Oh, yes.   This is the fourth.

Pt.   I can't determine it.   The two animals running down the trunk of a tree?   Maybe squirrels.

Dr.   Where do you see the two animals?   Oh, inside.

Pt.   In there, yes down the trunk of the tree.

Dr.   Down the trunk of the tree.   Go ahead.   This is the fifth one here.

Pt.   Looks like an animal.   It seems to me like the shape or a sea gull or bat.

Dr.   This is the sixth.

Pt.   Fur pelt.   A staff on top.   That's all.

Dr.   This is the seventh.

Pt.   The top of this are some mythological figures of some kind on a wall.

Dr.   This is the eighth.

Pt.   Two animals perched on some mountain.   A pair of lions.   Don't seem to see more.

Dr.   All right, and that's the ninth one, there.

Pt. This way there might be two buffaloes.

Dr. Those green ones?

Pt. Yes. I can't see anything else.

Dr. That's the last one.

Pt. It's a group of squirrels in trees, crabs, sea food.

(*It will be seen that there is a slight, but no remarkable change in his responses.*)

Dr. Fine. Now draw a picture of a man and a woman. (*There was practically no change in the crude drawings of the heads of a man and a woman as compared to the original drawings.*) As I explained to you once before, it is not merely the problem of your premature ejaculation, but rather that the premature ejaculation was the product of a lot of other things. Consequently you can benefit from treatments not only in terms of sexuality, but in the way you react towards other people and towards life in general. You have noticed a change in yourself other than sexual improvement.

Pt. Yes, definitely.

Dr. A stronger feeling about yourself.

Pt. That's right.

Dr. Good. How's the business?

Pt. Terrible.

Dr. So that is not the reason for your improvement.

Pt. No, no.

Dr. Fine. Now I'd like to have you sit back and go to sleep.

Pt. Yes, of course.

Dr. Put your hands down on your thighs, watch your fingers and begin to feel a sensation of lightness and drowsiness. (*Patient closes his eyes and sleeps.*) Now as you sit there I'm going to repeat to you what I've said before, and you will be able to integrate and absorb what I have to say to you and to utilize it in a constructive way for yourself.

The entire problem of your capacity to function in a sexual

relationship, seems partially to have been produced by a misconception about the damage that you presumably did to yourself through masturbation. Actually no physical hurt was done; but much psychological damage. It's fear that is your enemy and nothing else. The fact that you continued to masturbate against your judgment made you feel like a hypocrite. This had a damaging effect upon your aggressiveness and activity.

Why you reacted the way you did depended on the kind of parents and upbringing you had. The fact that you had to be good in order to feel secure and loved to some extent hampered your activity, and froze your feelings in spite of yourself. You felt no right to be expressive or aggressive. But it hasn't really hurt you.

Fortunately your upbringing impaired but did not destroy you. That's the important thing, it has not hurt you permanently. You have the seeds of everything it takes to function. You've been able to proceed to marriage; you are in love with your wife; you are able to derive pleasure out of sex. And your capacity to feel pleasure out of sex will increase. Again you must not look upon it as a marathon; you must regard it as a casual experience in which you can derive pleasure. Sex should not be used to prove that you're a man or that you're not a man. It must not be utilized for that purpose. Use sex as a source of pleasure for yourself. The urgency of performing perfectly will then vanish. You have noticed that as you've been less and less concerned with the urgency to have an erection for a long time, that you've succeeded better and better. You will continue to succeed better and better. Your sense of confidence will return and you will feel stronger and more capable, not only in terms of sexuality, but in terms of a capacity to take a stand in life, to engage in aggressive, productive activities.

As you sit here now, I am going to give you a strong suggestion that the gains you've shown up to this time will continue. Even if there are slip-backs, you must not be upset. The less concern you show, the better you will be able to function. Again I am going to repeat that when you engage in sexual relations, do it from the standpoint of pleasure and not from the standpoint of having to perform. A misconception may still be residual in you that there's something fundamentally wrong with your sexual organs. There is nothing fundamentally wrong with your sexual organs. It is your attitude that has been twisted by unfortunate early experiences. Your attitude will change, and you will get better and stronger. Perhaps you will decide to go deeper into your problems.

I am going to count now from one to five. At the count of five, open your eyes and wake up. One, two, three, four, five. (*Patient awakens.*) How do you feel?

Pt. Fine.

Dr. Now supposing we discuss your coming back for further treatments. How do you feel about this?

Pt. Maybe on the basis of once in two weeks we could accomplish something.

Dr. Would that be better for you?

Pt. Yes, it would be better because it's very difficult for me to get away.

Dr. At this particular period?

Pt. At this particular period, the business crisis and all.

Dr. All right, we can then continue on this basis. We could make it two weeks from today or sooner if you telephone.

Pt. Fine.

> (*This was the last session. Telephone messages from the patient indicated a consistent improvement. He was certain that he had conquered his sexual problem and that he was functioning in a normal manner. Because of this, and because he had no desire to probe deeper into his personality problem, he stopped treatments indicating that he might return at a later date.*)

REFERENCES

[1]PAYOT, J.: The Education of the Will. New York, Funk & Wagnalls, 1909.

[2]BARRETT, E. B.: Strength of Will. New York, P. J. Kennedy, 1915.

[3]——: The New Psychology. New York, P. J. Kennedy, 1925.

[4]VITOZ, R.: Treatment of Neurasthenia by Means of Brain Control (Translated by H. B. Brooks). London, Longmans, Green, 1913.

[5]EYMIEW, A.: Le Gouvernement de Soi-Même. Paris, Perrin, 1922.

[6]WALSH, J. J.: Psychotherapy. New York, Appleton Century, 1913.

[7]——: Health through Will Power. Boston, Stratford, 1931.

[8]DUBOIS, P.: The Psychic Treatment of Mental Disorders. New York, Funk & Wagnalls, 1909.

[9]——: Education of Self. New York, Funk & Wagnalls, 1911.

[10]DEJERINE, J. AND GAUKLER, E.: Psychoneurosis and Psychotherapy. Philadelphia, Lippincott, 1913.

[11]RIGGS, A. F.: Just Nerves. New York, Doubleday & Doran, 1922.

[12]——: Intelligent Living. New York, Doubleday & Doran, 1929.

[13]OSLER, W.: A Way of Life. Baltimore, Norman Remington, 1932.

[14]RIGGS, A. F.: op. cit., reference 11.

[15]STRECKER, E. A. AND APPEL, K. E.: Discovering Ourselves. New York, Macmillan, 1931.

[16]SAYLES, M. B.: The Problem Child at Home. New York, Commonwealth Fund, 1928.

[17]THOM, D. A.: Normal Youth and Its Everyday Problems. New York, Appleton Century, 1932.

[18]WILLIAMS, F. E.: Adolescence—Studies in Mental Hygiene. New York, Farrar & Rinehart, 1930.

[19]LEVY, J., AND MUNROE, R.: The Happy Family. New York, Knopf, 1938.

[20]HORNEY, K.: The Neurotic Personality of Our Time. New York, W. W. Norton, 1937.

[21]ROBINSON, J. H.: The Mind in the Making. New York, Harper, 1921.

[22]EDMAN, I.: The Candle in the Dark. New York, Viking Press, 1939.

[23]TWYEFFORT, L. H.: Therapy in psycho-neuroses (bibliotherapy). In PIERSOL, G. M., AND BORTZ, E. L.: The Encyclopedia of Medicine, Surgery and Specialties. Philadelphia, F. A. Davis, 1940.

[24]BRADLEY, C., AND BOSQUET, S.: The use of books for psychotherapy with children. Am. J. Orthopsychiat. 6: 23, 1936.

[25]MUDD, E. H., AND WHITEHILL, J. L.: The use and misuse of books in counselling. Parent Educ. 14, Nos. 2, 3, 1938.

[26]APPEL, K. E.: Psychiatric Therapy in Personality and the Behavior Disorders. Vol. 11 (Ed. by J. McHunt). New York, Ronald Press, 1944.

[27]WOLBERG, L. R.: Goals and objectives in psychotherapy. New York State J. Med. 44: 1792–1796, 1944.

[28]JONES, M. C.: The case of Peter. Ped. Sem.: 31: 308–318, 1924.

[29]YATES, D. H.: An association set method in psychotherapy. Psychol. Bull. 36: 506, 1939.

[30]Max, L. M.: Conditioned reaction technique; a case study. Psychol. Bull. *32:* 734, 1935.

[31]Mowrer, O. H., and Mowrer, W. M.: Enuresis—A method for its study and treatment. Am. J. Orthopsychiat. *8:* 436–457, 1938.

[32]Leuba, C.: The use of hypnosis for controlling variables in psychological experiments. J. Abnor. & Soc. Psychol. *36:* 271–274, 1941.

[33]Platanow, K. I.: The word as a physiological and therapeutic factor. Psikhoterapiya *11:* 122, 1930.

Part Three

HYPNOSIS IN PSYCHOANALYTIC THERAPY (HYPNOANALYSIS)

PALLIATIVE psychotherapy reinforced by hypnosis may be eminently successful in certain cases. It may provide a patient with methods by which he can improve his relationships with people. It may teach him how to pattern his life around his weaknesses, expanding his latent talents and aptitudes. It may desensitize him to stress, and aid him in achieving a more peaceful and productive life.

In many patients the basic personality structure is not too abnormal and has permitted the individual to function efficiently up to the time of the current upheaval. In such cases the goal in therapy need not be too extensive. The aim is to restore the habitual personality patterns that existed prior to the breakdown. Often all the patient requires is simple advice regarding a situation in which he is so subjectively involved that he is unable "to see the forest because of the trees." An objective point of view given by an unbiased authority can suddenly clarify the issues and enable the person to face his problem in a mature manner. Where the ego structure is relatively intact, one may rightfully feel that the chances of readjustment to the customary life pattern are good with relatively short treatment, employing such technics as ventilation, reassurance, guidance, persuasion and desensitization.

Palliative psychotherapy is also indicated in persons with more profound personality disorders who are either unable or unwilling to undergo more extensive therapy. It is useful in psychotic conditions, prepsychotic states and in individuals whose personality structure is so weak that they are unable to tolerate the anxiety and stress associated with analytic treatment. The aim here is to enhance personality assets to a point where they overcome the liabilities, and to help the patient arrange his life so that his emotional problems will neither handicap nor hurt him.

Yet in a considerable number of cases, palliative psychotherapy may fail to make a significant impression on the individual. There are many persons who seem incapable of adjusting themselves to their weaknesses, who cannot be desensitized to fearful situations no matter how judiciously the appropriate technics are applied, who get themselves into the same difficulties with people despite adroit guidance and environmental manipulation, who gain neither security nor self esteem, in the face of the most persistent and conscientious efforts on the part of the physician.

In such cases the personality problem is usually severe, the individual possessing so many contradictory character strivings that he is at the mercy of a never-ending psychic tug-of-war. He may, for instance, have inordinate expectations of himself, and possess perfectionistic impulses so pronounced that whenever he performs in any way below these expectations, he responds with panic. An investigation of his aptitudes may disclose that they fall far below his desired goals. His turmoil seems to be due to the disparity between his perfectionism and his performance abilities. As part of the therapeutic process, he may be advised to scale down his ambitions in order that he may attain success. It may then develop that success, in line with the more mediocre goals, is as devastating as complete failure—perhaps more so. Failure may actually be the lesser of two evils.

Discussion and ventilation may disclose inimical situations in the environment that call for immediate correction. Instead of making the patient more comfortable, this effort serves merely to plunge him into panic. The person may actually feel more comfortable in an environment that provides him with some objective excuse for his inner distress and permits him to rationalize his discomforts and to project his rage. Guidance and advice, may, in some cases, serve less to direct the patient toward a freer expression of his needs, than to precipitate an inner paralysis and a confounding helplessness that robs him of vitality and self-sufficiency. It may even provoke an anxiety reaction, the patient insisting that his independence is being taken from him. Attempts to externalize the individual and to divert his energies into social and recreational channels may strike a stubborn snag; the patient persisting in his detached, inhibited way of life.

No matter how thoroughly one tries to train some patients, they will be unable to master their symptoms. They may temporarily learn to conquer phobias, compulsions, and anxiety states by such technics and evasions as the recitation of certain formulas, the enactment of pseudoscientific rituals, the forceful substitution of joyous for painful thoughts, or the adoption of a spurious optimism. These devices may serve to keep them more comfortable for a short while. However, their symptoms will continue to weigh inexorably upon them, necessitating more and more vigorous neutralizing technics. Interpersonal relationships will remain disturbed, and attitudes toward the self will be distorted and contemptuous.

The reason palliative psychotherapy is so frequently unsuccessful is that the most important determinants of behavior are of unconscious origin. As a result of past inimical experiences and conditionings, the neurotic person harbors within himself impulses, attitudes, and emotions which are repressed because they conflict with accepted standards as embodied in the conscience. Although repressed, these attitudes and impulses constantly filter into the conscious life in a disguised form, influencing the person's feelings, values, and behavior.   To his consternation, the individual may be motivated to react in a way diametrically opposed to his rational self.

So long as destructive, unconscious motivations persist, maladaptive behavior will plague the person, will power and good resolutions to the contrary.   Assertiveness, activity, and creative self fulfillment will be impeded, preventing the ego from attaining proper strength and stature.   Fears of the world and of people will continue, conditioning compulsive strivings for dependency, submissiveness, affection, power, superiority, perfectionism and detachment, which will further complicate the person's relationship to others. The sole hope of bringing the person's destructive patterns to a halt lies in determining and enucleating their source. This is the primary aim of psychoanalysis.

In psychoanalysis the ultimate objective is to bring about a change in the ego which, up to this time, has been so involved in maintaining its defenses against anxiety that it is unable to mediate the legitimate psychobiologic needs of the person.   Wedged in between unconscious impulses, whose acknowledgment is dangerous or repulsive, and an overwhelming conscience, that supervises the person's actions with relentless vigilance and tyranny, the ego has elaborated a system of barriers and evasions to protect itself from hurt. The elaborated defenses, however, although calculated to protect the ego from anxiety, often prove to be a tremendous handicap to the individual, especially by interfering with normal relationships with people. Psychoanalysis strives to persuade the ego to give up its defenses against unconscious conflicts, or to modify its defenses to conform better with reality.   The eventual hope is that the ego will become more tolerant of the needs of the person, and more capable of entering into gratifying relationships with other human beings.

The medium in which ego change occurs is the inter-personal relationship with the analyst. This relationship is a two-edged sword, for, on the one hand, it precipitates destructive irrational transference feelings, and, on the other, it is the nucleus around which the person reintegrates his attitudes toward people and toward the world. The analyst becomes a living symbol onto whom the patient projects his fears, hopes and demands as well as his deepest strivings and impulses. The relationship with the analyst is surcharged with emotion as irrational attitudes and feelings precipitate out. The experiencing of such feelings, and the under-standing by the patient that they are the product, not of present day reality, but of previous conditionings acts as a fulcrum for insight. The tolerant attitude of the analyst eventually undermines the hypertrophied conscience and per-mits the individual to investigate repressed drives and memo-ries he could not acknowledge previously. Freed from the tyranny of his conscience, and from the threat of being overwhelmed by repressed fears and conflicts, the ego is strengthened to proportions where it no longer requires neurotic defenses and subterfuges in order to function. It can then attend to the legitimate demands of the individual, and can seek out in the environment the appropriate means of fulfilling basic biologic and social needs.

The therapeutic process, however, is constantly jeopardized by resistances which the patient mobilizes in his attempt to sabotage his progress. He comes to regard the analysis as a threat to the canalized system of defenses which constitute for him the sole means of bolstering his security and self esteem. The analyst becomes a foe, against whom he pits himself with facades and subterfuges to keep his system of values intact. The struggle which ensues between the pa-tient, who seeks to retain his compulsive neurotic trends, and the analyst, who strives to motivate him toward more mature reaction patterns, is intense and prolonged. As a consequence, psychoanalysis is apt to require many months, and in some cases years, of persistent work.

The time element is perhaps the chief drawback of psychoanalysis. Therapy is also extremely expensive, and the number of patients the psychiatrist can handle is restricted. Many persons who could derive benefits from psychoanalytic therapy are consequently unable to avail themselves of treatment.

In recent years a number of attempts have been made to cut down the time that is required for psychoanalysis. Brief psychotherapeutic methods have been evolved which employ the basic psychoanalytic principles. The question that may be rightfully raised is whether the dynamic psychic changes which are brought about by psychoanalysis can be accomplished by briefer psychotherapeutic methods.

In psychoanalysis we may distinguish two processes which go on side by side. The first is involved with "uncovering" those unconscious motivational patterns which determine the individual's values and behavior. The second phase of therapy is associated with reconditioning and re-education, and concerns the substitution of mature habit patterns for neurotic infantile ones. Because the ego is menaced by the unconscious material, and responds with resistance to the anxiety aroused by an awareness of unconscious trends, the uncovering process may extend over a long period of time. Resistances are manifested toward any influence that stimulates awareness of unconscious fears and conflicts. This is why the transference is so painful to the patient when it begins to precipitate out latent attitudes and feelings. Resistances will consequently be displayed toward the analyst in the attempt to ward him off or to discredit him. There will be efforts made to maintain control and bolster up the waning, repressive defenses.

An awareness of unconscious impulses and trends in itself does not guarantee recovery, since neurotic defenses and symptoms may possess values which dwarf normal psycho-biologic goals. The patient may be unwilling to relinquish the secondary gain in his neurosis even though he has insight into his illness. A long re-educational period may be necessary before the patient is willing to exchange his compulsive patterns for the happiness and security of normal interpersonal relationships.

Work by Erickson,[1-4] Erickson and Hill,[5] Erickson and Kubie,[6, 7] Eisenbud,[8] Kubie,[9] Lindner,[10] Gill and Brenman,[11] Fisher,[12] and Wolberg,[13] has indicated that hypnosis lends itself to a facilitation of the psychoanalytic process. A most important effect of hypnosis is its power to remove those resistances that prevent awareness of unconscious material. Whereas months may be consumed in attempting to remove such resistances during psychoanalysis, hypnosis is often able to achieve an almost surgical removal of barriers to the conscious appreciation of repressed elements of the personality.

A number of objections may be voiced against hypnosis as an aid to psychoanalysis. The first objection has to do with the matter of hypnotizability. Hypnoanalysis requires a deep and preferably somnambulistic trance. Not all patients can achieve somnambulism. This was the chief reason why Freud many years ago abandoned hypnosis as an avenue to the unconscious. The second objection involves the validity of the material brought up during hypnoanalysis. As is well known, a characteristic feature of hypnosis is the motivation to comply with the demands of the hypnotist. When the patient senses that he is expected to bring up things, he is apt to invent material in order to please the hypnotist. The third objection concerns the effect of hypnosis on the transference. One may suspect that hypnosis introduces a foreign element into the analysis which may interfere with the therapeutic aim. The last objection deals with the possible obliterating effect of posthypnotic amnesia on the hypnotic experiences.

The first objection, of hypnotizability, is an important one. Although most patients are probably hypnotizable, not all are capable of achieving a somnambulistic state. This puts definite limitations on the use of hypnosis in psychoanalysis. However, with an improved technic the number of somnambules may be materially increased. A slow systematic induction and the removal of resistances as they arise may produce desired results. Narcotic drugs also may be utilized as an adjunct for increasing hypnotic depth, posthypnotic suggestions being given the patient to the effect that he will be susceptible to ordinary hypnotic suggestions later on. Fortunately not all hypnoanalytic procedures require a somnambulistic trance. Free association during hypnagogic reverie is possible during a light trance. Dream induction and automatic writing can often be accomplished in a medium trance.

Replying to the second objection, it is, of course, possible that the patient may falsify material on the basis of complying with what is expected of him. One way of dealing with this problem is to get the patient to understand that the material he brings up is subject to his own evaluation, and that he can accept or reject it in accordance with whether he feels it to be true or false. During the final stages of hypnoanalysis, the dissolution of the last vestiges of the patient's dependency may have an important effect upon validating the material he has brought up.

The third objection, that of the possible obliterating influence of posthypnotic amnesia, may be answered by the simple statement that the amnesia, if it exists, is an artifact. The learning process, which a number of observers believe is accelerated during hypnosis, is not subject to annihilation on the resumption of waking life. This may be proven experimentally by establishing a conditioned hand withdrawal to a buzzer during the trance state and noting that hand withdrawal persists in the waking state in spite of amnesia for the experiment. Hypnotic experiences carry over into the waking state in a similar manner.

By far the strongest objection to hypnosis is its possible deleterious effect on the transference. In psychoanalysis the analyst assumes a passive role in order that the patient may project toward him various inner impulses and strivings which have no basis in reality. Rooted as it is in faith, hypnosis would seem to limit the patient's feelings and attitudes to those associated with the phenomenon of hypnotizability, namely, to dependency on the omnipotent hypnotist, to masochistic submissiveness, or to a desire to identify with the hypnotist thereby achieving magical power.

This objection is invalid because the patient always reacts to the hypnotist, not only with dependency and masochistic submissiveness, but with the full range of his inner wishes, demands, fears, and impulses which are the product of his character structure. When one analyzes the patient's free associations and dreams, one is convinced that the hypnotic situation does not eliminate spontaneous feelings or emotions which develop in a manner similar to their development during psychoanalysis. As a matter of fact, hypnosis catalyzes such feelings. However, in the traditional hypnotic induction, and where hypnosis is used as an adjunct to palliative psychotherapy, the patient is motivated to repress feelings as they develop in order to win bounties which he believes will accrue from the assumption of a passive state. In some forms of hypnoanalysis, an important innovation consists of the analysis of the patient's transference attitudes and feelings as they develop before he has had a chance to repress them.

During the orthodox employment of hypnosis, the subject maintains an inert role. This is unlike psychoanalysis in which the patient is expected to be active and assume the responsibility for much of the analytic work. As is well known, the activity of the patient is an aid to self growth. Hypnosis would presumably eliminate activity. The answer to this objection is that in hypnoanalysis the patient is not expected to be passive. Indeed, activity is encouraged during the hypnoanalytic procedures, and intellectual, emotional and motor functions are all vigorously enhanced. The patient engages in verbalization, dramatization, play therapy, writing and drawing without the inhibitions that exist in the waking state. This innovation in therapy has an important effect in opening up motor pathways which have, up to this time, been blocked to unconscious feelings and attitudes. It eliminates the intellectualization of the analytic process. Hypnoanalysis thus tends to stimulate expressiveness and assertiveness.

The dissolution of the hypnotic transference would seem difficult at first glance, since one would assume that the patient may, during hypnosis, render himself so dependent upon the analyst that he develops a need for prolonged guidance. Under the circumstances, we would expect that once hypnotic therapy is terminated, the patient will abandon his therapeutic gains and will take refuge in his customary neurotic defenses. This objection is not valid because the constant analysis of the hypnotic transference eventuates in the dissolution of the dependency ties, and results in a strengthening of the ego, enabling the patient to function under his own power. With a proper technic no difficulty will be encountered in the handling of the transference.

One of the chief drawbacks of hypnoanalysis is that the patient may not be motivated toward the analytic method. He may desire a directive authoritarian relationship in the form of guidance or persuasion. He may see no sense in connecting his symptoms with his personality problems, in investigating unconscious conflicts, or in participating actively in the therapeutic procedure. There are some persons who cannot be brought around to a point where they will accept the type of relationship or the technic essential in hypnoanalysis. They will refuse to work in a nondirective, nonauthoritarian medium, or to develop values or goals within themselves toward productivity and independence. In other patients the ego strength may not be sufficient to tolerate the anxieties liberated by the release of unconscious conflict. However, a skillful therapist will be able to create incentives for change, working within the boundaries of the existing ego strength toward preparing the patient for hypnoanalysis.

HYPNOANALYTIC PROCEDURES

HYPNOANALYSIS presupposes an aptitude on the part of the patient to enter a trance sufficiently deep to make possible the enployment of the various hypnoanalytic procedures. The ability to verbalize during hypnosis without awakening is mandatory. A somnambulistic trance is essential where such technics as drawing, play therapy, dramatics, mirror gazing, regression and revivification, and the creation of experimental conflicts are to be used. Free association, dream induction and automatic writing often require no more than a medium or light trance.

As has been indicated, not all patients are capable of being hypnoanalyzed because they cannot tolerate the anxiety associated with the release of unconscious material by the various hypnoanalytic processes. The strength of the ego must be carefully appraised before hypnoanalysis is attempted. Where the individual is unable to stand hypnoanalysis, palliative psychotherapy may be employed in the hope of building up adequate ego strength to make later hypnoanalysis possible.

GENERAL PROCEDURES

A daily training period for about one to two weeks usually precedes the beginning of therapy. During this time the patient is slowly and systematically inducted into deeper and deeper trance states with the object of reaching, if possible, somnambulism with posthypnotic amnesia. The patient should be trained to enter into a trance state immediately at a given signal. The last part of the training period is spent in teaching the patient to verbalize and to associate freely in the hypnotic state, to dream on suggestion, to write automatically, to revert memorially to earlier periods of life, and to engage in play therapy, drawing, dramatics and mirror gazing. Elsewhere directions for instituting these technics have been outlined in detail.[14]

Following the training period, the patient is instructed in the technic of free association, and he is reminded of the urgency of reporting his dreams and his attitudes and feelings toward the analyst. The patient may sit up in a chair at each session or, preferably, may lie down on a couch as in psychoanalysis. As a general rule, the first fifteen or twenty minutes of each session are spent in free association, the content of the patient's associations being noted for clues to the later framing of hypnotic suggestions. Hypnosis is then induced and the various hypnoanalytic procedures are employed as indicated. The actual period of hypnosis will range from twenty minutes to one half hour. Before awakening, the patient is instructed to sleep for five or ten minutes. This time may be used to induce dreams relating to important current problems. The remainder of the hour is spent discussing the patient's reactions or the material brought up during the trance. A one and one half hour treatment period is generally more satisfactory than the traditional hourly session, and, sometimes, an even longer period of time may have to be allotted to the patient.

Hypnosis and Free Association

Free association is an extremely important technical procedure. Unconscious trends usually manifest themselves in the stream of speech in a more or less discursive manner. However, many resistances may arise to waking free association, some of which are conscious and others unconscious in nature. Hypnosis can be used to facilitate free association. Hypnagogic reverie, as Kubie[15] has shown, may bring about a surprising elucidation of unconscious material. Lindner[16] makes use of hypnosis to overcome resistances to waking free association by inducing a trance whenever the patient manifests blocking in speech.

The mere induction of hypnosis may eliminate many resistances to free association. The material flows freely, and the results of one session are often equivalent to weeks of waking free association.   It is often helpful to have the patient visualize scenes in his mind as they appear.   He may become quite emotional and dramatic as he describes his thought images.   Hypnosis may also be used to analyze resistances that prevent waking free association.   The hypnotic state, however, cannot in itself dissolve all resistances to free association, and, in some cases, the patient will be unable to verbalize his thoughts even in the deepest somnambulism with the most persistent urging.   Occasionally material may be brought up by instructing the patient that, at the count of five, he will have a thought, or visualize an image.

The question may be asked as to what value free association during hypnosis can have, if, on the assumption of waking life, the usual resistances begin to function.   The ability to verbalize during hypnosis will not in itself produce an immediate change.   However, a corrosive process on the resistances seems to be set up which ultimately may result in a breaking through of unconscious impulses and feelings into awareness.

DREAM INDUCTION

Hypnotic stimulation and interpretation of dreams play a very important part in hypnoanalysis. As in psychoanalysis, the patient's dreams indicate the character of the repressed material, the nature of the transference, the manifold disguises that resistances assume, and the stages of therapeutic progress.

Dreams may be stimulated by suggestion under hypnosis, or they may be posthypnotically induced.   The nature of the problem to be dreamed about may also be suggested.   Hypnotic dreams have all the characteristics of spontaneous dreams and are dynamically as significant.

The dreams which spontaneously follow the first attempts at hypnosis are tremendously important and often contain the essence of the entire problem. Spontaneous dreams are stimulated by the material brought up during the trance, by resistance, and by the emotions aroused in the interpersonal relationship.

The ability to dream under hypnosis must be trained. A medium trance is usually required. Unconscious ideational processes of a purposeful nature may be stimulated by dream activity, and frequently the patient may work out an insight through dreaming when it is suggested that he do so. Dreaming under hypnosis or posthypnotically may also be used as a means of understanding attitudes and feelings that are not yet conscious and which cannot be verbalized. In this way attitudes may be divulged which reveal trends in the transference. Dream activity may also aid in the dissolution of resistance. An important use of hypnotic dreaming is in the recovery of dreams which have been forgotten, as well as specific portions of dreams which have either been repressed or have been subjected to secondary elaboration. Dreaming under hypnosis may also be used to help the recovery of forgotten memories and experiences.

Dreams revealed under hypnosis, as a general rule, should not be interpreted in the waking state. If an interpretation is indicated, it should be made during hypnosis, and the patient should be enjoined to accept or reject the interpretation in accordance with whether he feels it to be true or false. Frequently the patient will be able to interpret his own spontaneous or hypnotic dreams while in a trance, since the symbolic meaning is more apparent in hypnosis than in waking life.

AUTOMATIC WRITING

Automatic writing is a splendid means of gaining access to unconscious material that lies beyond the grasp of conscious recall. The technic of automatic writing is easily taught by placing a pencil in the hand of the patient during the trance and suggesting that his hand will move along automatically without his being aware of what he is writing. The product of such writing is usually an illegible jumble of letters and words which constitute a cryptic communication. Occasionally the writing is somewhat more coherent and will contain condensations, neologisms, phonetic spelling and other devices which can be translated only by the patient during hypnosis.

The patient is usually instructed to translate his automatic writing by opening his eyes during the hypnotic state and writing the full meaning of his communication underneath the automatic writing. Should he be unable to open his eyes without awakening, a posthypnotic suggestion may be given to him that the meaning of his automatic writing will be clear to him after he awakens. Because the automatic writing is so fragmented, it is best to permit the patient to do the translating himself in order to supply missing material that he has eliminated or condensed.

By an involved technic[13] it may be possible to create a hysterical dissociated personality through the medium of automatic writing which aids the physician in getting across to the patient important interpretations and insights. This artificially created personality usually lies closer to the unconscious and is capable of tolerating repressed material with less anxiety than the customary personality. The alter ego is highly protective of the patient and acts as an intermediary between the physician and the patient's habitual ego.

Hypnotic Drawing

Drawing may be stimulated under hypnosis and is another important way of getting at significant unconscious problems. Patients who have a resistance to draw in the waking state usually enter into hypnotic drawing with great enthusiasm. It is best that the patient be able to achieve a somnambulistic trance in order that he can open his eyes without awakening.

The topics to be drawn may be suggested to the patient, or he, himself, may be given free range to draw whatever subjects he desires.   He may delineate attitudes towards members of his family, toward his mate, or toward the physician, or he may illustrate an important dream or experience. Sometimes story-telling technics are combined with drawing, the patient being requested to make up a story about his drawing.   Hypnotic drawing can also be advantageously utilized during regression with reorientation to earlier age levels, the patient bringing up attitudes and feelings that are repressed at the adult level.

Play Therapy

The usual resistances that the adult displays toward play therapy may often be effectively eliminated during hypnosis. The patient usually plays with the materials with great vehemence as soon as he realizes that he is not expected to be inert, nor need wait for specific directions from the physician. Both active and passive play technics may be used.

Play therapy may be employed at both adult and regressed age levels, and, in the latter state, the physician may be able to recapture inklings of the conflicts the patient suffered as a child.   The directions given during play therapy must be specific and may have to be repeated several times.   If one has a general idea of the chief incidents in the patient's life, regression to the age level of these incidents, and setting the stage with appropriate materials, may facilitate the therapeutic process.

Dramatic Technics

Dramatization of inner feelings and important events in the past life may be readily effected during deep hypnosis.   The resistances to dramatization that exist in the waking state are readily removed under hypnosis when instructions are given the patient that he act out certain feelings or situations.

The emotional reaction elicited by such instructions may be intense and considerable abreaction may be achieved. One of the best examples of dramatization may be seen in the treatment of war neuroses when the patient is instructed under hypnosis to relive the battle scene. The response to such a suggestion may be extremely vivid, the patient reliving his intense rage, anxiety and fear in a most realistic manner. The analyst may play a passive role during dramatization, permitting the patient complete freedom, or he may play an active role becoming a part of the scene. In the latter instance, he may serve as a significant personage in the individual's life, encouraging the patient to express certain feelings, or else acting with him in the dramatization of an important event. Dramatic technics may sometimes be combined with story telling. These permit the patient to elaborate on his motor performances.

REGRESSION AND REVIVIFICATION

Two types of regression are encountered during hypnosis. The first type has to do with current conceptions of the patient toward an earlier age period, viewing the past with present day attitudes and judgments. There is here a simulated reproduction of a past period of life. The second type of regression is an actual return to a previous epoch with a reliving of the same pattern that existed originally. This is regression in the true sense, and in this state the individual is capable of recapturing and reliving events and impulses which have been forgotten or repressed.

To induce regression the patient is inducted into an extremely deep trance, and then he may slowly be disoriented to time and place. He is then reoriented to earlier and earlier age periods by appropriate suggestions. The specific age period to which regression is desired may be suggested to the patient, or he may, himself, be given a choice of a significant period. Where he displays a certain symptom, he may be instructed to remember and to live through the time when he first developed the symptom. Regression increases the hypermnesic effect of hypnosis to a marked degree, opening up pathways to forgotten memories and experiences which would not be available to the individual at an adult level. Many of the reports in recent literature have involved the utilization of this method.

Regression may be used in conjunction with other hypnoanalytic technics, such as in dream induction, play therapy, drawing, dramatics, automatic writing and mirror gazing.

Crystal and Mirror Gazing

Crystal and mirror gazing will require an extremely deep state of hypnosis inasmuch as the patient will have to open his eyes without awakening. Where a crystal is not available, a mirror may be used, so placed that it reflects the blank ceiling. Under hypnosis the patient is requested to gaze intently into the mirror and to see visions which he is to report to the physician. Visual hallucinations that come up by this technic frequently consist of forgotten or repressed incidents that have happened in the past. The visualization of these events often produces intense emotional reactions and considerable abreaction. Frequently the technic may be utilized to consolidate insights obtained through other psychoanalytic procedures which have not been fully absorbed and integrated.

Induction of Experimental Conflict

An experimental conflict offers a method of demonstrating to the patient the workings of his unconscious. Often it will inculcate insight where no other technic succeeds. Many resistances prevent the acknowledgment by the patient of certain unconscious drives. Only by experiencing them in actual operation can the patient realize how they are influencing his behavioral and attitudinal patterns. For instance, a person may have a problem involving an inability to express hostility which he turns on himself, with the development of a psychosomatic illness. During therapy, the patient may become aware of the fact that he feels hostile, but he may be unable to see how his hostility produces his somatic symptoms. An experimental neurosis created during the hypnotic state, in which a fictitious situation is suggested associated with feelings of hostility, serves to mobilize the same somatic patterns that develop when he spontaneously feels hostility. Under such circumstances it may be possible to demonstrate to the patient how certain emotions are responsible for his symptoms.

Experimental conflicts may involve significant incidents in the patient's life or may deal with the transference relationship. The wording of the experimental conflict is important as Erickson[17] has pointed out. The patient is told that he will remember an incident that actually occurred to him, but which he had forgotten because the memory of this incident had been frightening or painful. An incident is then elaborated which brings out the particular situation or pattern that is important at the time. The patient is then told that he will, when he awakens, remember the emotions relating to this situation, but he will completely forget the situation itself. Upon awakening, the reactions of the patient are carefully noted as are his spontaneous responses. Repetition of the experimental conflict may be essential. Eventually an explanation to the patient under hypnosis of the meaning of the experimental conflict, with directions to recall it in the waking state, may reinforce the understanding of his problem.

PRACTICAL APPLICATIONS OF HYPNOANALYSIS

For practical purposes hypnoanalysis may be employed in three ways. The first use permits the development of a transference neurosis with its analysis in the traditional psychoanalytic sense. The second use is for purposes of desensitization, allowing the patient to become aware of and to adjust to repressed elements of his personality. The third use involves the re-education of the patient through psychoanalytic insights. In hypnoanalytic desensitization and re-education, a neurotic transference is avoided as much as possible.

HYPNOANALYSIS WITH ANALYSIS
OF THE TRANSFERENCE

HYPNOANALYSIS lends itself admirably to the development and analysis of a transference relationship. The transference develops rapidly, and its significance may be studied in a facile way through the use of the various hypnoanalytic procedures. Through the analysis of the transference, the patient is brought to a realization of his deepest repressed conflicts, and the manner in which they distort his present day behavior. The relationship the physician attempts to establish with the patient here is as permissive and nondirective as possible.

Because hypnotic therapy has traditionally been associated with an authoritarian relationship, an analysis of the relationship may occasion some surprise, since it would seem to jeopardize the very foundations on which hypnosis depends. Nevertheless, such an analysis does not interfere with hypnotizability even though the motivations which condition trance susceptibility may be subjected to investigation.

Hypnosis is an intimate interpersonal relationship and is bound to incite profound emotional feelings in the patient. At the start the latter will display his customary demands, expectations and fears which he habitually demonstrates in his relationships with people. In addition to these habitual responses, he will experience an onrush of irrational transference feelings which frighten him and which he will strive to repress. The latter are the product of past experiences and conditionings so anxiety laden that they have been relegated to unconscious oblivion. In his ordinary interpersonal contacts, he is able to throw up various defenses against such feelings, to detach himself or to replace his strivings with those of a more acceptable nature. Resistance against these feelings is intense. In psychoanalysis a main task is dissipation of transference resistances. Many months may pass before the patient permits himself to come sufficiently close to the analyst to experience irrational attitudes and impulses.

In hypnoanalysis, the resistances to the deepest interpersonal feelings are cut through almost from the start, and these reveal themselves through the various hypnoanalytic procedures. The experiencing and the understanding of unconscious inner drives are of utmost importance in tracing the genetic development of the neurosis, and in demonstrating to the patient that his present symptoms are caused by them. As soon as the patient relieves himself of guilt and hostility, he becomes cognizant of a new element of congeniality and productiveness in his relationship with the analyst.

The ability of the patient to express himself freely during the trance, to utilize motor and ideational pathways which are not available to him in waking life, to vocalize and dramatize his trends and conflicts, acts as a stimulus to activity and self assertiveness. The ego, finding that it has not been devastated, is better capable of relinquishing repression and of permitting insight to filter into waking life. Above all the patient discovers in the intimate interpersonal relationship of hypnosis that he is not destroyed and that he does not destroy the physician. Instead he feels an element of peace and security which has been foreign to him in his habitual interpersonal contacts. This unique relationship experience acts as a bridge toward more vitalizing experiences with others. In detached and schizoid persons, especially, the hypnotic relationship may be the first close interpersonal experience, and may lead to a more realistic approach toward the world.

Trepidation may be expressed by some that the hypnotic relationship is bound to enhance dependency strivings. Such a fear is not at all justified because the hypnotic relationship is not utilized in an authoritarian way as it is during the various palliative hypnotic psychotherapies.

In hypnoanalysis, a most remarkable innovation in therapy is the directing of the patient toward activity and productiveness in both ideational and motor spheres. The release from the traditional restraints has a most important effect upon the individual's inner evaluation of authority as restrictive and condemning, and upon his own feelings of assertiveness and self confidence.

Resistance occurs in hypnoanalysis in the same way as in psychoanalysis, whenever the patient is confronted with anxiety, or is threatened with the loss of a gratification he values highly. The management of resistance during hypnoanalysis depends upon its character and function. Those resistances which oppose the penetration into awareness of repressed emotions and memories can often be dealt with surgically by urgent demands to the patient, during trance states at adult or regressed age levels, to talk about his inner conflicts or to remember a forgotten experience. The effect of this recall is to lessen conscious resistances to a point where the patient eventually brings up the material in the waking state, presenting it as the product of a spontaneous discovery. Resistances which issue out of the transference are much more difficult to deal with and call for a painstaking analysis along the lines of orthodox psychoanalytic technic, demonstrating to the patient the presence of resistance, its purpose, and, when possible, its historical origin. Various hypnoanalytic procedures may facilitate the dissolution of transference resistances. However, such dissolution may require a considerable period of time, particularly in the character disorders.

Psychic change is brought about not merely by a disgorging of unconscious material, but by a rational understanding and digestion of this material on the part of the ego. During psychoanalysis, insights are arrived at slowly as resistances are gradually resolved. The ability of the patient to tolerate his unconscious drives goes hand in hand with the strengthening of his ego. During hypnoanalysis, many resistances are swept aside. This effect is not at all automatic, but probably is due to the temporary strengthening of the ego during the trance as a result of an alliance with the hypnotist, and a replacing of the archaic tyrannical conscience with a more tolerant one patterned around the injunctions and commands of the hypnotist. One need not assume from this that the superego is entirely dissolved during the trance. Even in the deepest trance states it may continue to function, inhibiting the appearance of repressed unconscious material. The degree of superego replacement during the trance is an individual matter being most marked in hysterical conditions, and least apparent in the character disorders.

In the trance state, consequently, the individual may bring up emotions, conflicts, memories and strivings which are dynamically important in maintaining behavior patterns of a neurotic nature. The degree to which the patient becomes cognizant of these trends varies. In some cases important material may be directly verbalized. In other patients repressions prevent the accessibility of the material to speech. Here, indirect technics, such as play, drawing, automatic writing, and dramatics may disclose the material in a more or less symbolized form.

The manner in which the material is interpreted to the patient and its timing are tremendously important. As a general rule it is useless to present the patient in waking life with a verbatim account of his hypnotic productions. Unprepared as it is, the conscious ego will reject the validity of the material, will respond with resistance, or will, when the motivation to comply with the hypnotist is sufficiently strong, intellectually accept the material with no associated emotional benefit. Interpretations are given the patient during hypnosis, and in the waking state are phrased according to his awareness of a problem. Where he has an inkling of a trend, an interpretation will be beneficial. Where no such awareness exists, the interpretation may be worse than useless. It is especially essential to be cautious with interpretations where the patient is capable of bringing up the unconscious material only through the indirect hypnoanalytic procedures.

In some patients the elucidation of unconscious drives during hypnosis serves in itself to dissolve many conscious resistances to the acknowledgment of these drives. In the trance the patient lies closer to his unconscious. He will understand his dreams and his behavior patterns with much greater accuracy than in waking life. It is thus possible to be relatively active in interpretations, always tempering these to the existing degree of understanding. Authoritarian injunctions to accept material must be avoided. Rather the patient is enjoined to work on the interpretation and to accept it in the waking state only if and when he feels it to be true. In this way the patient participates in the analytic process and there is less chance that he will accept the interpretation on the basis of faith. Insight gained in a medium where the patient feels he can accept or reject an interpretation in accordance with whether he feels it to be true or false is usually irreversible.

Another important factor in hypnotic interpretation is to avoid regarding present day behavior as a stereotyped repetition of past happenings. Even though character traits and behavior patterns are evolved as a result of conditionings and experiences in relationship with important past personages, the individual does not carry on an automatic repetitive process in his interpersonal relationships. Character traits determine present needs and strivings and generate reaction tendencies of a compulsive nature. All behavior, however, is dynamically motivated to propitiate essential needs, and it is essential to see what needs the individual seeks to fulfill in his present day setting. What we desire to interpret is the purpose behind the patient's present behavior rather than its genetic determinants.

The matter of the handling of the symbolisms which emerge from the unconscious mental strata is also important. The language of the unconscious is frequently couched in terms of organ functions—in feeding, excretory, and sexual activities.   Phallic symbolism is extremely common, and one may get the erroneous impression that the patient's difficulties are entirely centered in a sexual sphere.   One can easily be led astray if he accepts such unconscious symbolisms at their face value.   It is essential to understand and to reinterpret the symbolisms in terms of basic motivational activities.   To bombard the patient with symbolisms usually does little except confuse him, inasmuch as the language of the unconscious may be inscrutable to his conscious mind.

An important aid in the interpretive process is the creation of an experimental conflict which is patterned around the patient's personal conflict and arouses emotions and behavior such as he customarily experiences.   Many patients are able to gain insight through the medium of real experience when they would be unable to understand their difficulties intellectually.   Another technic is to urge the patient during hypnosis to work out a certain problem in detail until he understands it thoroughly.   Much activity of an unconscious nature may be stimulated by this method.

Unfortunately, the use of hypnoanalysis with analysis of the transference requires special skills in the physician that can be gained only through training in the psychoanalytic method, including a personal psychoanalysis and supervised control work.   This is necessary in order to analyze the most significant trends in the interpersonal relationship, to avoid the pitfalls of countertransference, to handle resistance, and to make appropriate interpretations.

While a personal psychoanalysis with adequate supervised control work is essential for the physician in those forms of hypnoanalysis which depend upon the analysis of the transference as the predominant technic, there are some technics of hypnoanalysis which the unanalyzed physician may use, which restrict the development of a neurotic transference. These technics are first, desensitization, with revival of repressed memories and conflicts; and second, re-education utilizing psychoanalytic insights.

HYPNOANALYTIC
DESENSITIZATION

IN HYPNOANALYTIC desensitization, the patient, through hypnoanalytic technics, becomes aware of unconscious foci of difficulty, such as repressed fears, conflicts, and memories. Awareness of repressed material is aided by interpretation on the part of the physician who confronts the patient's conscious ego with the implications of his repression. The ego may, at first, be unable to accept that which has been repressed, and the patient may be inclined to deny its validity. However, as the conflicts or memories are brought up in manifold forms, the ego becomes inured to them, and the patient is more capable of accepting them as part of himself. The understanding of how and why the repression developed makes it possible for the person to liberate himself from the influence of unconscious foci.

Hypnosis is extremely effective for the recall of traumatic memories and experiences which have been repressed. Repression is dynamically motivated by a need to avoid anxiety which would be aroused by the forgotten memories and experiences. Many mechanisms are used to reinforce repression and these may constitute various neurotic symptoms, particular phobias, hysterical inhibitory symptoms and compulsions. Such symptoms often represent the surface manifestations of a neurosis.

The hypermnesic effect of hypnosis has long been recognized. Originally Breuer and Freud[18] utilized hypnosis as a means of recovering forgotten experiences and their associated emotions which they believed acted as potent founts of conflict. Research has demonstrated that hypnosis can facilitate recall as much as sixty-five percent. During the first world war this facilitating influence of hypnosis on memory was utilized by Brown,[19] Wingfield,[20] Hadfield,[21] and

Karup[22] who discovered that when shell-shocked soldiers remembered and lived through the traumatic war scene their symptoms vanished. Since then regression and reorientation of the patient to an earlier age level has been found to reinforce the hypermnesic effect. Therapeutic use of increased hypnotic recall has been employed by Taylor,[23] Smith,[24] Erickson,[25, 26] Erickson and Kubie,[27,28] and Lindner.[29] During the second world war, the method was extensively used and barbiturates were intravenously injected to expedite hypnotic induction.[30, 31] Lindner[32] recorded the productions of a man during hypnoanalysis, obtaining memories dating to the first year of life. As a result of the recall of these memories, the patient demonstrated a material improvement in his condition.

Various technics may be utilized to elicit unconscious memories. In some patients the simple command to remember incidents in the past may bring out an amazing amount of material. In others resistances function to keep the material repressed even in the somnambulistic state. Indirect technics, such as automatic writing, are frequently successful in recalling repressed memories. Sometimes the technic of delayed recall, such as described by Livingood,[33] is efficacious, permitting the ego to prepare itself for the memory. "Narcoanalysis" is also a helpful adjunct.[34] Regression and revivification may be utilized as a means of remembering events that have occurred at earlier age levels. Crystal or mirror gazing may similarly be of help.

As in psychoanalysis, the transference acts as a tremendous catalyst to forgotten memories and experiences, activating intense emotional reactions which are conditioned by previous happenings. The individual under the impact of such emotions will remember the genetic determinents of his neurosis far better than where no such emotion exists.

Since one is dealing with intensely traumatic material, it may be best to protect the patient by urging him under hypnosis to remember only certain aspects of forgotten past events and experiences, and to bring these up only when he feels sufficiently strong to tolerate their meaning. In this way the patient will recover piecemeal forgotten material which he can put together later on.

An important question is the exact effect of hypnotic recall on waking recall. Forgotten memories and experiences are repressed because the individual is unable to tolerate the anxiety related to the memories and experiences. During hypnosis the subject's ego appears to be strengthened temporarily by an alliance with the hypnotist, and it may be possible for him to master some anxiety and to tolerate material that he could not bring up in the waking state. This does not necessarily mean that the patient will remember such experiences in waking life even though he has discussed them during hypnosis. Nevertheless, experience has shown that where hypnotic recall occurs, resistance to waking recall is to some extent shattered. Eventually the patient may spontaneously remember the hypnotically remembered material on a waking level some weeks later. By observing the patient's dreams and free associations, one may sometimes detect less and less distortion in symbolic disguises until the material erupts into consciousness.

How hypnosis can recover a memory of a repressed traumatic experience is illustrated by the case of a man of forty-eight who applied for therapy to relieve anxiety, compulsive and psychosomatic symptoms. Although sexually potent, it developed that he had never, in the many years of his marriage, been able to have successful sexual relations with his wife. Puzzled by this fact, he was certain it created many of his symptoms. Three transcribed sessions follow, consisting of selected treatment hours over a three week period.

In the initial session the patient describes his problem in detail.

Pt. You see, doctor, I have many difficulties. For years I have had a stomach ulcer. I had a complete check-up.

They never were able to demonstrate the ulcer radiologically, but they assumed this overall ulcer. I took six months or a year off and it got better, but I always had a bad stomach which I feel sure now is due to my—the tremendous amount of tension that I have. Incidentally I have a number of compulsive symptoms that I want to tell you about. And in the army it just came back, but just worse—all the stomach symptoms, plus a new compulsive symptom. I come from out of town, Georgia, and I thought you could help me.

Dr. Tell me about your new compulsive symptom.

Pt. That while I drive a car at forty or fifty miles an hour, I have to close my eyes and see how high I can count. And I've had a compulsive cough for years which I know how it developed, and I know the time it developed, and the connection of its development. I don't know its psychic causes and I have other compulsive symptoms.

Dr. Can you tell me about them?

Pt. Oh, of course. If I write a check, I must always give an excuse to see it back after I've handed it; I want to see the right date. Actually I want to see it because I'm afraid that instead of writing it for fifteen dollars I'll have written it for fifteen hundred dollars. I know damn well I haven't written it for fifteen hundred dollars. I'm sure I wrote it for fifteen dollars, but if I don't get it back, I'm very much upset that maybe I did.

Dr. I see. And what other compulsions do you have?

Pt. Oh, I get quite a few sore throats and I have a very silly one. I mean if I'm gargling with hot salt water, I have to count on my fingers, gargle with counts. I have to count and repeat.

Dr. How often do you do that?

Pt. Oh, I do it often. Oh, God all the time during the day. It seems to be worse if I'm tense. I mean I can definitely see a connection with my tension.

Dr. When you're tense you find that it's essential to count.

Pt. To count and repeat.

Dr. Have you ever had any tics?

Pt. You mean a twitch? No, I never had anything like that.

Dr. Have you ever been preoccupied with fears of death?

Pt. Well, I have had definite hypochondriacal fears in the past. I seem to be much better about that. I have another peculiar compulsion. I'm very fond of cats ever since I was a little boy. We had a Siamese cat. We lived in Georgia. We were walking down the street, and we saw a couple in a car parked in a garage, and they had an old cat. I stopped to pet it as I invariably will, and they said, "Oh, we happened to find it. He is very old and very sick." So I felt very sorry for the cat. About three or four days later I walked by and they were sitting and they were alone. I said, "How's your cat?" The old man said, "Oh, he's in heaven." I said, "What do you mean?" He said, "Well, we had to have him gassed because he was suffering too much." Well, that depressed me so. I felt an actual weight on my chest. For days and days I'd go to my office and just sit there. I got so terribly depressed. I mean I realize that it was completely abnormal. No reason why a business man should be depressed because a cat has died. Even now if I see homeless cats on the street in the cold, I have to do something about it. And if I don't, I feel terribly depressed about it. I mean compulsive thinking about that. I just can't stop thinking about it.

Dr. And does it come to your mind constantly?

Pt. Oh, I can't get it out of my mind about the sick cat on the street.

Dr. When you don't see a sick cat on the street, do you think about cats?

Pt. Well, I like cats. That's all. I mean—

Dr. Do you get any obsessions, ideas crowding in on your mind that are difficult to control? And what about depressions now?

Pt. Yes, I do, also I will get depressions, not so often. I get a feeling of weight on my chest.

Dr. Do you feel tense?

Pt. You mean generally? Yes.

Dr. How about insomnia?

Pt. I sleep badly. I take a lot of nembutal. I sleep badly.

Dr. You take a lot of sedatives?

Pt. Yes. They help.

Dr. How many sedatives do you take?

Pt. I take, it depends, sometimes I'll get to bed, and I'll have to take one nembutal. I never take more than one. Maybe two or three nights in a row, and then I may go a week or two without any.

Dr. Any alcohol?

Pt. I practically don't drink at all, not because I don't like the effect of it. I enjoy the relaxation, but I find that it makes my stomach like acid, certain slight pain and burning. You see I'm tired all the time. Everything is an effort. I have an unfortunate tendency to procrastinate on certain things I don't like to face up to, and the fact that I'm moderately successful in business is due to whipping myself along.

Dr. And what do you feel is the cause of all this?

Pt. I feel it is some background there of my whole attitude towards sexual intercourse. I think the whole thing is wrong. I think it might perhaps be epitomized in a poem that I used to like very well when I was a young boy in my teens, of Kipling's "The Lady." "I wouldn't do such because I liked her too much." I used to have fantasies about my wife before I married her that maybe I would have sexual intercourse with her, and she would become pregnant, and I would be run over crossing the street, and she would be left to face the hostile world pregnant at seventeen or eighteen. I mean that I feel that I have the background to give me a wrong sexual slant.

Dr. Can you tell me something about your mother and father?

Pt. My mother and father are English. They had a very unhappy life apparently. My mother would awaken myself and my sister at two or three o'clock in the morning. I have a sister four years older than myself. My mother would be in a hysterical state, screaming at father. For years I didn't know what it was about, I just felt terribly sorry for my father. She was apparently making him so unhappy and upsetting him when he had to work the next day.

Dr. How old were you at this time?

Pt. I was very nearly fourteen or fifteen before I understood she was accusing him of going with other women. It was incredible to me. I didn't believe he wasn't true to her. I think that I resented the idea. I thought it was a figment of her imagination. It was incredible. To this day I don't know if he was or not.

Dr. What about your early life?

Pt. Well, my father was wealthy, and I had a nurse until I was eleven years old. I hardly knew either of my parents. The nurse brought me up, and she left when I was eleven. I was in a terrible depression for months. Maybe that's normal for a child, I don't know, I doubt if it was. My degree of affection was abnormal, maybe not in view of the fact that probably because she was more my mother than my own mother.

Dr. How old were you then?

Pt. Eleven.

Dr. At eleven you became depressed?

Pt. Terribly depressed.

Dr. And what do you relate the depression to?

Pt. To my nurse's leaving. They thought that I was old enough, also that was the time that my father was not so well situated and they thought the expense was not so necessary.

Dr. What is your feeling about your mother?

Pt. Noncommittal. I didn't like her so much.

Dr. What about your sister?

Pt. Very little feeling toward her.

Dr. How about your father?

Pt. When I became fifteen or sixteen, I was terribly attached to him. In fact he had a rather tragic death, and I thought my father was like a brother. I know he was a sort of the idealized image of a person. I pitied him the way he was treated by mother.

Dr. How long ago did he die?

Pt. He died when I was nineteen.

Dr. Let us get back to your wife.

Pt. That is the real hub of the neurosis, at least it's how it manifested itself. I met my wife when she was sixteen, and I was seventeen. I had only one sexual experience up to that time, I had gone to a house when I was sixteen with some boys and was impotent at that time. It disgusted me, it nauseated me. I met my wife as I say when she was sixteen, and I was seventeen, and I fell terrifically in love with her. There was an enormous amount of parental opposition. She was quite too young, and, of course, I was too young. And I think perhaps her family thought my family wasn't wealthy enough, and certainly we were too young. There was a tremendous amount of resistance to it. As it developed, we were married when I was nineteen and she was eighteen, I was a few months short of twenty. I had felt that I must suppress all sexual feeling towards her. And it was wrong, terribly wrong to allow myself to even think about it in that manner. We would kiss and fondle each other, and get terrifically excited; and I would not allow myself to ever think of having intercourse with her. In other words when I look back on it now, I see the sexual excitement I had with her was not normal. At least with me normal sexual excitement envisages the end of sexual intercourse. With my relations with her I wouldn't allow myself to envisage that end.

Dr. You felt you should restrain yourself.

Pt. And with this opposition, I remember the first sum-
mer when she told me she couldn't see so much of me. I
got a terrible depression. Terrible; I never had felt anything like it. In fact it was very peculiar, we were having
dinner at the hotel where we lived. At eight o'clock I
couldn't keep my head up at the dinner table. I felt I had
to sleep, an overpowering fatigue.

Dr. Before you got married?

Pt. Oh yes, this was about the first three or four months
that I knew my wife. And I went up stairs at eight-thirty
and went to bed. I slept until almost noontime the next
day, a thing I have never done since or before; it was almost
as if I was in a coma.

Dr. You then were reconciled.

Pt. Yes, but I had to keep my sexual feelings down. I
thought I must be strong. I musn't let myself think about
such things. We didn't know when we were going to be
able to get married. I would wake up, and I'd find I'd been
crying in my sleep, my pillow would be soaking wet.

Dr. This is before you were married?

Pt. Before we were married, it upset me completely.
I thought this was marvelous, this was wonderful. You've
now gotten control over yourself, you're being strong. I
was proud of that, you may imagine. Of course, I figured
when I was married, the power would all come back. Well
my father died and we had set a date to be married anyway
against parental opposition. And we got married and went
on our honeymoon, and to my astonishment I was able to
get sexually excited that night. But I wasn't able to have
intercourse with her. I was just unable to penetrate.
And I, the erection, I thought I just didn't get excited
enough.

Dr. You never had intercourse with your wife in all the
years you were married?

Pt. In all these intervening years, the only time I had

intercourse with her was when I was asleep. Half asleep
and half awake, and I didn't think it was her. I thought it
was something wrong. I couldn't bring myself to ever
think; and yet I was very fond of her, terribly fond of her.

Dr. Her as somebody else?

Pt. With some one else I could have intercourse. That
is why I thought there was something wrong, but definitely
wrong about it. I have had an improvement in recent years,
the last few years. I can think of having sexual intercourse with her, but I cannot bring it about. My wife is
sweet and willing. I mean she is attractive. She is an
amazingly young looking woman. She looks ten years
younger than she is. I love to kiss her, fondle her; but I
don't get sufficiently excited to have intercourse with her.

Dr. Do you have an erection?

Pt. Yes, not a complete erection, but it's better in the
past few years.

Dr. You feel you could function with another woman?

Pt. There is no question about it, but I couldn't leave
my wife. It is just as though you would ask me, or you
would say to me: "Here all the happiness in the world will
be yours if you just step into the next room. There is a
little girl there, and take this knife and stab her with it."
In other words the little girl would be my wife. I mean
facing her and telling her I didn't love her would be the
equivalent of doing that.

Dr. Any strong anxiety about this?

Pt. Well, I'm always in a state, I worry. I have nothing
in the world really to worry about. I mean my wife and
I go over, I mean our whole situation and everything, and
we should be the happiest people. There is nothing we
have to worry about. We have everything except a normal
sex life, which is of paramount importance. Everything
else we have, and yet I worry about every damn thing under
the sun.

Dr.   How does you wife feel about this?

Pt.   She is in love with me.   She wants sex.   I can't conceive of her being interested in it, but she is.   I just have a feeling it is just completely wrong.   But as I say, I am able in the last year or two to think about it, intercourse with her, which I was completely unable to do for all these years.   I mean, if she even wanted to discuss the subject, I wouldn't let her discuss it.   It was too painful to think of.

Dr.   Are you interested in having a normal sex life with her?

Pt.   Yes, if it is possible, I want it more than anything else.

Dr.   There are reasons why you are unable to have sexual relations with your wife.   We may be able to understand these reasons through hypnosis.   Once you understand them, you will have a better chance to straighten out your life.   Have you had repetitive dreams of any kind?

Pt.   Oh yes I have, I haven't had it lately, but I had it for many, many years.   It was a dream of some one coming for me, and I tried to shoot at them, and the damned gun, there was always something wrong with it, and it wouldn't fire.

After several sessions, during which the patient was trained to achieve a deep trance, material is brought in which lends itself to hypnoanalytic manipulation.

Pt.   I slept a little better last night.   Saturday night I dreamed I was with a woman, a dark woman, and I wanted to have intercourse with her.   I can remember that I was surprised that she agreed fairly readily.   Next thing I know, I was standing off with a group of people watching this woman have somebody else, having intercourse.   I was trying to justify the fact that they were doing such a thing in public, on the street, to the people who, in one way or another, were watching them more or less indifferently

But I felt criticism.   And that's all of the dream that I can remember.

Dr. Were there any other dreams besides that?

Pt. There probably were, although I don't know. I had another last night.

Dr. Supposing you associate to the first dream.

Pt. The woman, my wife is dark.

Dr. Any other associations?

Pt. No.

Dr. All right, and then last night?

Pt. That was very funny.   An elephant was chasing me. I can associate with that very easily, I think.   Chasing me through apparently back yards, I was so much afraid.   It came out of a building like a mirage, and in the back yards, and I saw a house.   It was a back entrance, but it looked like a front entrance with glass doors.   I knew if I went through this house, I would be able to come out on the street, right through the building, and come out on the street. It was Sixty-ninth, or Seventieth, or Seventy-first (*laughs*), and I ran through these glass doors, and the back of the building looked like the front.   I went in the back hoping to go through the building and come out in the front and escape the elephant.   A man was in there.   We got pleasant, and he introduced me to his daughters; there were three or four of them.   Two looked like twins.   One of them was lying on a bed, and I was talking to her.   Finally, they wanted me to play bridge on a little bit of a table—it was all out of proportion to the size of table you play bridge on— with these girls and myself.   I said, "Well I'd very much like to do it, but I have to call my wife and tell her.   How could I justify being away a few hours?"   Then I realized that I couldn't justify it at all, she would never believe I was playing bridge.   That was the end of the dream.

As a little boy I used to call my father "Elly."   He was a great big, stout man.   It was short for "Elephant."   I remember one of my neighbors used to tell me, "Your father doesn't like you to call him that. It isn't very nice, you shouldn't do that anymore." I didn't call him that after that time. I didn't realize; all of a sudden it dawned on me, that was in later years when I looked back and I remembered, it was very unkind of me to have done that. I think that the girl being sick in bed was my cousin. I may be wrong in that, but my cousin has been out sick and I called to see how she was last Friday, and I remarked jestingly that if she stayed home much longer, I would have to come up and see her. And she made a few facetious remarks about it. That's the only direct associations I can make with the dreams.

Dr. Now the back door entrance, back yards, an elephant chasing you around this area of the city.

Pt. Yes, it was around Sixty-ninth, Seventieth, or Seventy-first.

Dr. It sounds rather significant, since my office is on Seventy-first Street.

Pt. Of course.

Dr. And what does that suggest to you?

Pt. Well, I was expecting you to save me from the elephant, I suppose. He was chasing me, and you opened the door to me, which is—I mean I was pleased to see you. I mean I felt that it was typical, the man in the house was kind.

Dr. At any rate an elephant associated with a powerful figure, like your father may once have seemed to you, was chasing you.

Pt. Oh, I see.

Dr. Perhaps threatening you and threatening you in a specific way.

Pt. Would it be you or my father threatening me? Which would it be?

Dr. Perhaps both.

Pt. Both.

Dr. Threatening you in a specific way, you're running away.

Pt. Yes.

Dr. Your rear is toward the pursuer, isn't it?

Pt. Yes, yes.

Dr. The back and the front seem to be significant. Back yards, back door, what does that suggest to you?

Pt. Homosexual, ah, I can't think.

Dr. A homosexual fear of some sort may be present.

Pt. Really?

Dr. Perhaps you do fear an attack from somebody. And that attack and fear may unconsciously represent a fear of a homosexual attack. The fear of a homosexual attack may be countered by a need to protect yourself. In one of your dreams you mentioned trying to protect yourself with a gun. What does that suggest?

Pt. Maybe a penis, but it didn't work, it wasn't good.

Dr. Perhaps you feel your penis, or virility, symbolized by a gun, is defective.

Pt. I want to tell you a funny thing that happened. Incidentally a friend of my parents was in to see me this morning. She knew me when I was little. She was like another mother. I have an amnesia toward my sister, particularly the time when we lived in, the time when my father was poor and we lived in a hotel. And I knew that we couldn't have had many rooms because he was poor, and I asked this friend how many rooms we had. She said two rooms at that time. And I said: "Where did my sister sleep?" And she said: "She slept in the room with you." I can't remember that, and that's one of the periods when I particularly felt I should have remembered my sister. I knew we lived in a very small two or three room hotel apartment; yet I can't remember a single thing about it even though I was about eleven years old.

Dr. She slept in the room with you?

Pt. Tw'n beds, of course.

Dr. Twin beds?

Pt. Uh huh.

Dr. Well, maybe in hypnosis we can recapture some of those memories.

Pt. I forgot to tell you, this friend was scolding me this morning; I mean she scolded me as though I were a little boy (*laughs*) and instead of saying her name, I called her by the pet name that I have for my wife. I started to call her by it and instantly stopped, it didn't come out. I thought that, I thought that might have some interest. I know a slip of the tongue has some significance.

Dr. You feel that you are misidentifying your wife with other persons or members of your family.

Pt. Years ago I went to a psychiatrist a couple of visits, and I would tell him I felt about my wife like a combination of a sister and a daughter. I always remember I used the term "like a sister."

Dr. Yes, now another thing, in that dream where the man opens the door for you there are several children around.

Pt. I was introduced to three or four, they all looked somewhat alike.

Dr. And where were these children?

Pt. Downstairs. I remember the one was sick upstairs in bed, and I went up to see her.

Dr. Was she a little girl?

Pt. No, she looked like a woman, not a little girl, a young woman.

Dr. A young woman who was the daughter of this man?

Pt. Yes, that's right. Apparently she was his daughter, two or three of them, they looked alike. They looked wan.

Dr. How many children do I have?

Pt. I don't know, I'm not sure that I follow you.

Dr. Well, how many children do you think I have?

Pt. I've never thought about it. In one of your books I do remember the dedication, I did read it, by gosh. I remember that well now, I forgot, it was to your children, two I think. Wasn't it?

Dr. And sexuality may be a part of that dream?

Pt. Well, I'm sure it was that. I know that I had that feeling towards this girl in the bed, I definitely had that feeling.

Dr. And if I am the man that opens up the door, it would seem to indicate that she is my daughter.

Pt. Yes, I felt sure in the dream that she was your daughter, I have to tell you. Didn't I tell you that?

Dr. As you know, one of the reasons you came to me was to find out why you couldn't have sex relations with your wife. In your coming to me, the motive might be to be permitted to have sexual relations. In the dream you enter my house and seem to want sexual relations with a childlike person who may be my daughter. As if you seek permission to have sex relations with someone's daughter.

Pt. Oh? Well, I, of course, I can't—I . . . .

Dr. And in escaping from the elephant there may be a threat that actually preceded what should have gone before. In other words, both components of the dream may have been twisted around in the dream. In the desire for a sexual experience, there may be residual punishment in the nature of being attacked.

Pt. The elephant was chasing me. He'd be up on his hind legs and had a club or something I think. You don't think my father, thinking of him as "Elly," might have something to do with the elephant, you don't think that has any connection?

Dr. What do you think happened to you when you were a little boy? Do you think something possibly happened to you which made you fear that you might be attacked by your father?

Pt. Sexually?

Dr. Sexually or in any way.

Pt. I don't know.

Dr. Something possibly happened to you with your sister, too. It is quite unusual for an amnesia to extend to the eleventh year. You remember nothing about living in the hotel and sleeping in a room with your sister. Now it is possible that the amnesia is a means of masking a real or fantasied experience so repugnant to you that you envisage an attack or hurt.

Pt. I'm sure that nothing ever happened, because we each had our own nurse when small. And, of course, when during the teens, thirteen, or fourteen, I was very crazy about my sister, it may very well be that I had incestuous thoughts, but I don't remember them.

Dr. Well, we don't want to guess about such things. Now I should like to have you relax and sleep.

> (*A deep trance is induced with the object of regressing the patient to the period of his boyhood. There are indications from his dreams that he identifies his wife with his mother or sister, and that he fears a homosexual attack from a powerful personage symbolically linked with his father. It is possible that his fear of attack is both a fancied retaliation for incestuous desires, as well as a passive wish for homosexuality with a repudiation of the desire by flight into heterosexuality. As will be seen from a later session, the patient in regression recaptures the memory of an incident of sexual play with his sister during which he is interrupted and frightened by his mother. There is little question that he identifies his wife with his sister, and that his inability to consummate the sexual act with her masks an incestuous wish and fear.*)

Dr. Now as you sleep, you will get very, very little. You're going to regress to a point where you are small, to the time when you lived in that two room apartment. When I talk to you next, you'll be back in that two room apartment, and it will be just as it was in those days.

You're going to be able to see what was in the apartment. It is not necessary to reconstruct anything today,
but merely to get the feeling and the sensation that you
catch a glimpse of that which you had forgotten, during
the period when you have no memory of being with your
sister. I want you to go back, back, back into your life,
and when I talk to you next, you will be able to have gone
back to that age period. You will visualize yourself as being
in that room, or actually know that you are there. I want
you to go back, back, and recapture something that you
thought you had forgotten. Go back, far back, and be
small. As soon as you have gotten back when you forgot
important things and recaptured them, you will indicate
it by your left hand rising. Go ahead, now, go back, get
little. Your head is shrinking, your legs are shrinking,
your body is shrinking, you're getting little and your hand,
as soon as you get there, will start rising. (*Pause*) Now
your hand rises. I'm going to bring it down and I want you
to tell me how old you are.

    Pt. Eleven.
    Dr. And do you see yourself somewhere?
    Pt. Yes.
    Dr. Where are you?
    Pt. In a little room.
    Dr. Tell me everything that's there, everything you see.
    Pt. My father is playing the piano.
    Dr. What else?
    Pt. My mother is there.
    Dr. Yes, who else is there?
    Pt. I don't see anyone.

    Dr. You don't see anybody there except your mother
and father. You are going to have a dream, and in that
dream you are going to see some other person. As soon as
you've had that dream, indicate it by your hand rising.
Go ahead, have that dream, you're eleven years of age, and

you'll see another person besides your mother and father.
(*Long pause, but hand does not rise. Apparently the repression
is too strong to permit recapture of memories at this time.
The patient is asked what he is thinking about.*)   Tell me what
you've been thinking about.

Pt. Nothing.

Dr. Now listen carefully to me. You're going to be
here tomorrow. Before you come, you will get a flash, or
a memory, suddenly, during the daytime, without any
warning, of your sister, as you knew her when you were little.
You may perhaps remember the incident or the place, but
you will be able to experience a feeling that you actually
recall something. Suddenly it will occur without any
warning.

Now, I'm going to give you a suggestion that when you
wake up, you will have forgotten everything, except a few
insignificant things here and there. When you wake up,
it will be as if you actually wake out of a sound sleep. You'll
walk over to the chair opposite me, and sit down. Then
you'll lift your head up and look at me. You will notice
that it will be impossible to keep from blinking. Your eyes
will actually go into a spasm, and they will continue until
I rap on the side of the desk near me three times, like this
(*rap, rap, rap*). When you hear the third rap your eyes
will suddenly stop quivering and blinking. You will have
forgotten most or all of the incidents that have happened
here today, but nevertheless you will follow the suggestions
I've given you.

If you have a desire to get well, to be a happy person,
to achieve the objectives that you're driving for, you will
have the desire to understand and analyze those factors,
fears, anxieties and terrors that have kept you from your
objectives. With the understanding of those factors, you
will better be able to work through your problem. You
will then be able to achieve those goals and desires that you

want. As you achieve those objectives, as we work through and analyze your problems, you are going to be a stronger and healthier person.

In a moment, I'm going to wake you up, by counting from one to five. When I reach the count of five, open your eyes, wake up, walk over to the chair, look at me, and then your eyes will begin blinking. It will be impossible to control them, until I rap. One, two, three, four, five. (*Patient follows these suggestions and blinks compulsively.*) Good. You have found it impossible to control the blinking. It's impossible to control it no matter how hard you try, until I rap. (*Rap, rap, rap.*) Now you can look at me steadily. Now you can look at me without blinking. How do you feel?

Pt. All right.

Dr. Good.

> *At the next session the patient revealed that he had gotten a glimpse of his sister in a nightgown. Following this he entered a state of resistance which lasted for a number of days and was terminated by a dream as indicated in the following session.*

Pt. I felt a little better, but didn't sleep much. I'm always worn out in the morning. When I get up in the morning, I feel as though I had an hour's sleep. Every once in a while, I'll have a few good days where I really feel as though I slept deeply, and I'll feel like a different person, but they're few and far between.

Dr. Yes.

Pt. There are just enough of them to make me realize what it would feel like to really feel well. I had some sex dreams, and the part that I remember was being in a hotel room with this girl. I remember looking out the window. There was an awful storm coming up. Then I had sexual intercourse with her, I was sitting there on the edge of the bed, and I was partially undressed, and I had an erection, and all of a sudden the door opened, and several elderly women came in, looked at me and uttered the most piercing screams. I knew of course this was disapproval, a lot of trouble if I was caught in intercourse with the girl. After all I'm certainly in a most compromising position especially as it seems as though I have an erection.

Dr. I see.

Pt. My association to the ladies I don't know. I know the girl seemed to remind me of a girl that worked for me eight years ago. I happened to speak of her the other evening. I remarked to my friend who was with me that she was still an attractive looking girl. She couldn't have been so young any more, but she was in the upper twenties or around thirty, seven or eight years ago.

Dr. I see. Now this scream, can you recall the nature of it?

Pt. Oh, it was a horrifying scream, it horrified me, too. As though she had witnessed the most terrifying scene, as though she had seen someone murdering somebody, or trying to murder somebody. It was all out of proportion to the thing, after all, after all; but it seems when the dream fades, it seems that it was almost not an abnormal reaction. You know what I mean?

Dr. Can you associate to the room now, this particular room ?

Pt. Small hotel room, something Spanish about it.

Dr. Can you see the furniture, as you visualize it?

Pt. Yes, something at the window, the window seat or something.

Dr. And in the room there were two beds?

Pt. It might have been a double bed. The storm I remember, there's a lot more to it I forgot.

Dr. What are your associations to the dream?

Pt. I know my penis was quite visible. I was facing the door when she walked in. It seems to me I had a premonition that somebody was running into what was the court. You know I had that feeling I was very worried in the dream that something was going to happen, and it did happen. Almost anticipated it happening, it seems to me, yet I don't know if I was expecting it or fearing it.

Dr. And this girl, was she undressed in the dream?

Pt. I don't remember.

Dr. Now the person who walked in, who might that person have been?

Pt. I can't imagine. She might keep the girls in line or something.

Dr. What about associations to women who wear glasses? What is the first thing that comes to your mind?

Pt. A school teacher, somebody who is a school teacher type.

Dr. School teacher type?

Pt. Yes, I remember a private school I went to. I went to private school except for one year. I went for one year to a public school, and I was most terribly unhappy in that school. I was afraid of the boys, the rough tough kids, Irish kids, and I was afraid of the teacher. The whole atmosphere of this school I went to, big classes of boys, fifty boys, I was always miserable and unhappy at that school.

Dr. What grade, what school?

Pt. Oh, I must have been about eleven when my nurse left. I remember in childhood, I remember things about my sister although it seems to me I remember very, very little even about my mother in this whole state. Of course, I did have this nurse, you see, from the time I was a boy until I was around eleven or after eleven. I remember very little about my mother, it seems I don't remember much about my father. And a lot of that I think is colored by my later associations with him. I can remember very little about the whole family.

Dr. What about this nurse, what sort of a person was she?

Pt. Well she was sort of an Irish type. I was terribly attached to her. I told you that when they let her go, I went to bed for many months, very depressed about it. Terribly depressed.

Dr. What did she look like, I mean what about her appearance?

Pt. Oh, she had brown hair and blue eyes, an Irish coloring, and there's not very much else about her.

Dr. Did she wear glasses?

Pt. I don't think so, I'm not sure.

Dr. Was she harsh, was she kindly?

Pt. I don't know, I think she was very kind and generous. Very fine, I believe.

Dr. Yes, and did anybody else in your family wear glasses?

Pt. No.

Dr. Nobody, your father, mother?

Pt. My father wore them, my mother didn't wear glasses. Father used to wear them for reading, and sometimes he wore glasses and the rim was sort of. . . . It couldn't have been my father, could it?

Dr. We don't know about that.

Pt. Is it possible?

Dr. Possible, yes, but we're not sure. Now, did you notice any sensations or feelings yesterday and today? You didn't sleep well last night you say.

Pt. No. I woke up quite early, and I actually don't feel rested. I feel so much better if I take naps in the afternoon or at lunch time, you know. I haven't been able to do it, I have been too busy lately. It used to pick me up no end. I always feel worn out, completely worn out. I have to whip myself. I don't remember at all about my sister. I can remember one boy I went with in public school.

He was much older, fourteen or fifteen when I was eleven. And he was epileptic incidentally. He used to get fits right on the street. I felt sorry for him; he was a very poor boy. I remember a fellow who used to go with him. He would admire my sister when he was up at the hotel. He made some remark, I don't know what it was, but I was shocked and horrified at the idea.

Dr. When he was at the hotel?

Pt. Yes, this boy; I can't remember my sister, but he had met her. I know he remarked to me that she was a good looking girl, and he made some sort of a remark which horrified me. After all he was an epileptic.

Dr. How old were you then?

Pt. I was about eleven or twelve.

Dr. Where did you live around that period.

Pt. Well at this time we lived at the hotel. Things were so bad that my father and mother used to send me down with the nurse to dine. The nurse remarked to me that when we were having dinner, my mother and father weren't going to eat because they were afraid they wouldn't have the money.

Dr. You lived at this hotel when you were around eleven?

Pt. Yes. To get back to the sleep. I'm preoccupied with my job. I worry and fret about it. Become preoccupied, wake up at two or three o'clock in the morning, and think about work. That makes me anxious. It's just impossible to put those thoughts out of my mind.

Dr. Well, those are usually covers for a much deeper anxiety.

Pt. That's right, it must be that because I see that there's no reason. I'm convinced of it, I'm positive of that, there's no doubt in my mind that it's covering up some other anxiety. Incidentally is it important that I understand the dream of you, of my coming to the house and the elephant chasing me? I imagine it's a type of dream that isn't important, but is it?

Dr. It may or may not be too significant at this point. What do you think?

Pt. I mean, through my relationship with you, I realize that I'm in a very difficult, I mean the only thing I might be able to say along those lines that I have felt when I came here was sort of an expectancy which was certainly not borne out. I mean there's no reason why I should have any present expectancy. I have noticed that I have looked forward to seeing you. Maybe it's just the relief of telling you these things; it might be important, I don't know.

Dr. It is very important for me to know how you feel about coming here.

Pt. Well that's what I wanted to tell you.

Dr. Now, supposing you go to sleep. (*Hypnosis is induced.*) As you sleep you are going to be able to dream the same dream that you had last night in all of its details. If you have forgotten any part of the dream, it will be possible for you to recall those parts. It will be as if you redream the same dream that you had in all details. And as soon as you've had the dream, indicate to me that you've had the dream by your hand, this hand, rising up a few inches. Dream the same dream all over again, and then tell it to me after your hand rises, tell it to me without waking up. Go to sleep very deeply, and then dream the same dream and tell it to me without waking up. (*Long pause.*)

Pt. The only thing I forgot was that after she screamed, she'd go to the door, and she was going to call everybody in the building.

Dr. I want you, as you lie there, to begin to associate to the dream. Tell me everything that comes to your mind.

Pt. The scream, the scream, she screamed, the person's terrible scream. I was scared, terrified. She screamed and she closed the door and made believe she was going to call everybody in the house and there was going to be lots of trouble.

Dr. I gave you a suggestion the other day that you would be able to remember an incident with your sister that had happened to you when you were little. I suggested that perhaps you'd remember or dream about it. In the dream you are in the hotel room, there is somebody in the room with you. Perhaps there is an association there, a fear of something that might have happened. Or perhaps this is merely a fantasy. I want you to know the truth, and you will be able to know the truth because you cannot hide the truth from yourself. Whatever happens to be the truth will come up. If it's true that you had, in the past, gone through a situation similar to that which you dreamed about, it will become apparent to you, you will know about it. It certainly is significant that there is no knowledge about what happened to you, no memory about what has occurred to you in your early life with your sister. As you lie there, I am going to give you suggestions that may begin a series of associations. I am going to suggest to you as you lie there that again you go back to a point when you were small, to the age of eleven, or around that period. It will be again as if you are back in that hotel. As soon as I talk to you next, you will get the impression, will feel that you are actually back to that period. Then, I am going to count from one to five rapidly. When I reach the count of five, a number will come to your mind. Speak it without even thinking about it. Whatever number comes that number will be the number of letters in a word, a significant word. That word will make it possible for you to recall something that happened. Then as soon as I get the number of letters in that word, I'm going to count rapidly from one to five, and every time you hear the count of five, a letter will come up. Perhaps the word will not be apparent to you; the letters may be in a jumbled order, that is they may not come consecutively. But after you have given me all the letters, it will be possible to reconstruct the word. I'm going to count rapidly from one to five. At the count of five, give me the first number that comes to your mind. One, two, three, four, five.

Pt. Six.

Dr. Now as I count from one to five, give me the letters that pop up into your mind. Don't repress them in any way. One, two, three, four, five.

Pt. N.

Dr. One, two, three, four, five.

Pt. E.

Dr. One, two, three, four, five.

Pt. A.

Dr. One, two, three, four, five.

Pt. J.

Dr. One, two, three, four, five.

Pt. N.

Dr. One, two, three, four, five.

Pt. E.

Dr. Are there any more letters?

Pt. I don't think so.

Dr. Now it's NEAJNE. I want you to bring them together in your mind, and when I count from one to five, let them rearrange themselves, and you'll see a word that will have meaning for you. One, two, three, four, five.

Pt. Jeanne.

Dr. Who is Jeanne?

Pt. I don't know.

Dr. Start associating. What was your sister's name? Do you know anybody with the name of Jeanne?

Pt. My mother's name was Jeanne.

Dr. Your mother's name was Jeanne. Listen carefully to me. When you wake up, I am going to put a pencil in your hand. The hand will then move as if it's being pushed by some outside force. You will pay no attention to what the hand writes; it will just move along. It will just move along as if it's been pushed by an outside force. You'll pay no attention to what the hand writes, it will just move along. It will just move along as if it's been pushed by an outside force. You'll pay no attention to what the hand writes. As soon as you wake up, you'll sit in the chair opposite me. I will put a pencil in your hand, and then the hand will write and elucidate on other important things that we're trying to solve. You will not be aware of what the hand is writing. It will move along, and it will write. Now start awakening. At the count of five, open your eyes and wake up. One, two, three, four, five. Wake up.

> (*Patient awakens and a pencil is put in his hand. His hand writes automatically, "mtherscrmd," a condensation of "mother screamed." It was apparent that his sexual problem with his wife stemmed from a fear of incest with associated guilt feelings and fear of punishment.*)

The foregoing case illustrates how inimical overwhelming experiences can shock the organism so that the ego may utilize the mechanism of repression in an attempt to blot out the experience. Traumatic incidents in early childhood are particularly damaging since the ego is so vulnerable that it cannot handle too much stress. All children undergo traumatic experiences as a part of the normal process of socialization. Not all children react to these experiences with pathologic repressions. Insecure children, and particularly those who have been rejected, are prone to respond catastrophically to such events as habit training, the birth of a sibling, the discovery of the differences of the sexes and early sexual experiences. The traumatic event acts upon sensitized soil and comes to symbolize the accumulated fears and tensions related to countless happenings which have preceded the traumatic event.

There are some conditions that improve or clear up on the basis of the ability of the individual to come to grips with the initial traumatic experience. The individual carries scars that relate to damaging experiences and conditionings at the hands of early authorities. On the basis of early traumatic experiences, either with the parents or with other important persons, the individual may develop certain patterns of behavior, certain defensive devices that disable him. For instance, he may repress a traumatic experience that happened very early in his life, and then go on attempting to repress all symbolic associations to that experience. His whole life will be mobilized around devices that intensify the repression. The bringing of the patient to a realization of his early traumatic experiences may rectify those symptoms that have as their basis a re-enforcing of repression. Some phobias, hysterical manifestations like amnesia, certain compulsions, and occasional psychosomatic symptoms fall into this category. In the traumatic war neuroses, recovery of the fantasies and fears related to the provocative traumatic incident may produce a cathartic reaction and a disappearance of symptoms.

However, for the most part one must not expect the recovery of a traumatic memory to remove all of the patient's symptoms, even when the latter are genetically related to the memory. The individual's attitudes and present day reaction patterns are to a large degree determined by previous conditionings. A countless number of experiences have occurred to make the individual what he is. It does not follow that the recall of early conflicts and inimical experiences will necessarily change the customary reaction patterns. It is as if a person is suffering from a focus of infection which damages other structures of the body. The removal of the original focus will ameliorate, but will not necessarily remove the secondary foci which must be dealt with individually.

Perhaps the most important effect of recall of memories is that it gives the patient the motivation to inquire further into the fallacies of his present reactions to people. If he can see that what he is doing now is a product of misconceptions gleaned from inimical past experiences, that present day reality is tinctured by his past, that many of his existing concepts are merely a carry-over of misinterpretations and fantasies that he had in early life, that he is a repository of anxieties that are rooted in past experiences, then he will have the motivation to want to change his attitudes toward people. The recovery of memories thus serves as a means of creating an incentive for change.

RE-EDUCATION THROUGH
PSYCHOANALYTIC INSIGHT

THE AIM of all rational psychotherapy is to get the patient to a point where he can deal more aggressively with life on the basis of increased inner strength and acceptance of himself as a wholesome human being.

In a re-educational approach utilizing psychoanalytic insight, an attempt is made to achieve this goal by bringing the patient to an understanding of the dynamic sources of his difficulty. The meaning of his symptoms is demonstrated to him as is their source in repressed conflicts. He is shown how his conflicts affect the state of his present psychobiologic functioning, the circumstances under which conflicts originated, and, finally, how he can change his prevailing attitudes and patterns of behavior toward a more realistic and productive adaptation.

The medium in which this reintegration of attitudes is brought about is a congenial relationship with the physician wherein a neurotic transference is kept at a minimum. Acceptance of insight is achieved by an appeal to the intelligent constructive forces in the personality. There must be an acceptance of the authority of the physician, and the relationship consequently is somewhat directive in nature. Hostility and other irrational emotions must be dissipated as they arise to keep the relationship on as realistic terms as possible.

The stages in therapy may roughly be divided into a number of categories. The first stage consists of establishing a relationship with the patient on the latter's own terms, provided these are not too unreasonable or neurotic. The patient usually seeks a directive relationship in which he can depend on the physician for guidance, and this may have to be respected temporarily.

Once the authority of the physician has been accepted by the patient, an effort is made to demonstrate to him that his symptoms are not fortuitous, but have their origin in fears and conflicts that condition difficulties in inter-personal relationships, with an inevitable generation of tension and anxiety. Hypnoanalytic technics may be utilized for the purpose of connecting the patient's symptoms with their dynamic source. He is shown that problems in his everyday existence have a disturbing effect upon him and that they aggravate his symptoms. His prevailing attitudes and fears are analyzed to demonstrate that they are a distortion of life. The reasons behind his interpersonal difficulties and their origin in experiences and conditionings with important past personages are constantly brought to his attention, in the effort to motivate him toward change.

Although an effort is made to maintain stability in the physician-patient relationship, the patient will always attempt to establish a neurotic transference. He does not deliberately and willfully engage in this drama; he cannot help himself from reacting to the physician with his customary strivings and demands, for he knows no other way of reacting. If the physician is astute and analyzes what the patient is trying to do in the immediate situation—his expectations, fears and fantasies—he will have an accurate blueprint of the patient's personality in operation, without having to speculate as to dynamics, and without having to dig up extensive past conditionings. Indeed, the past will be embodied in what he is doing in the present, for the patient's impulses and strivings contain the residue of his most important past experiences.

For instance, the patient may enter the physician's office and criticize a withering plant on his desk. He may then change the subject and proceed to reveal how victimized he is, and the misfortunes of his early upbringing at the hands of a neurotic parent. The physician may be lured into a snare by this talk, and if he does not follow up on the patient's casual comment, he may miss the fact that criticism of the plant is actually a projected repressed criticism of himself as an authority he believes is mishandling him as brutally as did his parent.

In re-education, the neurotic transference is not permitted to develop to disturbing proportions. Before it has gone too far, a clarification of the patient's attempts to wedge the relationship into the framework of his neurotic misconceptions usually brings the patient back to a realistic attitude toward the physician.

Therapy may be terminated on the basis of acceptance of the physician as a reasonable authority. On the other hand problems with authority may be so pronounced a part of the patient's neurosis, that it may be necessary to change the therapeutic relationship to a nondirective character, in order to permit the patient to develop strengths within himself. Only in this way will he be able to function without a parental prop.

When a nondirective relationship is necessary, a definition of the treatment situation will be needed. The patient may be told that the physician's directiveness and guidance may have the effect of infantilizing him. For one reason or another he has needed to depend on authority for security and direction more than has the average person. This has tended to make him feel weak and helpless. It will be necessary for him to develop assertiveness and independence before he can be liberated completely from his neurosis. He can do this by activity, and by making his own choices and decisions in the immediate therapeutic situation. He will probably be reluctant about doing this and may resent the physician for avoiding responsibility. He may see no sense in a therapeutic situation in which he has to carry the greatest burden of the work. However, so long as the physician tells him what to do and how to do it, he will continue to feel like a child in relation to a parent. He must learn how to plan and execute action through his own resources. This may be painful and take a long time, but the physician will help him understand why he feels he has no right to operate under his own power, why he is unable to develop his own values and goals. The physician, in asking him to make his own decisions and to think things out for himself, does so out of respect for the patient's right to grow.

Once a definition of the treatment situation is made in this way, the patient will be prepared to enter into a new kind of interpersonal experience that permits him to develop self confidence and assertiveness which will have an enhancing effect on his security and self esteem.

ILLUSTRATIVE CASE

THE FOLLOWING case illustrates the technic of re-education utilizing psychoanalytic insight.

FIRST SESSION (February 15)

The patient, a single man of thirty, applies for therapy with the complaint of a persistent headache which has been going on since the age of sixteen. In addition he complains of indecisiveness and fear of making mistakes. He believes his headache is responsible for his tension and for his inability to socialize freely. He is unaware of any personality problems or of any marked difficulties in his relationships with people. The initial interview reveals evidence of a fear of aggression and a resignation to the injunctions and demands of his parents. A neurologic examination is negative.

In this case the method differed from psychoanalysis in that the sessions were conducted along conversational lines, with little recourse to free association. No attempt was made to penetrate to the deeper unconscious strata, and interpretations were in interpersonal rather than libidinal terms. A method such as this is no substitute for orthodox psychoanalysis, but that structural alterations can be obtained in the personality is demonstrated by the Rorschach changes which were obtained at the end of therapy.

Pt. My trouble, doctor, is a headache I've had since I was sixteen, a terrible headache. I wonder if you can help.

Dr. You say that ever since the age of sixteen you've had a headache? Has that headache been constant?

Pt. All day long, when I go to sleep, when I wake up.

Dr. I see. Could you tell me where the headache is? Point it out to me.

Pt. It's hard to point out, Doc.

Dr. It goes across like a band?

Pt. Precisely.

Dr. As if a band is completely around your head?

Pt. Like that.

Dr. Does it extend into your eyes?

Pt. No.

Dr. Before you were sixteen, did you also have head-aches?

Pt. I had none. Well, I'd have them one day, say, then probably I wouldn't have them for months.

Dr. I see; can you recall the first headache that you had?

Pt. No, I can't recall it.

Dr. Tell me something about your work.

Pt. I was working very heavily as a clerk all my life in my father's hardware store.

Dr. How old were you when you started work?

Pt. I've been working ever since I can remember.

Dr. Did you resent working when you were little?

Pt. I don't know if I resented working.

Dr. But you resented not having time to yourself?

Pt. That's right.

Dr. Did you play with the other kids?

Pt. Not unless I sneaked out.

Dr. When you were able to get out and play with the other kids and have fun, did your parents resent your going out?

Pt. I don't know. They resented my going out; they wanted me to stay in all the time.

Dr. Could you tell me more about how you felt, about their wanting you to stay in all the time?

Pt. Well naturally, when you, when you do something that you actually don't want to do, naturally you resent it.

Dr. What did you do when you resented it? Did you show that you resented it?

Pt. Well, I'd blow my top.

Dr. What did you do?

Pt. I'd just holler, "I want to get out on time." Something like that.

Dr. Would they give in to you then?

Pt. No.

Dr. What would they do?

Pt. "Your job is still always here, that's all," they'd say.

Dr. What about your parents now, are they alive now?

Pt. Yes, they're both alive.

Dr. Are you living with them?

Pt. I am.

Dr. Do you have any brothers and sisters?

Pt. I have one brother and two sisters.

Dr. How old is the brother?

Pt. Twenty-seven. I am thirty years old.

Dr. And the sisters?

Pt. Twenty-five and thirty-five.

Dr. Can you describe for me the personality of your mother?

Pt. My mother? Well, I'd say she's a serious woman, likes things done right all the time, doesn't like any frivolity except let's say on Sundays when frivolity was to take place.

Dr. A serious woman who doesn't want frivolity.

Pt. Except at the proper times.

Dr. In other words she's inclined to be strict but not unbending.

Pt. Yes.

Dr. And your father? What sort of a person is he?

Pt. Well, he's a very gay fellow, he likes his fun. I get along swell with him, I'd say.

Dr. What about your brother and sisters, how do you get along with them?

Pt. Oh, fine.

Dr. You don't get in fights with them?

Pt. No, I haven't had a fight with them yet.

Dr. Do you get into fights with anybody?

Pt. No, I'd say I have an occasional argument with my brother, but it's more or less due to business problems, you know, things which we may or may not agree upon.

Dr. How do you get along with people in general?

Pt. Wonderful.

Dr. Tell me about that.

Pt. Well, so far as I know, I have no personal friends—enemies I mean, no actual personal enemies. I don't refuse anybody anything. I get along swell with everybody. I have as yet to hear any business man or personal friends of mine saying anything bad about me.

Dr. I see.

Pt. Not that I'm perfect, mind you, but essentially it is I don't bother any one. I go out of my way to make a friend of him, and it's happened in business already. My folks, as a matter of fact, didn't like the idea, but that's how I am.

Dr. You don't like to fight very much?

Pt. I don't like to fight at all.

Dr. And if somebody is pretty nasty or mean, you go out of your way to avoid trouble.

Pt. I go out of my way to sort of straighten things out.

Dr. I see, in other words you're a pretty equable sort of person?

Pt. I'd say that.

Dr. And you don't lose your temper very often?

Pt. Not very often, but occasionally I do.

Dr. What happens when you lose your temper?

Pt. Well, just say words, that's all.

Dr. Now I'd like to ask you about nervousness when you were little. When you were little, were you a nervous kid, or were you just an average youngster?

Pt. I think I was average.

Dr. Do you get depressed at the present time?

Pt. The depressions I have are mostly when I know I'm getting old, and I want to get married, and I don't want to get married because I have a headache.

Dr. You don't want to get married because you have a headache. Why does that enter into the picture?

Pt.   Well, I . . . now I'm thirty, and I find it very difficult to concentrate.   I notice I begin to get morbid all the time, so by the time I'm fifty, I won't be worth anything to anybody.

Dr.   Perhaps a great deal can be done to prevent that.

Pt.   (*Laughs*)   I hope so.

Dr.   Can you tell me about that dent you have on your forehead?   (*Patient has a slightly depressed area on his forehead.   A later x-ray, neurologic examination and electroencephalogram indicate no brain pathology.*)

Pt.   You see I had a fall when I was about ten or eleven years old.   Now I've had x-rays taken of that.

Dr.   I presume that you've gone to a lot of doctors about your headaches?

Pt.   Not very many, no, just a few.

Dr.   Did they x-ray your head?

Pt.   Yes.

Dr.   Did they give you a thorough examination?

Pt.   A thorough examination, scratched my feet, stuff like that.

Dr.   Did they look inside your eyes?

Pt.   Yes.

Dr.   Did they tell you what they thought the headaches might be due to?

Pt.   No, I never completed any doctor's treatment.

Dr.   Why was that?   Did you get impatient?

Pt.   Yes, I do get nervous very often.

Dr.   Well now, you must expect that you probably will get impatient here, too.

Pt.   Well, here's what I'm thinking now.   You say there is something that can be done for me?

Dr.   I shall have to complete my examination before I can tell you that.   Do you have fears of any kind?

Pt.   Yes.

Dr.   Tell me about them.

Pt. The biggest fear I have is the fear of making a mistake.

Dr. Can you describe that?

Pt. Sure I can. Let's say a salesman comes into the store and he wants to sell me something. Now from five minutes to another I can't remember the price of an article. I'm afraid to buy it, afraid it will be the wrong price. That's one thing. I'm afraid to make a decision that has anything to do with anybody else, business or my home. If it's only to do with me, it's different. But if it has to do with someone else, where someone else's voice must be heard, I'm afraid to make a decision. I know it's then that I actually start getting headaches. I mean headaches are what they are.

Dr. In other words when you have to make a decision that involves some other person, or for something for which you can be criticized, you get upset.

Pt. Exactly.

Dr. Then you begin to feel the headache increasing.

Pt. Exactly.

Dr. I see. Now what other fears might you have besides the fear of making a mistake?

Pt. There's nothing that I can think of.

Dr. Now how about dizziness?

Pt. I don't get frequent dizzy spells, doctor. I get dizzy while I'm on my feet, two or three times a year, probably that's normal.

Dr. Any stomach trouble?

Pt. No.

Dr. You mentioned that you were forgetful.

Pt. Well, it's this way. I've got to do two or three things, and I've got to keep concentrating all through, from the time I'm told to do it until the time I actually do it, in order for me not to forget.

Dr. Do people have to tell you to do it?

Pt. Well, if I'm supposed to do something, like, let's say if somebody goes to the store, gets a pound of nails, a bottle of shellac, and a brush let's say. If I keep concentrating on nails, shellac and so forth, from the moment they tell me until the time I actually get it in my hands, I remember. But let's say they tell me to get that thing, see. I say, "O.K. I'm going," and I leave and the list slips my mind, then when I get there, I find it hard to remember.

Dr. Without concentrating it's hard to remember.

Pt. Yes.

Dr. Can you remember things that you, yourself, tell yourself to remember, or is it only when somebody tells you to do certain things?

Pt. Well, it all depends upon the person. Now for instance your name I have never forgotten since the very first time I saw it in a book.

Dr. What about your relations with women?

Pt. I'm not looking to get married.

Dr. Because of the fact that you don't want to get involved with a person, due to the headaches? Do the headaches frighten you?

Pt. The only thing that I'm afraid of is getting old and feeble minded.

Dr. How do you sleep?

Pt. Well, I sleep fine.

Dr. Do you take any sedatives?

Pt. No.

Dr. Alcohol?

Pt. No.

Dr. Do you avoid people?

Pt. No.

Dr. Do you like people?

Pt. They're all right.

Dr. Now I'm going to briefly examine your eyes and nerves and then we'll go on from there. After this I will want to get some psychological tests.   (*A neurologic test is done which is negative.*)

REPORT OF PROJECTIVE TECHNICS (February 22)

Rorschach Record

Card I 10″	Reminds me of a map, the whole thing. It looks barren, deserted because of the black and the shading, also the shape. Reminds me of a polar region.	W FK map Additional FC′
	Could remind me of Jimmy Durante —caricature, shape.	D F Hd
Card II 30″	Looks like two dogs because of the shape. Looks like scotties. They have tongues.	D F AP
Card III 20″	Outside two men. Looks like they are trying to pull something apart.	W M HP
	Couple of kidneys because of the shape.	D F AT
	I don't see nothing.	
	Reminds me of the boot of Italy.	D F Geo.
	A stomach because of the shape, here is the tube and the color.	D FC At
Card IV	Is this supposed to remind me of something?	
29″ (Turns card)	Could be a crude form of family shield.	W F Embl.
	Looks like a rock formation with rugged edges.	D F Geo.
	X-ray of the spine in the center.	D FK X-ray
(Turns card sideways)	Two shoes because of the shape, the heel and the toe. They are all components of the shoe.	D F Clo.

Card V 3″	Butterfly or a bat. The whole thing because of the shape. That's all. The color reminds me of a bat.	W FC′ AP
	(Bottom looks like doctor's pincers or it could be a bean shooter.)	
Card VI 15″	Design on a carpet. The whole thing. Shape and shading.	W Fc Art
	(It looks like a black skin.)	
	(Looks like the shape of a cake like the Italians make. That is because of all the projections.)	
Card VII 35″ (Turns card)	Certain portions reminds me of the inside of a crab, near the eyes. The eyes of a crab look like that.	d F- Ad
Card VIII 17″ (Turns card)	Nice colors.	
	A corset because of the shape.	D F Clo.
	Couple of animals. Looks like a mixture of animals looking at their prey. They are tense ready to charge. A dog or buffalo.	D FM AP
	(Reminds me of an orchid. The whole thing.)	(W CF Flower)
Card IX 36″ (Turns card)	Heads of quadruplets. Prenatal because of the shape and the color.	D FC Hd
	Two hearts bisected or it could be one heart.	D FC m-Hd
	(The center looks like a flame thrower.)	
Card X 10″	Two caterpillars—green. Look like they are doing something.	D FM FC AP

Looks like a crab again. Shape and   D FM AP
motion.

An amoeba because of the color too. D FC A
I saw a picture of one.

That's all. There is nothing of
interest on this card.

Limits: accepts women as VII; Best, VIII; Least, X, IX.

R = 21 + 4
W = 5   M = 1   evasive content
D = 14   FM = 2   W: M = 5: 1
d = 2   Fm = 1   M: 2C = 1; 2½⁺⁺
                  F = 9 + 3   FM: Fc = 2: 2⁺
                  Fc = 1
                  Fc′ = 1
                  Fk = 1
                  FK = 1
                  FC = 5
                  CF = +1

Rorschach Analysis

The Rorschach is that of a constricted, "flattened out"
individual who is attempting to repress spontaneity and
responsivity.   There are a number of depressive, dysphoric
features which appear to be resulting in inhibition of ideational material.   Lack of productivity is apparently more
related to his present dysphoric, low mood than to dullness
of intellect.   The protocol itself is extremely meager, indicating lack of imagination, of creative urges and of constructive productivity.

Although he has an overt poise, the patient reveals much
underlying anxiety when he has to cope with a new and
seemingly unstructured situation.   He is a highly ambitious
person and seems to be under the pressure of strong "power
drives" so that his own recognition of the inadequacies of
his productions and his inability to overcome his anxiety,
are greatly perturbing to him.   However, he seems to have
little insight as to the basis of his perturbation and tends to

project onto the environment the results of his feelings of inadequacy.

He is at ease only in the most familiar, routinized situations and it is in such situations that he can bring his aggression to the fore. In relation to this it is felt that although he is a very passive person and has difficulty in handling his environment, he conceives of the environment, as he does of himself, as being empty and desolate. The experience of aggression seems very closely related to his own fear of attack and this may in part be the result of an attempt to keep from awareness of homosexual drives. His aggressive drives are repressed and kept in check and this is apparent in his sexual attitude as well. He cannot accept his libidinal urges, but it is felt that this is in part based upon his fearfulness of his inadequacy, and he attempts to cope with it by overemphasis on external factors such as social prestige.

Basically this is a dependent, passive man whose primary mechanisms are inhibition and repression, and these are being taken out on himself in the form of somatic symptoms.

His attitudes towards authoritative pressures are rather immature and he has not been able to develop a critical and rational approach in relation to authority. He is essentially a mother-tied person and dependency in his social and interpersonal relationships probably stem from his inability to break away from the mother surrogate.

He has a potential for warmth in his relationships, but it appears that he is so fearful of attack that he cannot relate his pleasurable affect with other people and that when he does it is very likely to be in a rather sadistic manner.

Reality testing is good. He can work effectively in the manipulation of pragmatic, everyday factors in living, but he has a great lack of awareness of what he is like in relation to others. He is having difficulty in accepting mature, heterosexual interaction and it is felt that this is due both to the fearfulness and to guilt which sexual activity arouses in him, and to the dependent relationship he has upon the mother.

On the whole this is the record of a neurotic individual with hysterical symptoms who at the present time is laboring under depressive moods.

Thematic Apperception Test Analysis

The T.A.T. reveals fluctuating forms of ego ideals. This is observed in the areas of his ambition, his desire to "reach the top," to be recognized and famous. It is almost as though he cannot accept such drives within himself and then indentifies with the lost, the displaced and those people who were never given an opportunity to show their worth.

The T.A.T. also confirms the Rorschach findings of an immature relationship to the mother. He tells a story in which a boy who "makes good" in a distant city constantly returns to his mother's home, attempts to get her to come with him, is never successful in this and is under constant conflict as to what to do about her. It is of note that in this story he conceives of the mother as highly dependent upon him. As a solution he leaves her a substitute and overcomes his guilt by hiring a man on the farm to take his place.

In response to a structured story he reveals a very beaten down attitude. When it was suggested to him that the individual in the picture might be a hopeless case et cetera although he did not adopt a completely hopeless attitude, it was one of: "Wait and see. Perhaps science will find something for him. I would just sit and wait." In this story, as in some of the others, there was indication of a rather high social awareness that could reach the point of moral masochism with him.

In regard to sex he seems to identify it with violence and he has so much guilt in this connection that in one story he consistently speaks of the man as: "He tried to lead a good life. He didn't do anything immoral. He tried not to get her into trouble. He was cautious and tried to be good, but he will have to call on the *family* to help him take care of her."

There is some suggestion that much of his conflict regarding his interpersonal relationships (on the level th t he is aware of them) is a resistance of his own dependence in that he feels that if he really wanted to get married, he would. This is both because he is not sure of his ability to love and also because of his expectations of support and push from the woman he might marry. He goes through a gyration of defenses regarding this need and ends up with a displacement of the whole problem onto a financial area. That is, it is necessary for him to make as much money as possible and to be as socially successful as possible so as to solve the problem of his interpersonal relationships.

It is the feeling of the examiner that there is much that is suggestive in these stories which would indicate that he has great difficulty in realizing that a multiplicity of factors are disturbing to him. Instead he seems to be seeking a single thing for an explanation.

Although there is so much emphasis on the passive, dependent aspects of his personality, he does show, on a peripheral level, the desire to do something positive about his problems, but is doubtful that this will be sustained.

In regard to therapy his underlying attitude appears to be somewhat skeptical. He has the feeling that it is quackery and seems to think he has reached the ultimate merely by coming here and expects an out-and-out cure. In relation to hypnosis he sees a man as being helpless on the couch and it is possible that he would consider hypnosis as an attack. His approach to therapy here seems to be a positive one.

SECOND SESSION (February 26)

*At this session the motivation is created for hypnosis and mis-
conceptions about hypnosis are removed.   Hypnosis is induced
and the patient turns out to be an excellent subject.   Because of
this an attempt is made to recover the incidents surrounding the
origin of his first headache.   The patient remembers an incident
at thirteen when, after attending a movie against his mother's wish,
he suffered an intense headache.   He is them reminded that there
may be reasons for the continuance of his headache at present, and
he is enjoined to inquire into their source.   Temporary posthypnotic removal of his headache is successful.*

Dr.   How are things?

Pt.   About the same as usual.

Dr.   Any dreams?

Pt.   Little ones.

Dr.   Suppose you tell me about them.

Pt.   I don't know if I can remember.   They were about girls.

Dr.   Could you tell me something about your adjustment with girls?

Pt.   I have no difficulty there.

Dr.   Are you interested in girls?

Pt.   Too much, if I'm interested.

Dr.   What have you been thinking of?

Pt.   About coming here.

Dr.   Supposing you tell me what you thi k about coming here.

Pt.   You see I suspected something was wrong, that's why I came here.

Dr.   You realize that there is a relationship between your headaches and other symptoms and things that happen to you day by day in your relations with people?

Pt.   I never really suspected that, doctor, but I can see what you mean.

Dr.   If it is true that your headaches are caused by some difficulty that exists in your everyday life, we must first find out what this difficulty is and then see if you can correct it. Only in this way will the headaches stop. Supposing you tell me what you have observed that aggravates your headaches.

Pt. I remember last time telling you about that, how I was afraid of making mistakes, remember. Also that I rarely get angry.

Dr. Under what circumstances do you get mad and do you show your anger?

Pt. Repetition of a mistake; if I do make a mistake or do something that's wrong, then my dad who sort of mentions it the first time, you see, he'll keep on repeating the same story, and repeating so that I lose my temper and I . . . see?

Dr. Is it that you get mad at him for keeping on picking on you?

Pt. Uh huh, I get angry at what he says.

Dr. When you have words with him, do you feel badly afterwards?

Pt. No, I feel relieved.

Dr. Does the headache feel a little bit relieved too?

Pt. No.

Dr. The headache is constantly with you. We have to find out what there is behind that headache. To do this we may use hypnosis. I'd like to work with you for a few sessions to see if we can make some headway. I'd like to work that way because I want to make sure that we are on the right trail. I don't like to work with a person unless I believe that I can help him. In other words, if by the fifth session you feel and I feel that we don't see any progress, I'll advise you to try a different kind of approach that may take longer. I want you to understand that if I feel that not enough progress is being made, I will tell you so. Do I make myself clear?

Pt. Yes, most clear.

Dr. Good. I want to tell you, before we go ahead with hypnosis, that dreams are very important. They can tell us a great deal about what has happened to you and what is affecting you right now, about the kind of a person you are, the kind of relations you have with people, and probably what is stimulating the headache. When you have a dream and you find it difficult to remember it, write it out for me. Bring me all the dreams that you remember. Now also you may possibly find that under certain circumstances the headache is better and under other circumstances, it's worse. I want you to see if you can get a relationship between events, emotions and your headaches.

Pt. All right.

Dr. Have you ever seen anybody hypnotized?

Pt. No, I haven't. Is it true that I will be at your mercy?

Dr. What are your feelings about hypnosis?

Pt. If it can help me, I want you to do it for me.

Dr. Good; however, I will help you help yourself get well. The way we are going to work is that you're going to feel that you, yourself, are participating and are therefore not at my mercy. I want you to feel that you, yourself, can work with me, that you are entering into the situation, and are not passive and helpless. With your kind of a problem there is a possibility that you may regard hypnosis as an attack on you. This idea will prevent you from going into a deep sleep. In other words if you are afraid of it, you are likely to resist going into a deep sleep.

Pt. Now I know, I won't be afraid of it. Now how will I know when I'm hypnotized?

Dr. When you are very deeply hypnotized, you'll find that you will be able to follow certain suggestions without effort. For instance, if I suggest that your hand is numb, and I touch your hand with a pin, you'll notice that there won't be any pain, while touching the other hand will produce normal pain.   Or you will notice that your lids get so heavy that they close and when I challenge you to open them, it will be impossible to open them.   Then you'll realize that you're hypnotized.

Pt.   I see.   There is one thing I want to ask you.   I just had it on my mind right now; supposing I know I'm not hypnotized, should I tell you?

Dr.   Of course.

Pt.   Um hum.

Dr.   Hypnosis is a state of drowsiness, not sleep.   You are not asleep.   You are conscious, fully conscious.   There is nothing miraculous or magical about it, and we don't want it to be that way because it is necessary for you not to feel as if you're a powerless person, at the mercy of someone.   That would make you feel as if you are a little boy and the doctor is the master.   We want the ultimate result to be that you are more assertive, more productive, more self confident.   We want you to be more of a grown-up person and less a child.

Now I'm going to ask you to sit back in your chair, lean back and clasp your hands in front of you.   Close your eyes and imagine that your hands are like the jaws of a vise. I am going to count slowly from one to five: at the count of five, your hands will be so firmly clasped together that it will be difficult or impossible to separate them.   One, tight; two, tight; three, tighter and tighter; four, very tight; five so tight that even though you try to separate them, it's difficult, extremely difficult.   The harder you try the tighter they seem, until I give you the command to separate them. Now, slowly open them, slowly separate them just like that; slowly pull them apart and bring your hands down on your thighs.

Watch your hands.   I want you to observe everything your hands do.   I want you to keep watching your hands, watching every movement, every feeling.   Become aware of

every sensation. Perhaps you'll begin to feel pressure in
your hands as they press down against your thighs. Perhaps you'll feel the weight of your hands as they press down
on your thighs. You may feel the roughness of the texture
of your trousers. Whatever you feel, I want you to keep
concentrating on your hands. You notice now that one of
the fingers is wiggling a little. Soon one of the other fingers
will wiggle and move, you don't know which one. Watch
the right hand. You don't know whether it will be the first
finger or the middle finger or the little finger or the ring
finger. The ring finger moves a little bit, you notice. Keep
watching your hand, and you will become aware of something very interesting. You notice that the hand will feel
light, and that it will get lighter and lighter. It will begin
to feel so light that it will slowly lift up from the thigh right
up in the air. It will lift and rise straight up in the air towards your face, lifting and moving and rising straight up
in the air, higher and higher and higher, straight up towards
your face.

As it rises, you become very tired and drowsy. As the
hand continues to rise, your breathing gets deeper and more
automatic. Your eyes get heavy, very heavy, and the hand
moves straight up towards your face. You get very tired
and drowsy. Your eyes are closing, closing. When your
hand touches your face, you'll be asleep, deeply asleep. The
palm of your hand will be up against your cheek, and you'll
rest your hand against your cheek, and you'll feel very
sleepy. You feel drowsier and drowsier and drowsier, very
sleepy, very tired. Everything seems to be floating in the
distance. Your eyelids are like lead. Your hand moves up,
up, up, right up towards your face, and when it reaches your
face, lean your head up against the palm of your hand and
go to sleep, go to sleep, go to sleep, just asleep. And as you
sleep, I want you to concentrate on a state of relaxation, a
state of tensionless relaxation, think of nothing else but

sleep, deep sleep.   (*Patient closes his eyes as his right hand touches his face.*)

I'm going to stroke the left arm.   It is going to get just as heavy as lead.   The heaviness will go from the shoulder, right down into the arm, elbow, wrist and fingers, so that the arm feels as heavy as lead.   I'm going to count from one to five, and at the count of five the arm will press down against your thigh.   One, two, three, four, five, as heavy as lead, as heavy as lead, as heavy as lead.   So heavy and so firm that it feels like lead.   As you sit there, it will get heavier and heavier and heavier, just like lead.   I'm going to lift it up in the air and you'll notice that it feels so heavy that it is just like a rock, stiff, and when you try to keep it up it comes right down.   It feels so heavy that it's just like lead.   Now it gets heavier and heavier, and stiffer and stiffer; the muscles stiffen up so that when I try to budge it, it is as stiff and rigid as a board—just like that.

> (*Patient seems so responsive to suggestions and in so deep a trance that it is decided to deepen the trance to somnambulism. This is, of course, exceptional for the first trance.*)

As you sit there, I'm going to suggest to you that you imagine yourself and myself walking out of the door.   We approach a church yard and you look directly overhead and notice the church's spire, and a church bell.   The bell moves You notice the movement of the bell.   Can you visualize that?

Pt. Yes.

Dr. As you visualize that I want you to hear the sound of the bell.   Listen and you'll hear the sound of the bell. As soon as you hear the bell, indicate it by your left hand rising about an inch, like that.   (*Hand rises.*)

Your hand comes down now and the next thing we do is walk into a school yard, and then into the school building. We enter a school room and you notice a blackboard.   Walk over to the blackboard and put down a series of numbers—

eight, seven, nine, four, three, seven, five. Then pick up
the eraser and remove these letters on the blackboard so
that the entire blackboard is blank. Can you visualize the
blank blackboard now?

Pt. Yes.

Dr. Good. Now listen to me, try to repeat the numbers.

Pt. (*Pause*) I can't think of them.

Dr. The fact that you have forgotten the numbers does
not mean they are not there. I will prove it to you. When
I rap on this table three times, the numbers will suddenly
return to you. (*Rap, rap, rap.*)

Pt. I remember now—eight, seven, nine, four, three,
seven, five.

Dr. That's right. You see you remembered. Important things are never forgotten. Every person has within
himself a residue of everything that's happened to him before.
In other words when you were a little boy, you had many
experiences that you cannot obliterate from your mind because they are a part of you. And it is possible through
hypnosis to revive these, to bring them up, even those things
that you believe you have forgotten.

I am going to demonstrate to you how that works. For
instance, imagine that you are getting very little, imagine
that you are getting smaller and smaller. Imagine that you
are getting so small that you're like a tiny child. As you
sit there, you'll notice that you get smaller and smaller.
Your head grows small, your legs grow small, your arms grow
small, you grow small all over, from your head right down
to your feet. You are getting smaller and smaller, so small
that when I talk to you next, you'll be exactly six years of
age. Possibly it will be at the time of your birthday, or
when you are at school. When I talk to you next, it will
be as if you are exactly six years of age. You will remember
things that occurred when you were exactly six years of age.
You'll be little, six years of age. When I talk to you next,

you'll be exactly six years old, and you'll be able to talk to me and not wake up. Now you are exactly six years old; when I talk to you and you answer me, you're exactly six. How old are you now? Talk to me without waking up.

Pt. I'm six.

Dr. And what grade are you in?

Pt. One.

Dr. Who's your teacher? Do you know your teacher's name?

Pt. Yes.

Dr. Do you have any friends at school?

Pt. Yes.

Dr. What are their names?

Pt. Frank, Jack.

Dr. And what about your mother and father? Do you like them?

Pt. Yes.

Dr. Are they good to you?

Pt. Yes.

> (*Because the patient is an excellent hypnotic subject, regression is decided on as a technic to recover memories associated with the onset of headaches. The rationale of the procedure is to acquaint the patient with the fact that his headaches have a cause and that they may now be produced by symbolically similar situations. This may promote the incentive for the patient to inquire into his present interpersonal experiences to discern reasons for his symptoms.*)

Dr. All right, now you are going to grow a little older. You're going to be seven years old. When I talk to you next, you'll be exactly seven years of age. You're seven years old now. How old are you?

Pt. I'm seven.

Dr. Do you get any headaches?

Pt. No.

Dr. Now you are going to grow older, you are going to

be at the age when you got your first headache, no matter
when that may be. When I talk to you, you must speak
very clearly and tell me what happened to you. When I
talk to you, you'll live through again what actually happened
when you got your first severe headache, no matter how old
you were, no matter when it occurred. When I talk to you
next, you'll be able to tell me all about it, how it happened.
(*Pause*) Now, how old are you?

Pt. Thirteen.

Dr. Do you have a headache?

Pt. I feel like as though I have a bad one.

Dr. What's happened to you?

Pt. I've just come back from a show.

Dr. Tell me all about it.

Pt. I was told not to go to a show and I went.

Dr. Who told you to go?

Pt. Nobody.

Dr. Did you want to go to the show?

Pt. I wanted to go. They wouldn't let me.

Dr. Who wouldn't let you?

Pt. My mother.

Dr. Why wouldn't she let you?

Pt. I don't know.

Dr. Well, did you go to the show anyway?

Pt. Yes.

Dr. And when you came back, you had a headache?

Pt. Yes.

Dr. Do you always do what your mother wants you to
do?

Pt. Yes.

Dr. Why?

Pt. I don't know, maybe I'm afraid.

Dr. Afraid of what?

Pt. I dunno—afraid I'll be punished.

Dr. Now grow older, to your adult age. As you grow

older, you must see if you still feel deep down that life is exactly the way it was when you were little, when you wanted to do what you wanted to do, but your mother said it was wrong and you felt it was wrong. You may not remember this when you wake up. Perhaps you will not remember it, but gradually you will be able to see and to understand how it was that your headache developed, and why it is that your headaches actually continue at the present time. You will see that better and better. Grow older, you are all grown up now. Do you understand what I said to you?

Pt. Yes.

Dr. Good; now when you wake up, you will notice a relief of the headache. Even though you may not remember what happened here, the fact that you have probed the sources of your problem will produce a lightness in your head and a beginning of disappearance of your headache. You will feel, perhaps for the first time in years, that it's all right for you to have done what you did. That you have a right to be happy and free, and you will experience considerable relief because of that. This will be the first step in breaking up your headache. You will realize that the headaches have a cause, and you will want to inquire into what causes them now.

I am going to count from one to five, and then suddenly you will open your eyes and feel yourself to be awake. Perhaps you will have forgotten everything that happened there, but you will definitely have a feeling of lightness in your head and a feeling that the headache is beginning to leave you, even though you may not remember what happened, do you understand me?

Pt. Yes.

Dr. Good; at the count of five open your eyes and wake up. One, two, three, four, five. (*Patient opens his eyes.*) How do you feel?

Pt. Dizzy.

Dr. Feel a little dizzy.

Pt. My head.

Dr. What do you notice in your head?

Pt. Ah, it's gone away now, the headache.

Dr. The headache is leaving you? Good; do you feel a lightness in the head?

Pt. Yes.

Dr. What do you remember?

Pt. I just can't think, it's hard.

Dr. All right, we'll make an appointment for next time.

THIRD SESSION (March 5)

The response to the last session was good and patient is able to recall the repressed memory he brought up with hypnotic regression. The memory is utilized to demonstrate to the patient the fact that many of his difficulties are rooted in problems in his relations with people. The dynamics of the patient's headache are illustrated by dream induction, and the patient is given a further explanation of his neurosis.

Pt. The afternoon I left here last time my morale was so high I could have licked a dragon.

Dr. Supposing you describe to me how you felt.

Pt. Well, I noticed I wasn't as tense as I used to be; I noted I wasn't tense at all; I noticed my headache was better, in fact it was gone for a while.

Dr. Were you afraid?

Pt. No, I wasn't afraid. I felt good inside.

Dr. I see.

Pt. I felt I could conquer the world.

Dr. How about the headache?

Pt. Well that was still there, but very much better. I still have a bad headache now.

Dr. Did you have any dreams last night?

Pt. No.

Dr. Do you remember much of what happened last time?

Pt. Well. . . .

Dr. It's sort of hazy?

Pt. I remember that I went to sleep and had a dream.

Dr. You had a dream while you were asleep here?

Pt. Sort of a dream.

Dr. What was that about?

Pt. Oh, first I saw an image, first my mother and then my sister. Oh, no, the first thing I felt was as though I was going skiing. Then I saw the image of my mother, and then I felt as though I was going up a hill and using, using my penis coasting up an icy hill.

> (*The oedipal nature of the dream is obvious. Recovery of the traumatic memory and expression of his resentment may have had a releasing effect on his aggressive masculine strivings. The icy hill may represent the feelings of coldness inherent in what he believes is his mother's response.*)

Dr. Up an icy hill. Now last time—I don't know if you recall it—but while you were in a trance we talked about your feelings when you were a little boy.

Pt. I seem to remember something about it.

Dr. We went back to an incident that happened when you were thirteen. You mentioned going to a movie. Can you tell me more about that?

> (*An effort is made here to see whether the patient has been able to master anxiety sufficiently to recall the experience on a waking level. The fact that he had no posthypnotic anxiety or anxiety dreams would indicate that he may be able to tolerate the implications of the memory consciously.*)

Pt. As it happened? Yes, I can remember now. Well, I was going to school at the time. Somehow I think it was some holiday, and we had half a day off, so my mother knew I was going to come back early. Instead I went to a show, and made some excuses that I stayed in school. But I happened to stay in the movie later than the regular hour that I should be home. It was about four-thirty when I got out of the show.   I was walking back from the show and while I was walking from the show I was thinking now what am I going to tell her.   She knows very well that I'm not in school as late as that, and I was thinking about it and worried about it.   And then I got this awful headache.   It's funny that I forgot all about that.

Dr.   She didn't know that you actually had gone to the movies?

Pt.   No sir, no.

Dr.   In fact, she warned you not to go?

Pt.   That's right.

Dr.   What about other members of the family.   Do you have sisters?

Pt.   Two.

Dr.   Brothers?

Pt.   One brother.

Dr.   How old is your brother?

Pt.   Twenty-seven.

Dr.   And you are how old?

Pt.   Thirty.

Dr.   What are your feelings about your sisters, what sort of people are they?

Pt.   Well, I got two sisters.   They are the type that could be talked to.   They won't ridicule you, they'll listen to you, and they in turn would talk to me, and to anyone else up there.   They're very sociable.   They don't get angry, and they just lead a pretty healthy, happy life.

Dr.   Now your feelings towards your mother?

Pt.   There's a difference.

Dr.   What are your feelings toward your mother?

Pt.   She likes to keep her thumb on you.

Dr.   What happens when some of the children do something she doesn't like?   What is her reaction?

Pt.   So far as I know, whenever the children do something she doesn't like, she just talks about it and says it's no good, or something like that.

Dr. What happens when you do something against your mother's desires?

Pt. Well, it's about the same thing, see, only I take it very bad when she talks to me that way.

Dr. What does she say to you?

Pt. She says, "Didn't I tell you you shouldn't have gone out," or something like that. "Why don't you come home early at night?" See? Then the following day when she gets out of patience: "Why did you come so late for? What did you do?"

Dr. I see, do you fight with her?

Pt. Well, we have occasional words.

Dr. To return to your headache for which you sought treatment, you must get to realize that the headache is a product of certain important emotional factors that exist in you, that are operating today, that possibly had an origin far back in your childhood. The headaches probably are associated with certain attitudes toward people. In order to get rid of the headache, it will be necessary to change those attitudes toward people that are responsible for the headache. When you do this not only will it take your headache away, but it will make you a more normal, capable person. Your tests show that you've got certain potentialities and some artistic ability. However your creativeness is being interfered with constantly. Do you have any interest in art or music?

Pt. Well I play the piano, by ear that is.

Dr. Have you taken any lessons in piano?

Pt. No, I just picked it up mostly.

Dr. You've never taken any lessons in piano? You're interested in the piano though?

Pt. I like it.

Dr. Have you done any art work, sculpturing, painting, or anything like that?

Pt. Nothing bordering on the arts.

Dr. Have you had any desire for that at all?

Pt. Well, when I was—I must have just started to go to high school—I was taking these lessons on the side, taking piano lessons on the side. I took about two lessons.

Dr. What happened then?

Pt. Well, I couldn't get, couldn't rob enough to pay for the lessons. My mother disapproved.

Dr. I see. Your mother didn't want you to.

Pt. No.

Dr. Did your father ever take your side in an argument with your mother?

Pt. No, my mother and father always stick together, no matter what.

Dr. I see, perhaps you will want to start music lessons.

Pt. I should start music lessons?

Dr. If you want to.

Pt. Ye gods, when am I going to get time to start music lessons?

Dr. At the time when you were little and stopped those lessons, you wanted them. They were something you wanted to do; but you were blocked. We haven't got all the answers to your problem yet, but we know a few things about you. One thing is that whenever you wanted to do what you wanted to do, a vague kind of punishment hung over you. Your mother perhaps is a domineering, rather overpowering person, but you wouldn't permit yourself to knuckle down to her completely. You did what you wanted to do, but you did it on the sly, and you punished yourself afterward. It was as if you said, "Boy, you are doing what you want, but it may be the wrong thing. You don't know when the ax is going to fall." In other words, your conscience tortured you for doing what you wanted to do when you wanted to do it. Do you get what I mean?

Pt. Yes, yes. I know you are right because that's the way I felt.

Dr. All right, now when a thing like that gets started in early life, it continues later on very insidiously. It is as if you say, "Life is so that if I do what I want I also have to make it appear that I am doing what my mother wants me to do. However, if I do what I want to do and my mother doesn't like it, I'm being bad and I've got to punish myself for it." Then you get mad inside and tension piles up. Now the absence of tension that you noticed yesterday is possibly explicable on the basis that you felt, as a result of our session, that maybe you have the right to be a free person, maybe you have the right to do what you want to do.

Pt. It was my mother that prevented me from doing what I wanted to do and I punished myself. Yes, yes, I see what you mean.

Dr. You were in a terrific state of rage inside with a fear you weren't doing the right thing. The rage and tension could have built up inside of you and created a headache. Let us assume this is what caused your headache originally. Now we have to ask ourselves why the headache continues and why it is constant with you. Do you still feel the same way? Do you feel that you have to inhibit yourself, prevent yourself from doing what you want out of fear of condemnation? Or do you sometimes do what you want and punish yourself later?

This sort of reaction is not uncommon. For instance, one of my patients had the same problem of headaches. He remembered an incident that happened to him when he was a child. On one occasion, he wanted to go roller skating with the other boys, but his mother refused to permit him to do this. She was afraid he'd be run over. She was an overprotective, domineering mother who was so insecure herself that she wanted to keep him home and watch him almost every minute of the day for fear something terrible would happen to him. But he wanted to be like all the other fellows. He saw the kids skating and wanted to do the same, but his mother refused to permit him to skate. He went around the corner and put on roller skates and skated along the road. As he skated, it occurred to him that his mother could see him from the window. So he took his skates off and sat on his stoop. As he brooded, he developed the most excruciating headache. However, he decided to skate nevertheless and did so in spite of his headache. From that time on, whenever he did anything that he knew his mother disapproved of, he had a very bad headache. He kept on doing what he wanted to do, he kept on defying his mother even openly, but he still punished himself with a headache. Do you see what I mean?

Pt. Yes, yes.

Dr. In other words, a parent, very early in a child's life, exercises great authority over the child. In the case of a boy, fear of the parent and a need to comply with the parent can create dependency and a fear to develop into a man. The person still feels like a child even when he grows up. He is afraid of being hurt. He feels tied down to the parent, and has the idea he is completely done in and licked. Do you believe you are dependent on your folks?

Pt. I don't know.

Dr. You continue to live with them, don't you?

Pt. I've got a bed there, get my meals, sleep there.

Dr. Did you ever leave home?

Pt. Yes, when I was in the Army.

Dr. What was your rank?

Pt. I was sergeant.

Dr. How did you like the Army?

Pt. I got along all right. The thing is whatever I was supposed to do, I did it well. Except that the fellows with the rank over you—well they sometimes abused the rank.

Dr. Did you feel at all compelled to do certain things that you, yourself, felt you could do better if you used your own judgment?

Pt. I'll tell you something, there was a first sergeant, and we were both on the same job, I was his assistant. Well, I had my way of doing things, and he had his way, see. And somehow or other, though eventually the work would turn out right anyhow, no matter who did it, he didn't like my work so much. He thought that I was trying to chisel in somehow or other, see? So he came to a point where knowing that I could do the job, see, he'd leave for a day or so, and come back any time he pleased. Work had to be done immediately, get it out, see, and I would do the work myself.

Dr. So he tried to take advantage of you?

Pt. He did take advantage, but I did what I was supposed to do.

Dr. Did you ever say anything to him about that?

Pt. Never did.

Dr. What about headaches in the Army?

Pt. They were pretty bad, constant.

Dr. Does it occur to you that possibly the same sort of situation was going on in the Army that had gone on in your own home, that exactly the same sort of situation might have existed in your relationship to the authorities in the Army, existed and exists right now in your relationship with your parents? You had to be a good boy, do your job, but inwardly you wanted to do certain things your own way.

Pt. Taking care of the laundry department at one time, I devised a method where, whereas we can tell who is ship ping out and who wasn't shipping out, you see, and have all the men in the squadron, that even though they did ship we could keep a good check on things. Well it was a pretty good system. And I brought it over to the officer in charge of arms, and he liked it very much, so he told me: "You keep on that system that you just picked up, and we'll see whether or not we can use it." For about six months they had me, just me alone, doing that particular system, but they wouldn't change the entire field although they liked it.

They wouldn't change the entire field, but they made me use that system, that system of mine.

Dr. I see, how did that make you feel?

Pt. Well, somehow or other I didn't feel too badly about it. You discount a lot of things you see in the Army.

Dr. Did you get mad?

Pt. No.

Dr. I want you to observe what happens to you at home, to see what causes your headaches to increase.

(It is apparent from this material that a repression of aggression is a component part of the patient's difficulties.)

All right now, supposing you lean back in your chair and go to sleep. Just relax yourself, watch your fingers, just keep gazing at your fingers, until finally you begin to notice that the fingers spread apart. This time, things will come faster. You notice that your eyes get heavy, become tired, and that very rapidly your fingers spread apart. Then they spread apart, lift, rise, and move right up to your face and touch your face. Lean your head against the palm of your hand, and go to sleep. When I talk to you next you will be deeply asleep. *(Pause)*

As you sit there, I'm going to give you a suggestion that you have a dream. The dream will indicate your greatest fear. As soon as you've had that dream, indicate it to me by your left hand rising about two inches. *(Pause)* Your hand rises, and you've had a dream. I want you to tell me about your dream without waking up. You've had a dream?

Pt. Yes.

Dr. Tell me about it.

Pt. I am going with a girl. We're going out in a storm. It's not real lightning. I'm afraid sort of what will happen to us if we go out and do something and get caught.

Dr. And now, as you sit there, you are going suddenly to feel as if you were in a theater visualizing a scene on a stage. When I say "Now," the curtains will spread apart and you will see what actually could happen to you if you were caught with a girl, doing something. You may see other people in that role, as if another person is with a girl, and that person will act exactly as you. The thing that you fear most will happen. When I say "Now," you notice that the curtain is spreading apart. You'll visualize it directly, and tell me about it without waking up. Now.

Pt. I was shot in the head.

Dr. You were shot?

Pt. Yes.

Dr. Who shot you?

Pt. I don't know.

Dr. Now I am going to take you back there to that scene. I will count to five. As I reach the count of five, an image will come into your mind. You have no idea what that image is now, but as soon as I count five, the image will come into your mind. Tell me the first thing that comes into your mind without keeping it back.

Tell me who that person is that shot you. It will come to you like a flash, don't repress it. Tell me the first thing that comes to your mind. One, two, three, four, five.

Pt. My mother.

Dr. Your mother. Here again is an example, as you can very well see, of how restrained you feel in doing what you want. Your headaches are apparently related to this problem of being restrained. You were shot in the head for doing something you wanted.

All people love their parents, but parents also can have a hindering effect on a person. They can prevent a person from growing up by certain things that happen in the early relationship. A person may even be impeded in achieving masculinity, in feeling like a man. Could this have happened to you? Perhaps a deep fear is like in the dream, a fear of being hurt or killed for doing what you want to do when you want to do it. Not only may this involve sexual activities, but also other activities.

More and more clearly you will see what it is that causes your headaches and other symptoms. If you correct the causes of your problem, not only will your headache leave you, but your relationships with people will become more aggressive and realistic. You will then become more assertive in everything you do.

I suggested to you when you were awake, that you might possibly benefit by taking music lessons. If you, yourself, feel that that is something you'd like to do, it would be very helpful if you went ahead with lessons. Now, if you do not desire to do that, you will analyze and understand why it is that you do not wish to take lessons.

I am going to count from one to five again, and at the count of five, slowly wake up. Then tell me exactly how you feel. At the count of five, open your eyes and wake up. One, two, three, four, five. Wake up. How do you feel?

Pt. Tired.

Dr. What is the last thing you remember?

Pt. I was to wake up.

Dr. And before then?

Pt. That I'm going to get better, that the headache will go away.

Dr. Eventually.

Pt. Eventually (*laughs*).

Dr. Well, now you understand that our objective is not only to remove your headaches, but to find out what bigger problems you have with people that need correction. How about the music lessons?

Pt. I really feel as though I haven't the time. I have enough relaxation if I go downstairs and play on the piano without taking lessons.

Dr. This is your own project. The only reason I suggested it was to see if you want to continue something that was stopped when you were little.

Pt.   I have little time, you see I work all the time except when I see my girl.

Dr.   All right, we will talk about that next time.

Fourth Session (March 11)

The patient, in observing his reactions during the week, reports discovering an increase of his headache whenever he entered an argument with a person. He reveals the fact that he has a girl friend seven years his senior, and that he maintains a detached relationship with her at the same time that he resents his bondage. It is obvious that he desires a dependent relationship with the physician. A strongly directive re-educational approach is utilized in the attempt to inculcate insight. An attempt is also made to begin to change the character of the therapeutic relationship so that the patient is more participating.

Dr.   What's been happening to you, since I saw you last?

Pt.   Well, what's been happening? You said last time you wanted to know when my headaches seemed to increase or not.

Dr.   Yes.

Pt.   They seemed to increase most always when I was in trouble, in an argument.

Dr.   When you had some sort of argument?

Pt.   That's right. I noticed that the day after I left you.

Dr.   You got into an argument with somebody?

Pt.   That's right.

Dr.   And you noticed your headaches increased?

Pt.   Yes, automatically.

Dr.   Did you have any dreams since I saw you last?

Pt.   Well, I had two dreams, but they don't have anything to do with the story.

Dr.   Suppose you tell me about them.

Pt.   Well, one is that a customer had to come into the store. She prices an article, and though she is not right, we let her have it at her price, and she ups and says, "I don't want it any more," and walks out. That's all.

Dr.   Did you react to that?

Pt.   No I didn't react to it, except that I answered her back and didn't get a headache.

Dr.   And the other dream?

Pt.   That generally is something on the same style. Some one came into the store, paid for something, and the old man refused to give it to her.

Dr.   What does that bring to your mind.

Pt.   Nothing.

Dr.   The last time you started talking about your girl friend.   Supposing we carry on from that point.

Pt.   Well, you want to know from the beginning, or what?

Dr.   Yes, from the beginning.

Pt.   Well, I met her at the store.

Dr.   Your store?

Pt.   My store.   She seemed like a very nice girl and we got acquainted.   I put the question to her when I felt she wanted me to.

Dr.   How long did you know her before you put the question to her?

Pt.   About a month, I'd say.   I found enough nerve to ask her.   I actually didn't have enough nerve to ask her. I thought that she was above me.   She speaks well, and carries herself well, she looks wonderful—a nice girl.   And we've been together for about seven years now.   She lives in the neighborhood.   We've been getting along fine.   She used to take a fit when I'd say that sometime we'd have to part.   So I just talked kind of love talk.   The way she looks at it, she'd keep on going with me until we both die. She's perfectly satisfied the way things are.

Dr.   What does she do?

Pt.   She's a clothes designer.   She was married and divorced.

Dr.   She doesn't want to get married?

Pt.   No, so it seems; that's the way she talks anyway.

Dr.   How old a woman is she?

Pt.   Seven years older than myself.

Dr.   Does the age disparity make any difference to you?

Pt.   No, some, no, not too much now, I mean.

Dr.   Is there anything about this situation that gets on your nerves?

Pt.   Well, one thing, I like her to a certain extent in that she's more or less convenient to have around.   She's a good person to talk to; she's very understanding.   She's more or less the encouraging type, you know, doesn't knock you down, always keeps on encouraging you and things like that. When the first time I went with her, I did have to set her back from feeling that I wanted to protect her against anything, you know.   I wanted to be sure she wouldn't get in trouble, as well as keeping myself out of trouble.

Dr.   In the years that you've gone out with her, have you gone out with other women?

Pt.   Actually we both have a complete confident faith in each other.   We know we won't hurt each other.   She won't go with other men and I won't go out with other women just as long as she's around.   And she's there any time I want.

Dr.   How often do you see her?

Pt.   I see her only once a week.

Dr.   Do you have a desire to go out with other women?

Pt.   It's not necessary.

Dr.   You haven't met any other woman that particularly appealed to you?

Pt.   No, I wish I had.   You see a beautiful girl come into the place, you know, and, well naturally, you look at her, and she's nice; but that's as far as it goes.   I wouldn't think of asking her out.

Dr.   Why?

Pt.   I don't know, I'm pretty well satisfied the way I am.

Dr.   But are you satisfied with things the way they are?

Pt. I think I am.

Dr. Then what fault do you have to find with your present friend?

Pt. The fault that it's still on the Q. T. We still have to sort of hide. That's why I can't take her out. I can't walk with her in my home. My mother would shoot her down in the street. I don't want anybody to know about her.

Dr. Why not?

Pt. Why should I? Now why should I have anybody think that she's been going with someone else? Understand? On the chance that someone actually does ask her to marry, well her chances of—shall I say the fact that she's been going out with me would limit her chances of having someone take her over.

Dr. In other words, if another man came into her life and wanted to marry her you wouldn't object.

Pt. No, I wouldn't.

Dr. So you couldn't be too much in love with her.

Pt. I don't love her, I said I liked her.

Dr. If she weren't around, would you then go out with another woman?

Pt. I think I would, yes.

Dr. What would happen if she found you going with another woman?

Pt. Well, so long as we're together, naturally I don't think she'd like it. In fact I know she wouldn't like it.

Dr. But if you did go out with someone else?

Pt. I don't know. I intimated if the relationship would break up what would she do? She said, "When you think that you're going to break up, that you want to get married, let me know."

Dr. In other words she's willing to let it go along on this basis?

Pt. That's right.

Dr. I see, she lets you lead your own life and you see her on your own terms.

Pt. That's right.

Dr. Now what do you do with yourself all the rest of the week?

Pt. We've got a neighborhood show on the corner, and I go every other day or so. Otherwise I stay home, play the radio, read. I'd like to read more, but somehow when I do read I read just words.

Dr. You can't concentrate?

Pt. I can't concentrate.

Dr. How far in school did you go?

Pt. I graduated high school.

Dr. Do you feel that you just can't absorb what you read, or what?

Pt. I can't absorb it.

Dr. Well, now, let's get back to the headaches. What have you learned about your headaches, so far, since you've been coming to see me?

Pt. Well, the only thing I've learned about my headache is that now I seem to know how to fight it off. I mean if I know I'm going to do something, I just go and do it, and sort of control my emotions to the extent that I prevent myself from getting headaches.

Dr. For instance, can you describe that more clearly?

Pt. Well, for instance, before I came here, see, I used to be afraid to do what I wanted. Take my brother who works with me. He's funny type of fellow, I mean hard to explain. And he has no expression on his face, you know. The only expression that he has is a growl. When you tell him that you're going to leave the place for a while and he's going to remain there, he more or less, shall I say, resents it, see. Well, I used to be afraid to leave the store for a cup of coffee, see; but now I just tell him, "Look, I'm going for a cup of coffee down the street, I'll be back a little later."

Dr. In other words you go ahead and do what you want to anyway. And when you go ahead and do what you want, do you stew within yourself?

Pt. No, I don't, but I used to.

Dr. You're able to be more aggressive in what you want to do. You go ahead and do it.

Pt. Yes.

Dr. What about the headaches, has that made any difference, have there been any periods when you've been clear of headaches?

Pt. I haven't been clear of headaches, but there are many days that it seems to me as though it's slightly lessened, shall I say?

Dr. The intensity?

Pt. The intensity is lessened. As a matter of fact I used to talk with some salesmen, see. I used to be afraid to talk to them because I couldn't concentrate well and my speech would come out in stutters. I noticed that for this past week I more or less controlled my speech even better. And I talk more fluently, and it wasn't too difficult to concentrate.

Dr. Possibly you feel we are getting closer and closer to the cause of your headaches which was bound down originally with the fact that you were not permitted to do what you wanted to do. You remember our discussing that?

Pt. Yes.

Dr. The last time, you said you felt that you could not, of your own free will, do things that would make yourself happy, that you had to keep them secret. You remarked that you felt that if you wanted to do certain things something terrible would happen to you. This probably caused feelings of rage that exaggerated the headaches. Now, learning about the first experience when you had a headache teaches us that there is a relationship between your headaches and a fear of doing something wrong. The fact that you felt that something bad would happen to you, if you did what was opposed to what your mother wanted, caused you much difficulty. What may be going on now is that there is a repetition of that same thing, not only with your mother, but with everybody. You have to be retiring whenever you are in an argument, and when you want to assert yourself, you feel that you cannot. This may cause much resentment and contribute to the headaches. Last week you noticed that you could express and assert yourself with your brother and the salesmen and that you felt better, not worse. However, there probably is still a need to hold on to your neurosis.

Pt. Why should I want to?

Dr. There is a part of every person that does not want to get well, that wants to hold on to his neurosis. This is because the neurosis yields certain dividends for him. You probably will want to hold onto your neurosis the way everybody else does. You can't get away from it because there are elements of your neurosis that are valuable for you. You want to get rid of your symptoms, of course, since they cause you difficulty, but the things that create your symptoms may continue for a while. As a result of your early life and relations to your parents, you felt powerless to do what you wanted to do. You feared your mother and possibly your father. When you defied them, you were punished; but even when you did something forbidden they knew nothing about, you punished yourself. This condition by now has become a habit. Part of you now continues to have a childish attitude toward your mother and toward all authority. You have a feeling like you had when you were little, as if you haven't yet grown up. You hold on to the idea that it is wrong for you to express your own mind, to do as you want to do, to be aggressive, assertive and to lead your own life.

It is unfortunate that economically you're tied down to

your family even though you obviously earn your living in
the business.   To work elsewhere would give you a better
chance of overcoming this problem.   In the eyes of your
mother, you are still the little boy.   It takes a long time for
mothers to realize that their baby has grown up.   You
cannot depend on her to arrive at this idea.   You will
have to force her to accept the fact that you are grown.
This is your own problem now and you will have to take
steps to overcome it.   As a result of experiences with your
mother, you've built up a conscience that is very, very strong
and that punishes you and makes you want to act like a
little boy and do what he is told.   Part of you probably
wants to be dependent on your folks.

Gradually you will discover that you have the right to be
grown up, to be free, to do what you want to do.   You will
say, "I will be a free man if it's the last thing I do."   When
you do, your headaches will start getting better because you
will not be afraid nor filled with rage.   However, the resistance to getting well will try to stop you.   You may say
"My God, if I do that then nobody will like me.   My mother
won't like me, my father won't like me.   I won't even like
myself.   I'd better not do that; it's dangerous.   I'd better
be a little boy and hang onto my mother's apron strings.
I'd better just restrict myself and not be aggressive."   It is
going to be a fight for you to overcome these ideas.

With your girl friend, you may be working through some
of these same patterns.   After all, she is not your mother,
but part of your attitude toward her is as if she were a mother
figure.   What makes the relationship difficult for you is
that you may feel restricted by her and tied down.   You've
got to be faithful to her, and at the same time you don't
want to go too far with her.   You are in a trap there, as
much as you are in a trap with your family and in your work.

So far as your work is concerned, you don't have to give
up your job if you don't want to.   If, for instance, you went

out and got yourself another job, you might find it easier to work out the problem.   But mind you, you probably still would adopt the same attitude toward your boss and toward the people you work with that you have towards your folks. As a matter of fact, there might be some advantage in your tackling this thing at home.

Pt.   Even though I do what I want to do, I still have that feeling that what I do is wrong, as if I should be punished.

Dr.   If a child gets spanked for doing something wrong, then sometimes a child will want to be spanked if he does something wrong, to get the punishment over with.   If a person with a strong conscience like yours does something he thinks is wrong, he may punish himself as you probably do with headaches.

Pt.   But the thing is, how can I stop it?

Dr.   All right, that's our job.   It may seem tough, but we can do it.   We've got to do it, haven't we?

Pt.   Perhaps.

Dr.   You just can't go along the rest of your life with this thing.   Not only is it a matter of your headaches alone, but it is your whole life that's involved.   The headaches are just like the smoke from fire.   The fire that is causing the smoke is the pattern of your living.

Pt.   Do you think if I got married, there'd be any difference?

Dr.   Possibly not, because the kind of a woman that would appeal to you most might not be the one to whom you could best make a good relationship.   When your relations with people straighten out, your marriage will more likely be a success.

Pt.   You mean to tell me that if I got rid of this headache, my taste for women would change?   I would like a different type of woman?

Dr.   More probably when your taste for women changes, your headache will go too.   Involved in your neurosis is a special attitude toward women. That attitude possibly gets you into a jam.

Pt. Do you think so?

Dr. Do you?

Pt. I don't know.

Dr. All right, now supposing you lean back in your chair and go to sleep.

Pt. Give me a little help this time, will you? Just don't sit back and let me do it all (*laughs*).

Dr. We will have to figure out what that means. Perhaps you resent taking an active role and want me to take over all the work and make you well. You will see that should I do this for you, you would feel as if you were being treated like a child. You would resent it very much.

Supposing you gaze at your hands, just gaze at them, and as you do, you will begin to feel a sensation of drowsiness sweep over you from your head right down to your feet. Go to sleep, deeply asleep. Your hand rises, touches your face and you are asleep. When I talk to you next, you will be deeply asleep. (*Pause*) What is puzzling you most?

Pt. I can't figure out how I got the way I am. Tell me more.

Dr. From what we know now it seems that when you were little you developed a kind of relationship to your mother in which you felt that you were obligated to do what she wanted you to do, in which you were more dependent upon her than you should have been. It is likely that you had to repress yourself from doing certain things that you wanted to do for two reasons; first, to avoid punishment, second, to avoid losing the affection of your mother. Later on this kind of reaction was transferred to people in general, and your own conscience became as severe as if your parents continued to supervise you. The consequences are that you think you must do the right thing at all times. And when you do what you feel to be the improper thing, you suffer.

Let us try an experiment. Suppose you try to be more aggressive this week. You are going to become more aggressive this week, even more aggressive and outspoken than last week. You're going to be able to do things that you didn't do last week, things that will help you become stronger and more self confident. You can utilize the following suggestions if you so desire. You, yourself, must be the judge of what you want to do. If you want to go out more with your girl friend you can also adopt a more realistic stand. You will want to break out of this little, tiny shell that surrounds you. You will want to be more self expressive and assertive.

Now I am going to give you a suggestion. I want you to dream of what happens to a person if he does what he wants to do. As soon as you've had that dream, wake up and tell me about it. (*Pause, following which patient awakens.*)

Pt. I just had a dream. In the dream I feel I'm doing what's right to be happy, getting better. I can get married and be happy. But there is some one on the corner. On the corner of that dream I can see mother looking down at me. I am very, very small like. She is just looking down at me.

Dr. Your mother is big and you are small. This may be one of the kernels of your neurosis.

FIFTH SESSION (March 18)

The patient reports remarkable progress in the past week in his relations with his parents and girl friend toward whom he is acting in a much more assertive manner. He is a great deal more talkative in the session and participates more actively in the therapeutic work. His aggressiveness extends into the relationship with the physician. He is encouraged to observe the dynamics of his neurosis and warned about a possible relapse.

Pt. I've improved this week.
Dr. You have improved.
Pt. How've *you* been feeling this week?

Dr. You got the drop on me this week (*laughter*). How are things?

Pt. As far as I am concerned it's better than it ever has been.

Dr. Yes?

Pt. I find that the headache has disappeared for long periods. It never happened before.

Dr. I see.

Pt. And so far as doing anything is concerned, I feel I have more confidence all the time. Not afraid to speak, not afraid to face people. I seem to be putting up all right, making a fight for it.

Dr. You won't take it lying down?

Pt. No.

Dr. Good. How have you noticed that this confidence has expressed itself in relation to your family?

Pt. Well, so far as I know they don't seem to feel hurt about it, and I don't seem to feel as though I'm depending on anyone.

Dr. Fine. In other words they're able to take the activity on your part without blowing up.

Pt. Nothing happens.

Dr. Nothing happens; were you afraid that it might?

Pt. Very much.

Dr. Tell me about that.

Pt. Well that was before I came here.

Dr. Before you started treatments?

Pt. Yup, I was afraid to do most anything. I was afraid of what they thought of me. I didn't think that they'd like my way of doing things, and I was afraid to do it because I was afraid they'd have some talk about it. I'd hold myself back when I wanted to do something, and when I did want to do something, I was afraid and I'd go around and scratch my head and be bewildered. Now it's more or less getting to where I can do what I want.

Dr. Now that we've made a little progress, we're going

to have to take another step forward. Treatment will be a process of steps. Now what about your relations with your girl friend? Has anything happened there?

Pt. As a matter of fact this week somehow I got to like her even better.

Dr. Perhaps you adopt a different attitude toward her.

Pt. I used to be a little afraid of the association. I thought that it was wrong—wrong to a certain extent. But I'm not as afraid as I used to be of that.

Dr. Have you had any dreams?

Pt. Well, one dream that I kept on my mind purposely that I dreamt this Saturday night. I felt as though I was in a room with another woman, and we were making a display in the center of the room with oil cans, see?

Dr. You were making a display in the center of the room?

Pt. Exactly, with oil cans, on a shaft-work, sort of, on a counter in the center of the room. To make my display we were cutting up cardboard, then making one complete cardboard and pasting it on top of three or four cans, so that we can place the other cans on top of that, so that the other cans can't topple over. We're cutting them in strips, sort of. I make a long strip before the entire length of the cans of oil and then another strip. And I make a couple of strips in quarter inch pieces, and I make those strips a little longer. I don't know this woman, I never saw the girl, but somehow there was something in our mind, panic about something, panic, I don't know. So when we had the display finished, she heard someone coming to the door. There's three doors in this room, one, there, exactly where that is there. One right where that is, and one right about here. Now when she heard the knock at this door, she immediately goes into that room there, goes through that door, and a man comes in. And right away I know there's something between me and this man. I don't know what it is, but there's something between us. Just when he comes in another lady comes in through this door. So as soon as both of them come into the room, I get in back of the counter. When I get in back of the counter, he gets over on this side, see. I was on one side of the counter, he was on the other side, and he picks me up, lifts me right up, see. He's a big strapping fellow and picks me right up with one hand and takes me over to the other side of the counter and says, "I'm going to break your neck." So I says, "Go ahead, do what you want to do with me afterwards, kill me, break my neck, but that woman" I said, "well she, she'll make up for it in court. She'll take you to court and win besides, and make you pay for what you're doing to her and what you're going to do to me now." And that's all.

Dr. Does that make any sense to you?

Pt. Well, I tried to analyze it. Somehow or other I got the impression that this other woman was my girl. That's the impression I got, that she was my girl.

Dr. And this other girl?

Pt. The other girl I somehow or other don't know.

Dr. Were you attracted to this other girl?

Pt. No, I wasn't. This fellow I know had something against her.

Dr. You were not afraid of him even when he was capable of vanquishing you?

Pt. It's true, it's true, I wasn't afraid of him.

Dr. You weren't afraid of him.

Pt. I wasn't afraid. I knew he was holding me up in his arms and saying: "I'm going to kill you." I wasn't afraid, I actually said, "Go ahead and do what you want to do. What she's got on you, she'll take you to court, and by God they'll make you pay for both things."

(*As will be seen the dream points to fear of a powerful male in the face of activity, possibly of a sexual nature, with a woman. However, the patient does not feel entirely helpless and threatens his assailant with retribution for his malevolence.*)

Dr. Are you able to see any connection between the way you've been, your headaches, and your relations with your parents? Are you able to figure out any connections?

Pt. Well, I feel as though there is a direct connection between my parents and my headaches.

Dr. Supposing you elaborate on that.

Pt. Well, I mean that restriction they used to keep on me, that certain power they had over me that made me fear them, that power is more or less, that power I can feel it.

Dr. Has there ever been a man you've been afraid of, something like in the dream? Has there ever been a man that you were mortally afraid of?

Pt. No.

Dr. What about your father?

Pt. I've never been afraid of him, I mean afraid, of being afraid of my dad. Maybe I was afraid a little, before I mean. Now if this thing would have happened a couple of months ago, that happened today, I would have felt pretty low and blue and moody and all that stuff. I know damn well I would have got a terrific headache, too. You see, I ordered some twenty-five cases of paint. So as soon as they come into the place, he called me up to him and says, "You know, we've got a lot of paint today; why did you order twenty-five more?" I says, "So," I says, "I ordered them, I need them; take them and that's all." And that's all that happened. I didn't get no headache. I usually would, I wasn't afraid to talk back to him, and I usually am. That's exactly how I felt with my dad. Any time before I did something, he'd want to put the O.K. on it, and he'd have to put the O.K. on it, or I couldn't do it. Therefore when I did want to do something, to order something, I was afraid to do it because I was afraid of what he would say.

Dr. It's very necessary at some point in an individual's life for him to take a stand with his parents. If you were a little child who didn't have brain power and couldn't think as clearly as your parents, you'd want their advice and you might feel you were doing the wrong thing. But after all you do know the business, you know what is needed. You are no child any more. Your judgments are as good as anybody's.

Pt. I'll give you an instance.

Dr. Yes.

Pt. About a month ago I was reading the papers and I was talking to salesmen, and I was more or less convinced that all kinds of oils were either going up in price or they were going to be scarce in the market. I noticed every single day. I read in the paper that the prices were going up constantly, and the prices at wholesale still remained the same. I said eventually the market has got to break; I know damn well the price has got to go up eventually. So I put in an order with various companies for about two hundred cases of oil, all different kinds. Some came in. Those that did come in we gave away at a half way decent price. Well the fact is I wanted to keep the price down a bit so far as retail was concerned, and turn it over and buy again. So it happens that my father sees that as I predicted a couple of months back it is happening. Oil is getting scarce, and oil actually did go up this week and the week before. So he says, "Do you know what we'd better do," he says, "We'd better stop selling oil and keep it on the side for a while." (*Laughs*) Well, there you are, that goes to show you that it's a matter of making a good guess or not.

Dr. Yes, you can use your brain power.

Pt. See, the one store we have now, it's a pretty nice place now, but we're just barely making out here. So that we have to do something, expand.

Dr. Perhaps you want to start a store of your own and break away from the folks.

Pt. I thought of going in for myself, but then I think of the fact that my folks actually have been sacrificing. No

two ways about it; they have been good to me. I couldn't
say that I wanted a pair of shoes and couldn't buy them. I
couldn't say that I wanted a suit and couldn't get it.
They've been all right all the way around. As a matter of
fact, we attribute our success to the unity in the family.

Dr. Still you have a decisive step to make, an objective
to look forward to, and that is for you to plan your life in
accordance with what you feel you want to do. Do you
have any ambitions for your future?

Pt. Yes, of course.

Dr. Supposing we discuss that.

Pt. Primarily, I'd like to make a little dough so that I
could marry. If I get married I'll be happy. I think I will
be. But I won't have any going here and going there. I
like home life. I like to stay home occasionally and just
listen to the radio and things like that. I do those things
at home, but I mean it's not the same thing as a marriage.

Dr. Marriage is a final objective for you?

Pt. I would like to have two, three, four, five, six daughters, maybe seven, I can handle it. And make my people
proud of me, have my wife get the life from me she needs,
have children and give them what I didn't have as a child.

Dr. What can we do to take a step forward to getting
those objectives?

Pt. Oh, how I'd go about it? First I'd get the store,
which is a very difficult thing to do nowadays, but I'm sure
I could find one. And then naturally I'd set it up right, the
right merchandise matters, I mean, take your store seriously,
let people know that you're there, get your business in.

Dr. Do you have the initial capital?

Pt. Oh, you can borrow it, sure.

Dr. It would be your project rather than your family's?

Pt. I—we always work together.

Dr. Perhaps you could be the motor behind things.

Pt. I could be the motor. My father is very conservative. He wants to make sure that when he puts his foot down there's no quicksand. He is very conservative. He wants to make sure that the thing is going to turn out his way, no two ways about it. He can't go wrong when he makes a decision. He makes it because he knows it is going to turn out as he said it would, see. Whereas I, myself, I'm a little different, I gamble. I'll take a step; if it comes out, it comes out; if it doesn't, so what? But why does that scare me?

Dr. It does scare you?

Pt. Not so much now, no.

Dr. The other business of getting married. There's no reason in the world why you shouldn't, but you've got to have one thing in mind: if you enter into the wrong kind of relationship with your wife, you're going to be in the same boat as you were with your mother.

Pt. Well how will I know which is which when I find her?

Dr. You'll be better able to understand and sense that as time goes on. When you find a woman who wants to wear the pants, you'll feel more comfortable, but you will also pay a penalty. You have to wear the pants.

Pt. It's better to do things to please myself?

Dr. Absolutely; you're the fellow that's not on the bottom then.

Pt. But I was always impressed with the fact that it's the motherly type of woman that is a successful wife.

Dr. A maternal type of woman need not be domineering. I am thinking more in terms of a person who is going to take you over and direct your life. If you permit that you will suffer. If you marry the wrong kind of woman, you are apt to enter the same kind of relationship with her as you did with your mother. You will find yourself obeying her, doing what she wants you to do, and it's not going to work for you. It will take longer to find the right kind of woman, but you can do it.

Pt. Then you recommend that I get married?

Dr. If you think you want to get married.

Pt. I do.

Dr. It will take courage to break out of your home; because your folks may not like letting you leave home.

Pt. There was an argument at my house Sunday night.

Dr. What happened?

Pt. My brother, John, as I told you before, he's the dead pan type, he started to talk to me and I didn't bother answering. I didn't talk to my father, too. He's nobody's fool; there ain't nobody going to take him over. As far as business is concerned, he's better than I am. He fights for his point. He isn't going to be made a sucker out of for nobody. Well, it just happens that when my brother comes home, he's always gloomy. He's always gloomy. Sits down or sort of stands there and doesn't talk to nobody. Doesn't even start the conversation in all the years I've known him. So my mother is wondering why is it he's like that, see. And so my father starts to ask, "What could be the matter, boy, what could be the matter," he says. There's no use getting mad about it, no use getting mad at him, because it's not going to do anybody any good. So my mother right away, she thinks of me, that I'm coming to you. And once a person goes to a psychiatrist, he's got to be crazy. That's what they figure. So I go into the room where my brother is and say, "What do you say? Why are you this way?" And the first thing he tells me is, "Well," he says, "you made Mom unhappy. You talked back to her." So I said, "Well I can't help that." I said, "That's not the only reason why she's crying. It's because she sees you this way," I said, "and she doesn't like it." I said, "Well, while we're talking about this, what's eating you up?" So he says, "Don't bother me. When I'm in the mood I'll talk to you." So he gets up out of the couch and walks out. Naturally he came back in time to eat. Now I noticed that when my mother was crying, I sort of felt so helpless, and I noticed at that very minute that I got a headache.   Actually it became intense.

Dr.   When your mother began crying?

Pt.   Exactly.

Dr.   That's interesting, isn't it?   Almost as if her hurt is your hurt.   Almost as if you were guilty.

Pt.   I guess so.

Dr.   All right now supposing you go to sleep, deeply asleep.   Gaze at your hand until you are asleep.   When I talk to you next you will be asleep.   (*Pause*)   Now have a dream and tell me about it without awakening.   (*Pause*)

Pt.   For no reason at all my mother is scowling at me. And I was telling her "Why, I didn't do anything," I kept on repeating, "Why, I didn't do anything."

Dr.   Now, you're going to have another dream which will explain to you a little better what is behind your headache. You have been making good progress.   You have been able to see the connection, to some extent, between your headaches and your relations with people.   You have not yet discovered all the things that keep the headache going.   Is it due to guilt feelings on your part in relation to your mother, as if in some way you are hurting your mother?   Is it a restriction of your assertiveness, your self confidence, your ability to do what you want to do?   You are beginning to feel more assertive, still with some trepidation, still with some fear that you are not doing the right thing.   You find that you're capable of getting away with it.   You must go one step further.   You must find out why you bind yourself down to your family so that you deny your own masculinity, assertiveness and desire to be independent.   It is necessary for you to grow because you have the capacity. You want to go forward, be more assertive, more aggressive, more self confident.   You want to get better and rid yourself of headaches, and to advance in your own development, don't you?

Pt.   Yes.

Dr. If you do, you need feel no guilt about it. You must liberate yourself from that neurotic feeling.

Now I'm going to count from one to five, and at the count of five open your eyes and awaken. As soon as you wake up, a scene will appear in front of you. You remember the dream you had about setting up the oil cans, and cutting the cardboard into strips? As soon as you wake up, the activity of that dream will become more clear to you. Just don't force it, let it come spontaneously. One, at the count of five wake up; two, three, four, five. Open your eyes.

Pt. I saw, saw the cans when I was fixing, when I was displaying this week. I remember cutting up strips of cardboard and bending something into shape, about the same size as the strips on the oil can.

Dr. Yes, and are the oil cans just like the oil you mentioned to me that you ordered?

Pt. Yes.

Dr. So it may have something to do with your own activity. Doing something you want to do.

Pt. Yes.

Dr. How do you feel?

Pt. All right.

Dr. Good, then we'll see each other next week.

Pt. I'll tell you another thing. Just when I first started to dream, an object did come to my presence. A boy whose head suddenly grew big, like this, see. And somebody was beating him on the head with an ax, with a hammer sort of, or else that all of a sudden he was engulfed. He disappeared, then he'd pop up again, see, with his big head, he'd pop again and then was engulfed in a fog.

Dr. A little boy who was being beaten over the head with an ax may really be you.

Pt. You know, doctor, I meant to ask you. Doctors usually at times fool their patients to make them believe certain things. For instance, I know very well that I need some sort of intelligence and also need some sort of lessons to get ahead. And you know I need them, yet you told me that I had both. Have I really, or are you kidding me?

Dr. If I were kidding you, we couldn't make any progress. If you didn't have intelligence, I couldn't talk to you the way I do. I would tell you frankly, "I don't think I can do anything for you." What is the sense of my wasting my time and you wasting your money, if we don't feel you had the potentialities for development and growth? My own professional integrity would prevent me from doing this because I want to see results. I don't like to treat a person forever.

Pt. On the other hand how would I know that you actually put your professional integrity before money, shall I say?

(It will be noted that the patient is displaying the same type of aggressiveness with the physician that he has displayed at home with his family.)

Dr. That's a good question. I think the only thing that can teach you that is experience and the feeling that you are making progress. Have you been making progress with me?

Pt. Sure.

Dr. Where do you think the progress came from, by magic?

Pt. No, I've got to do my own concentrating, put my mind to it.

Dr. Yes, don't you think you know you are on the right track?

Pt. Sure

Dr. Of course ups and downs are to be expected. You might have a relapse and suddenly give in to your mother. You may be afraid that you've done something wrong and have a terrific headache. You may want to stop being assertive. You may have set backs but you will learn from each set back.   Set backs are to be expected, and you cannot let them get you down.   You've got to go forward in spite of any relapse.   You have no other alternative.   You can't go backwards any more, can you?

Pt.   Of course not, actually when I put my mind to it.

SIXTH SESSION (March 25)

Patient reports further progress in that he decided to stay out late one night in order to go to a dance. In spite of having a good time, he responded with a headache. The dynamic significance of this symptom is pointed out to him. He discusses an inability to stand up to his father, and a great part of the session is spent in elaborating on his relationship to his father. Under hypnosis he arrives at the idea that he may harbor death wishes toward his father.

Dr.   What's happened in the past week?

Pt.   Well, for the first time since I got out of the Army, I went, I went dancing.   Well, I spent a time, had a good time, let go.   I stayed until about three o'clock.   As I was coming home, I didn't feel nothing; all I knew was that I was getting a headache because I was out too late.   I got home. The minute I was at my door I had the same feeling that I had before.   I was going to get hell because I was so late, you know.   They expected me to be out late, and yet there I was having a headache.

Dr.   That should be a very good demonstration to you of what actually goes on.   Previously you accepted the headache without even thinking about it.   Now, even though you expect it and know why, it will still be there because such things don't change immediately.   But your knowledge and insight of the connection between your headaches and a feeling of doing wrong will give you the best chance of adjusting your life so that your symptoms need not be with you.

Pt.   Outside of that I had no other trouble.

Dr.   Did the headache get bad?

Pt. It wasn't bad. I met a girl there, a friend of the family, see, and I had a few dances with her. I just hung around for an hour before I even danced. And then after she left, well, I still wanted to dance, so I just picked on anybody, see. But I mean, I've just got to have my right type of girl or I can't dance.

Dr. What type do you like?

Pt. Well, she's got to be lovely.

Dr. You mean very good looking?

Pt. That's right.

Dr. Older or younger?

Pt. Just so she's good looking, that's all.

Dr. There are lots of good looking women around.

Pt. I know, but where are they?

Dr. If you go around enough, you'll probably find one.

Pt. I seldom want to go anywhere. Now, the last night a woman asked me if I wanted to go to the fights with her. I more or less didn't care to.

Dr. Maybe we can work on that; maybe we can find out why it is you don't like to go out.

Pt. Well, my family don't restrict me now, they don't hold me back. That can't be why I stay home.

Dr. Perhaps we can find out why. How have you been feeling in general?

Pt. Pretty good, but I noticed that Sunday and yesterday and even today I had that headache, probably from staying out too late.

Dr. Did you have any dreams?

Pt. I remember having a dream, but it's so vague, I just couldn't remember it now. But it was a pleasant dream, I know that. I know if it was something very bad, I'd remember it. I'd awake and try to remember it. It was something half-way decent. There's no connection anywhere; at least I don't think of any connection.

Dr. It is quite an amazing thing that the headache will

stay with you, so long.   Almost as if you expect something
bad to happen.   You must be convinced by this time that
the headaches have a definite connection with right and
wrong.

Pt.   I was going to say also that yesterday and today that
something happened that I didn't like, you understand?   It
happened between my father and myself.   I find it very
difficult to fight it off, to say, well the heck with it.   I find
it very difficult these two days.

Dr.   Can you be more explicit about that?

Pt.   Ah, for instance, we're, we're putting up some cases,
you know, one on top of the other, and I didn't like the way
my dad was doing it.   I didn't tell him that I'd rather work
alone and do it my way.   At least I'd know where I can
find the various articles, see.   So he insists on doing it his
way and naturally we started arguing.   And I didn't give
him an argument there, so I said, "Go ahead, do it your way,
ɔut I don't like it," and I just didn't fight at all.

Dr.   You wanted to do it your way?

Pt.   Now it actually, actually did come out my way you
see.   He did find out that it was better to put it in straight
as I said than to put it one here and one there as he decided.
But, nevertheless, although it was done that way, I sort of
find it difficult to fight off that feeling that he wanted to do
it his way.

Dr.   In other words, even though he did it the way you
wanted, it was very difficult to fight off the feeling that
maybe it would have been better his way?

Pt.   Yeah.

Dr.   What do you figure that's due to?   It must have
some sort of significance.

Pt.   I don't know.

Dr.   Maybe you still feel that your parents are right, and
that you must be wrong, even though you know darn well
that your judgment is as good as theirs.   Maybe you expect
that they still treat you like they treated you as a little boy.

Pt. You mean I actually expect them to treat me that way yet? I don't feel as though I expect it. But here's the other thing. They're getting on in years. It gets to a point now where I hate to hurt them for anything at all. I'm trying, I try my best, although I'm doing a very poor job at it, I'm trying my best, to try to eliminate as much worry as possible from their minds and body. That's what I'm trying to do. Somehow or other it just doesn't work out like that. See, when I try to do something, there's a conflict of minds.

(These rationalizations serve obviously to reinforce the patient's resistances.)

Dr. When you do something, you immediately begin to feel that there's a conflict of minds. You have two alternatives, you can alter what you think they expect of you, or you can still go forward. I talked about resistance before, resistance against moving out of your neurosis. One of the elements of that resistance is inertia and lack of ambition, a little voice inside that says, "Why do you want to do anything? You might as well stay home. What good is it going to do you to get out with the boys?" And one reason for that inertia is that part of you is afraid of exposing yourself to a headache. Your parents did not slap you down, but your own conscience punished you. It's not pleasant. Since Saturday night you've had a terrible headache. Now the memory of that may be enough to make you want to stay home and not get into any more messes. The way the resistance disguises its motives is to tell you, "What the heck are you going to get out of it? All you'll get is a headache." And you may say to yourself, "What the heck do I want to get myself involved in anything that will cause me a headache?"

Pt. As a matter of fact, I know it's bad myself. For instance, my Dad—I work for my Dad and he does certain things I know is wrong, and he knows is wrong, see—now,

I tell him, "Pop, it's no good, it's wrong. Do you notice it's not right?" He won't admit that it's wrong. Although he can see he's wrong, he won't admit it. And yet I want to make him see where he's wrong. Somehow or other I get a sort of satisfaction out of telling him he's wrong. Now it's only with him. In the store there's a couple of boys working there. They're complete strangers. I know when they do something wrong, I do not assume the same attitude as I do with my father. If they're wrong, at times I even overlook it; but when I do see it's wrong it's got to be corrected. I do it in a very good way that they don't have no offense, see, and I show them where they're wrong, and I show them the right way. But to my father, if he does something wrong, I have to show him where he's wrong even if I hurt him doing it. I don't go on to be diplomatic like.

Dr. Perhaps we can clarify some of your unconscious attitudes towards your father, what possibly may underlie a feeling of that kind. There might somewhere be a fear of him. You may not know it, and it may take a disguised form in your getting in the first lick before he comes back at you. Let's tackle it and see if there's something going on in your attitude toward your father.

Now supposing you go to sleep. I want you to lean back in your chair, make yourself comfortable, put your hands on your thighs, watch your hands, keep gazing at them, and as you gaze at them, slowly your hands will rise and lift, and you'll go into a deep, restful, relaxed, comfortable sleep. Keep watching your fingers, and your eyes will get tired, the fingers will spread apart, the hand will move up, will rise and lift. When it touches your face you'll be asleep. Your hand rises, your breathing gets deeper, and you go into a deep restful, relaxed, comfortable sleep. Go to sleep, go to sleep. (*Pause*)

Now that you're asleep I am going to talk to you. I am going to repeat what I said before. You have gone a long way towards finding out what is behind your headaches, and you've been able to see that there is a fear of punishment when you feel you are doing the wrong thing. The fear of punishment originally may have existed in some other form. Perhaps the fear was of doing something that you wanted to do when you were very little, even before the time when you went to the movies.

You've been able to see that finding pleasures in things you think will be interpreted as wrong has an effect upon you of causing a headache that persists, just like the dancing on Saturday. You have also noticed that you have an inertia about leaving the house. We have to understand what that inertia is. It may be in some way connected with a feeling of anticipation that if you go out, you're doing the wrong thing for which you'll be punished.

Now a problem that we have to solve is what still makes you feel it necessary to do the right thing all the time. You will be able to solve this partially here, partially through your experiences outside in your relationships with people. Do not get discouraged. It is important for you to do what you want to do, like going to the fights tonight if there is any pleasure in it for you.

We have now several things we must solve. One is about the fear of doing what you would like to do. The second is about your relationship with your father. We want to know what factor your father plays in your life, and why it is that you want to prove him wrong.

As you sit there begin to feel yourself getting very, very little. Feel your whole body getting little. Your head shrinks, your body shrinks, and your arms get small. Your legs get small, your feet get small, almost as if you're returning back to childhood. Return to a period in your life when you did something you wanted to do and felt it was wrong. Now as soon as you regress back, as soon as you get little, indicate it by raising the left hand. (*Pause*) Your hand has risen. How old do you feel now?

Pt. I'm eight.

Dr. Tell me exactly what you were thinking about.

Pt. With the boys, the swimming hole, I used to go swimming there. I might as well go from the place.

Dr. What would happen if you didn't?

Pt. I'd probably get hell.

Dr. I see, did you want to go?

Pt. Yes, I wanted to go.

Dr. Now as you sit there, imagine that your father walks through the door. Do you observe him? Do you notice him? Tell me what that feeling is.

Pt. Feel I don't want to go near him.

Dr. Do you have any idea why?

Pt. He seems to be very angry.

Dr. He is angry?

Pt. Yeah.

Dr. Why?

Pt. He was going to work. He had a little, little wagon, and I'd take the wagon up and go down the street with the boys. One day as I was coming down, the wagon sort of took off. the wagon shoved me off, and he began hounding me. He started to holler at me and hit me.

Dr. Now, as you sit there, dream about your father. Have a dream which involves your father; no matter what the dream may be, as soon as you've had that dream tell me about it without waking up. (*Pause*)

Pt. Now dad came from a very poor family.

Dr. Yes?

Pt. He knows the value of working and making money. There's no two ways about that. And the boy is to stop school and working out, and he can't see any reason why he shouldn't stay at this time to make some money and help the family out.

Dr. That's your father?

Pt. Says I should work.

Dr. And you like to play?

Pt. Yeah.

Dr. Now, listen to me. Start growing up. You are grown up now, asleep. Even though you are grown up, you probably still have with you the conscience of a child who has absorbed the prohibitions of its parents. That conscience tortures you; that conscience makes it very hard for you right now. It's necessary to break it up a bit. No harm can come to you. Your father and your mother really want you to be happy now. It's not necessary for you to work all the time. Your father may imply that, but you know it is not necessary. You've got to have pleasure, you've got to do what you want to do because you have a very rigid, a very punishing conscience, and we have to undermine it a bit so it won't torture you so much.

Now, as you sit there imagine that the pressure of your mother and fahter on you lifts a bit and that you can do exactly what you want to do. I want you to have a dream which will signify and indicate what it is that you want to do deep down underneath. As soon as you've had this dream, tell me about it without waking up. (*Pause*)

Pt. I see my mother and father very happy.

Dr. Yes.

Pt. I can see them going off. Don't do that to me. I want to get married myself and have a family, also have my own business and be happy. I have a right to it, to it.

Dr. There is no earthly reason in the world why these objectives, which are reasonable and part of the right of every human being, cannot be achieved. There is no reason in the world why you can't be happy, why you cannot have fun from life, why you cannot do those things that are so necessary for you to do in order to make yourself happy. If you so wish it, it will be easier to express your own desires and wishes, to feel that you are no longer a child who's being victimized by his parents.

I'm slowly going to count from one to five. At the count

of five, wake up and you'll have a flash in your mind.   A
thought will come to your mind.   The minute you wake up,
a thought will come to your mind that will be quite significant to you.   As soon as this thought comes to you, tell me
about it.   One, two, three, four, five.   Open your eyes, wake
up.

Pt.   (*Pause*)   I hate to say it.

Dr.   What?

Pt.   It's very bad.

Dr.   Tell me about it.

Pt.   I almost wish my father was dead.

Dr.   We should understand why.   We should learn a
little more about it, why you might possibly wish he weren't
around.

Pt.   I'd be free to do what I please.

Dr.   Does he weigh you down, does he inhibit you?

Pt.   He never gives me credit for doing something that
he could not have done better.   If it is bad, it's the usual
thing.

Dr.   That makes you angry at him.

Pt.   I'll tell you one thing, though.   I know that a few
months after I'd been out of the Army, we had a little discussion at the table, sort of argument with my father, my
mother and myself.   I felt they would be happy if I died and
got away.   I actually, I went inside and started to cry, like
a baby, actually sobbing.   It actually did hurt me that
much.   My mother naturally came out and comforted me,
and told me he didn't mean it the things he said.

Dr.   All boys go through a period when they wish their
father weren't around.   They don't really want to kill their
fathers, but feel like it or wish he were dead.   It's just a
feeling, that's all.   You can't be blamed for a feeling, but
you can't run away from it, either.

Pt.   Well, deep down my father, I tell you he's really all
right, but he's hard to live with.

Seventh Session (April 1)

Progress continues in the patient's ability to express aggressiveness and to experience himself more as a person with rights and capacities. Guilt feelings that he may be hurting his father through his increased independence produces some resistance to change. Under hypnosis re-educational therapy is continued. A dream under hypnosis to do something he wants to do and to notice the reaction of his parents, produces a headache. The opportunity is taken to explain the mechanism of his symptom, and a strongly directive approach is utilized to get him to make a decision about his right to come for therapy without needing the permission of his parents.

Pt. I feel a lot better.

Dr. Do you? In what respect?

Pt. I could also be a lot better. I used to bring you pretty big problems in the beginning, and all of a sudden it is bogging down somewheres.

Dr. Supposing we discuss what is happening, and in which way you bog down.

Pt. For instance, my mother says, she says, are you still going there? Going to see you. "Don't tell me you're going there again," she says. Then she adds on that, "I don't see any improvement. You're going there wasting your time, and he's taking your money, and you don't seem any better." She says that because this week I was arguing with my father and standing up to him.

Dr. And she considers that a sign of lack of improvement?

Pt. Why would she consider that a lack of improvement? I always argue with my dad now and she figures my coming here I should be improving.

Dr. In other words she feels that in order to get well you should accept everything. Just like that.

Pt. Uh hum, just like that.

Dr. Well, in what way are you bogged down? By that you mean that you slipped back?

Pt. No, it isn't that I slipped back; there's no further improvement this week.

Dr. I see, in other words you have been consistently, week after week, showing improvement, and this week you retained your gain but showed no further improvement?

Pt. Exactly.

Dr. What about the headaches?

Pt. Well it's just that they seem as though they're gone from here. (*Patient points to the back of his head.*)

Dr. They're gone?

Pt. They're gone from back here, but a dull feeling is in front.

Dr. There's a dull feeling still that remains on the front?

Pt. Exactly.

Dr. Were there periods this week when that headache became more extreme?

Pt. I can't remember any, except when I argue with my father. I control that headache now better, though.

Dr. What about other areas in your life?

Pt. Well, this is the first week that I didn't see my girl friend. I decided to go dancing once. Not too much fun.

Dr. You stayed mostly at home during the week?

Pt. Yes.

Dr. Do you think your mother is going to affect your attitude about coming here?

Pt. No.

Dr. Why not?

Pt. Why should it? I want to get well.

Dr. Good. Do you think you've got the desire to fight for your health?

Pt. I just, well, doc. . . .

Dr. We'd better lay our cards on the table, because we've got to know what we are heading for and where we're going. There's no sense in you're coming here and wasting your money. You have a lot of good fighting stuff in you, and you want to get well; but you also have a problem that wants to tie you down and prevent you from progressing.

Pt. Well, that's what I want to know. What should I do to prevent that?

Dr. You can't do it by sheer force. All you can do is work at it patiently. You must not expect consistent improvement. The resistances will keep trying to pull you back. Eventually you will convince yourself that whatever ties your family have on you, they are ties you felt as a child. They don't have to apply now. As an adult you are a different person than you were as a child. As a child when you wanted to do what you wanted to do, you were strapped down, prevented. Now you have the right to your own life.

Pt. There's a lot of child in me yet.

Dr. There is still in you the child that wants to hold on to your family, that is afraid to be assertive. Did you have any dreams last week?

Pt. No. I sleep heavy now, I never slept heavy before. The least little noise would wake me up, like that. When I was angry at father, I couldn't sleep.

Dr. Last week we took up your relations with your father, and we brought up the fact that your father seems to make demands upon you. He has an attitude that infuriates you. It seemed that you swallowed your resentment towards him and took it on the chin. Recently you've been more expressive towards him. You've been arguing with him more, since you've been coming here.

Pt. Well, in only one respect I don't want to hurt him. He's an old man.

Dr. How old a man is he?

Pt. Sixty-eight.

Dr. What was his attitude as you were growing up?

Pt. The attitude? Well, there was really only one attitude. There was no room for play, just do your work, and that's all. In most everything else we get along swell. Anybody would like him.

Dr. Did you resent his insistence that you work constantly?

Pt. Well, naturally. Like when I see those kids out in front, I'd like to go out and play, too.

Dr. Did you?

Pt. No, I couldn't, I had to work.

Dr. You had to stay in the store?

Pt. Or sneak out, and then worry about the consequences.

Dr. Well, are you sneaking out now?

Pt. There's no necessity for it, somehow.

Dr. Good, and you'd like to do that more and more and more.

Pt. (*Laughs*) Two things happened last week that made up my mind. One was when I left here, I went down to the cafeteria, the little luncheonette there, a block and a half away. I was having a cup of coffee and a piece of pie. Just then about three young girls came in, probably of high school age and they wanted to play the juke box. Well, they said they didn't have any nickels, so they sat down near that juke box. Did I tell you this?

Dr. No.

Pt. So, somehow or other I had a feeling as though I wanted to go ahead and put a nickel in it for them, see? So I got up, put a nickel for them and I asked them what song they'd like to play and I played it for 'em. I sat down and I was feeling pretty good, see. Now this week I went to the show, the movie. Two seats away from me there was a lady sleeping there. The movie was over and I wanted to shake her to tell her, "Wake up, it's time to go home, see?" But somehow I couldn't get the courage to wake her up. And when I left I felt bad about it, I should have told her to get up, see, I mean that I set my mind, I should have acted there, but I didn't.

Dr. That's something you wanted to do.

Pt. I think I wanted to when I put a nickel in the slot

for the girl. But in the movie I wanted to do it, but I didn't do it. And I felt badly about the second one, as I felt good about the first. Now I've made up my mind when I think I should go and do something, I'm going to do it.

Dr. You feel you have the right to do it.

Pt. Well, why didn't I ask that lady to get up?

Dr. Perhaps you were afraid or shy toward her as you may be toward many people. How do you feel about me? What about your attitudes toward me? What have you been thinking about that?

Pt. Well, (*cough*) frankly, the minute I leave here I don't even think about you. What I do know is that when I expect to come here I anticipate it. Somehow or other I am getting plenty of confidence.

Dr. Remember you've got a life pattern we're trying to break up. You will get the formula here that will show you what has happened to you. That will help you take steps to make you well and keep you well. But you must understand thoroughly the nature of your problem. You came to see me because of headaches. Supposing you tell me what you believe has caused your headaches and is causing them now.

Pt. Well, I think it mostly is a fear of making a mistake. I'd say, that caused the headache and then the not being able to do what you want to do.

Dr. How do you explain the fact that your headache became more exaggerated when you fought with your father?

Pt. Well, actually it became exaggerated when he'd blame me. For instance, we argue about little things that don't matter, or something I know has been done one way and it's the best way, and yet he did it another way, see. And, I don't like it; it upsets me inside. I know what he did I've got to do over again. That aggravates me. And the fear of making a mistake, that's really terrific.

Dr. The fear of making a mistake.

Pt. A mistake. I'm afraid to actually do things, you know, do things that have some bearing on some one else. I'm afraid that person is liable to get hurt by it.

Dr. How far back does that fear of making a mistake go?

Pt. Well, it goes back a long, long ways. I'd say about when I was fifteen.

Dr. You always had to do the right and proper thing, because if you made a mistake that would mean, what?

Pt. If I made a mistake, well, I wouldn't get hit or anything, but they'd start in on me with words, my father mostly, especially when we're in the store, see?

Dr. He'd just keep picking at you?

Pt. Yes, looking for mistakes.

Dr. What sort of a mistake would be the worst kind to make?

Pt. Just now? Now let's say that you were buying an article. If the price isn't just right, if I happen to buy at a price and it goes up, well all right. But if it goes down, goodnight. "Didn't I tell you not to buy it? What's the matter, you can't wait?" and so forth. Stuff like that. "Do you want them to take you for a fool? Do you want the salesmen to take you for a fool?" I hate the word, fool. Gosh, do I hate that word. I hate to be called a fool. I think I'd jump anybody more that called me a fool than anything else.

Dr. I see.

Pt. And I hate to be taken for a fool. Like there are some people who come into the store and they work on until finally they're fired, see. Or at the time that they go home take something out, and say that we were short. Now, my father insists that I act tough so as not to be taken for a fool, see. When they come back and pretend that they took nothing, although I'd like to give it to them, I feel it's a sign of weakness if I gave it to them. Now for myself I think I would give it to them because it amounts to practically nothing. But I got to do what father says.

Dr. Well, we come right back again to that old fundamental problem that you are still that little boy in short
pants and your father the fellow who rules. Perhaps we
can investigate this further. Supposing you go to sleep now.

Pt. All right.

Dr. Keep gazing at your fingers. Breathe in deeply and
go to sleep. As you sit there, have the experience of feeling
very drowsy, and tired. The hand will start getting light
and rise, slowly rise, up, up, straight up in the air. It will
lift and rise, up, up, up, higher, higher, higher, straight up,
lifting, lifting up, rising, and as it reaches your face, you'll
get sleepier, and sleepier and sleepier. You're so tired and
drowsy and sleepy that you'll go into a deep, restful, relaxed
sleep. (*Pause*)

I'm going to review what we've learned about yourself.
You came to me originally because you had headaches that
were constant and severe, but that had no apparent organic
basis as a number of physical examinations finally convinced
you. We were able through hypnosis to trace the origin of
one of those headaches to an early experience in which you
felt you were doing something wrong, in which you felt that
it was not proper or right for you to do what you wanted to
do. We discovered that there was a relationship between
your headaches and doing something that you wanted to do.
As we examined your problem further, it appeared that you
had a fear of your parents, and that your fear of your parents
had persisted longer than it should. Your father enters into
that picture in some way. Perhaps you have a desire to
express yourself through defeating your father. Now this is
more or less the case in every boy, but in your case you may
have feared acknowledging this impulse out of fear that you
might really hurt or kill your father.

I am going to suggest that you begin utilizing the insight
that you've gained here toward a real understanding of your
difficulty to a point where you can gradually liberate your-

self from your family, from your father and from your mother.

Now coming to see me plays into the picture. It is something you want to do, it is something you believe in. But your mother, in opposing your coming here, is likely to cause you a great deal of anxiety and conflict. Now if you accept the expressed criticism of your mother in your coming here, you are likely either to have headaches, or to find that your progress is blocked. This will happen unless you liberate yourself from her. I should like to have you consider your coming here as your own private project, something that you yourself can do entirely apart from your mother, that has nothing to do with your mother. It is extremely important to you to be able to do things on your own.

Now as you sit there, I am going to suggest that you begin seeing your way clear to working this problem through. Next week you may want to test the things that we have worked on even more to see if you can possibly do things you want, knowing that they are apt to cause a headache, knowing that they are apt to make you feel fearful. You still have the right to do what you want to do when you want to do it. That is the inalienable right of every human being, the right that comes with being grown up. You are a grown man; you have the capacities for happiness, and the very fact that you are blocked by a childish relationship to your parents is causing you no end of resentment and grief.

I am going to suggest now that you have a dream. In the dream see yourself going ahead, working, doing, and playing in such a way as you yourself desire. In other words, you will see yourself doing exactly what you want to do. Go to sleep sufficiently deeply so that you dream, and in that dream you see yourself doing exactly what you want to do. See your parents reacting to it, and see yourself handling your parents so that they adjust to the situation. Have the dream and as soon as you've had the dream, wake up. Perhaps you won't have any recollection of the dream at first, but it will come to you, the significance of the dream will come to you, then tell me about it.   So first have the dream and then wake up.   (*Pause, following which patient awakens.*)

Pt.   Got a headache.   Right here.

Dr.   Right there, what were you thinking about?

Pt.   I was thinking that I was doing my work.

Dr.   Anything else?

Pt.   No.

Dr.   Did you have a dream?

Pt.   I had a dream, yes, yes, I did.

Dr.   Tell me about the dream.

Pt.   I felt somehow I was doing what I wanted to do, for instance like taking care of the store without direction, and my mother and father were both there, and I was not too bad, and my father says, "No, it's not too bad," and, ah, ah, he didn't mean it though.   You could see, well, I don't know though.   And my father says, "Come on, let's go away for a little while."   And I think we could go away, but my mother had an eye on the door, you know.

> (*The dream and the patient's response to the situation with a headache demonstrates that he is not yet desensitized to the domineering attitudes of his parents.*)

Dr.   She had an eye on the door?   You felt you could go away and that your father would approve, but your mother had an eye on the door.   Then you woke up with a headache. I think we see the connection much more clearly now, the feeling within you that she still is too powerful to cope with, that your mother still isn't letting you sneak through the door, and that you still, therefore, are afraid and respond with a headache.   Now, what about the treatments here with me?   Does she have to know anything about what goes on?

Pt.   She doesn't have to know everything.

Dr. This is your own private affair, as far as she's concerned or your father. This should be your own project and you can tell them that.

Pt. I'll mow 'em down, is that what?

Dr. What do you care what they think?

Pt. (*Laughs*) I mean you can't defy them that way. I mean you just can't say "I'm going away, that's all there's to it." I've got to tell them every place I go.

Dr. How old are you?

Pt. Thirty.

Dr. Why do you?

Pt. I dunno, I mean aren't you supposed to respect your father and mother?

Dr. When a person gets to be thirty years of age, it's about time that his folks had sufficient confidence in him to feel that he knows where he is going and that he is not going to get into any trouble. Part of your treatment process is to make your folks accept you and trust you so that you don't have to give them a report of where you go. Of course they don't have a right to know where you're going. You're no baby, you don't owe them a verbatim report of everything you do.

Pt. Don't I owe them a little responsibility?

Dr. Yes you do, but you owe yourself the chance to live your own life.

Pt. I guess you are right.

Eighth Session (April 9)

The patient states that although he was more aggressive and active this week, his headache persisted without let-up. He demonstrates keen interest in solving his problem and he appears to be making a genuine effort to master his fear of standing up to his parents.

(*Patient comes in late today*)

Dr. You're late, twenty minutes. What happened?

Pt. Well, it just happens that when I leave the place I ust have time enough to make it here, you see. This time when I was home the ceiling was leaking, and no one was home. So I had to locate my folks.

Dr. It was an emergency then. How have things been going with you?

Pt. I don't know. All right, I guess, although last week I couldn't, I couldn't see any improvement in the headache. I had a very bad headache all week, off and on.

Dr. You had a bad headache all week?

Pt. Yes.

Dr. How have other things been?

Pt. I felt much better. And I want to tell you this—and I wouldn't tell it to anybody but you—but I happened to go to a show one night last week. There were two boys next to me. They must have been about sixteen, seventeen years old. They were annoying the girl in front. I tell them to stop. Three times that happened. There were two fellows there. Another boy said "All right let him talk, we'll fix him later." I don't know whether I'm mad or not. One of the boys leaves, the fellow I'd said things to. He was the big one. So about then, this other fellow leaves. So I figured they went home.

Well after I saw the show completely, I went to go out, and I find one of the boys standing right by the back of the theater as though he was looking for me. I felt they actually are, actually going after me. I actually started to get frightened more. I thought maybe they have four or five fellows. Who knows what they'll do? Well I started to walk down the street, and as I was walking down I noticed footsteps in back of me, but I didn't want to turn and look back. If I did turn around they were liable to say I was afraid. Well, anyhow, I took out a cigarette and stopped to light my cigarette, and sort of cast my eye around to see who was following me. I stopped, lit my cigarette and saw who was following me—four fellows.   I went on and believe me I was actually afraid.   I started to walk, and suddenly I said to myself, "What are you afraid about?   They're not after you," I said.   "They're after that little guy, that little fellow the doctor was talking about, the little boy, not you, not you the big one.   What is going to happen to the little boy?   The little boy is scared.   Get him out of your system. You've got to do it yourself.   You're big enough to take them on."   And believe it or not, I walked another block or so, and I was getting enough courage, so that I didn't care if they all came after me.   Well, by the time they were actually right near me, on top of me, the fear I had of them was gone.   Then they passed me by, see, but by the time they got to me the fear was gone.

Dr.   Why did you say I'm the only one you would tell that to?

Pt.   Well, I mean, after all, I'm supposed to be a pretty big fellow.   I mean why should I be afraid of those kids for?

Dr.   You felt it was the little fellow who was afraid, not you.

Pt.   That is what I was trying to convince myself.

Dr.   Well, you did convince yourself and it worked.   But there was a realistic element too.   Four fellows could actually do some pretty foul stuff to a person.   You realize that.

Pt.   Sure they could.

Dr.   But the important thing is that it was mostly a neurotic fear, mostly it was this little fellow inside who trembled and shook, the same little guy who trembles and shakes in his shoes when he is home with his father and mother.   You react to your folks still as a little fellow. You're afraid of doing things you want to do, because that little fellow still may say, "Look you're a little boy and you've got to be good to your parents."   You can be good to them, but for pete sakes you've got to be good to yourself too.   They'll respect you more.   Your parents have to get

used to the fact that you have grown up. If you don't give
them that chance they never will permit you to spread your
wings and grow up. How have they been towards you and
how have you felt towards them this week?

Pt. All right. I think it's sort of, it seems to me as
though everything is loosening up.

Dr. How?

Pt. I feel more free. Like this Easter, I wanted to buy
my nieces and nephew a few presents, see. I used to buy
them presents, but somehow when I'd come home with that
present, I'd be so afraid that they were going to say something. I was afraid that they would say, "Why did you
spend the money for it? It's foolish." You know what I
mean? Well I didn't have that feeling this time. Every
time I had anything to do with money and I had to lay out
money, I was afraid they'd say something like that. I
didn't have it this Easter.

Dr. You think you are changing?

Pt. Yah, I hope so. There is one more thing too that
I wanted to tell you. Today, when I went home and I
found the ceiling was just dripping with water, and the floor
was all full of water, I knew very well that if I waited five
minutes there, I'd never make it here on time. So immediately—I didn't have a headache, mind you—I didn't
have that headache, but the minute I knew that I'd never be
able to see you on time, the headache just came just like that.

Dr. That's very interesting, isn't it? Let's see if we can
make the connection and figure out why that headache
came. Supposing you try to figure it out, why the headache
could come when you felt you couldn't come here to see me.

Pt. Well, I knew I was supposed to come to see you, but
I couldn't.

Dr. Wasn't it also because there was something tying
you down to that house, that you were forced to attend to,
and you couldn't do something you wanted to do?

Pt. That's right.

Dr.   How did you think I would react to your not coming here, if you didn't come?

Pt.   Well, if I called you up, how should you react?

Dr.   I want your idea.

Pt.   I don't think you'd get angry. I don't think you'd get angry.

Dr.   Because you might expect the same kind of attitudes as with your mother and father, you may feel I'm the same kind of person, too.   And you might have the feeling that you have a certain sense of obligation; that I'm expecting you, and you can't come.   The headache may come as a result of that.   Another reason is that because of circumstances that you can't control, you are prevented from doing something you want to do.   Something like your mother holding you down, except that it is a leaky ceiling that is preventing you from doing what you want to do.   These are two reasons why you might have had that headache, and whichever reason is operating is the interesting thing. From what you say about your attitudes towards me and your feeling about me, it would seem to be more that you were prevented from doing what you wanted to do.   Maybe both of them are part of the picture.   Did you have any dreams this week?   Have you done anything more constructive with yourself?

Pt.   Well, last week I didn't do anything.   I mean I wasn't feeling up to par.   Besides I had nowheres to go.

Dr.   Is it that you have no outlets where you can meet the right sort of people?

Pt.   That's right.

Dr.   And no outlets where you can get the right kind of entertainment or find friends or do things which bring you into contact with other people?   If that is the problem maybe we can help you there.   We have a department here which has contact with different things going on in the city, where you can find outlets for your spare time.   Maybe you might get a few suggestions. If you'd like to utilize that service, tell me about it, and I'll see to it that they take care of you. It would be much better if you could do it on your own, but sometimes a person doesn't have the resources at his fingertips.

Pt. No, I'll do it for myself.

Dr. Good.

Pt. Is that a good sign?

Dr. That's a very good sign.

Pt. Has it ever occurred to you that maybe I'm sort of, I'm afraid to take that advice from you, to take that information from you?

Dr. About where to go?

Pt. Yes.

Dr. Maybe you are afraid because then you'll have to do it?

Pt. Exactly. And I may not be able to do it.

Dr. Why wouldn't you be able to do it?

Pt. Maybe during the weekend I could do it, see, but not during the week days, or anything like that. I wouldn't want to go out. I need sleep.

Dr. So long as you do something you want to do. So long as you don't stay in because you feel bound down to your folks, that is the important thing. It is not so much the fact that you have to do these things, but rather that you are doing something that you feel nobody is forcing you to do. If you want to stay in at night, if you feel that is the best thing for you, if you feel it is not because your folks expect you to stay in or because you're afraid of the folks, that's up to you. The same thing holds true with going out with women.

Pt. I know my kind, I know the type I like and if I see them I'm with them.

Dr. The important thing is that you don't see them.

Pt. (*Laughs*) The important thing is that I don't scc

them? The important thing is that I do see them, you should say.

Dr. Do you see them?

Pt. No.

Dr. We ought to see if there is any block in you still that prevents you from seeing them.

Pt. No, the only thing that prevents me from seeing them is the actual going out, the social life that I seem to neglect.

Dr. There aren't enough of those.

Pt. Exactly. It's not that I'm afraid of people, I like people. I actually do, and I don't mind actually talking to a strange girl. I can find conversation. I mean when I was dancing I met two different girls, both of them were two different types of women, and I was able to hold a conversation with both of them.

Dr. We are making progress, but we must be sure that you haven't just gotten to the half-way mark where you feel safe. You feel better, but you want to go forward and feel that you're not going to slip back.

Pt. I'll hold my own. I will make progress. If I make another slip back I'll make progress after that.

Dr. Good. Look, I'm not going to charge you for this session, because my payment is the fact that you were able to come here in spite of the fact that you were going to be late.

Pt. That's very nice of you, doctor.

Dr. Believe me, the greatest reward I can have is to see you get out of this muddle, see you get out of the stalemate that you've been in so long.

Pt. In a week or two from now, I think you'll really see something, some real action. I was talking to a fellow the other day and he told me, he said, "I'm going to have you meet a couple of women," he said, "and one of them I know you're going to like. They're both pretty good," he said, "but one of them I know you're going to like." I know very well I've got to get out before the closing of the business day, and I've got to see how I react to that. Because then I know very well there is going to be hell to pay, when I ask them that I want to leave to go somewheres.

Dr. Involved in this business about getting away from home is the way parents raise their children. They feel he's got to be a good son, and he's got to take care of his parents. They build up this idea to a point where a person gets tied down to his parents so that he never can get married and never can even break away. He's married to them. Even when he gets married, he always feels that he has done a terrible thing; he feels guilty about it.

Pt. I don't think that parents do it deliberately.

Dr. Many parents are so insecure in themselves, they always have a fear of the poorhouse. They try to train their children to be good to them, so that when they get old they will not starve. It is worse with people who are in business than with common working people, because working people usually shove their kids out to forage for themselves. They don't hem them in and overprotect them too much.

Pt. What's on the agenda?

Dr. On the agenda is that we have to see what forces there are that still tie you down. You'll notice again other experiences where this headache develops like you noticed today. The headache has been loosening up gradually, hasn't it?

Pt. That's right.

Dr. And getting better and better as time has gone on. You can see the connection between the headache and the situation at home as well as with people. Not only is it with your family, because the same thing can happen to you with other people. It is a pattern that repeats itself. It's not so much getting away from home, but breaking this pattern up so that no matter where you go, you will not get yourself new parents to take the place of the old ones you left behind.

Pt. I feel pretty well satisfied with what I've been doing somehow. I'm making progress.

NINTH SESSION (April 15)

The patient spends the greater part of the session talking about his girlfriend. He feels tied to her by a fear that she may harm him if he breaks the relationship. The relationship is one he apparently maintains out of habit, obligation and fear. It is not something he wants genuinely. He has much more insight into his condition and the genetic origin of his problem is explained to him in waking and hypnotic states. The patient mentions reading about an incident in the newspaper of a man being murdered by his mistress. He fears that the same thing may happen to him if he breaks off relations with his girl friend. He has a hypnotic dream which points to a desire for a close relationship with a girl of his choice.

Dr. How are things?

Pt. Fine, I think we're on the right track.

Dr. You do; what makes you say that?

Pt. Well, (*laughs*) I finally got the head pulled around that. I understand what it is and why. My headache was practically gone.

Dr. Did you have any dreams last week?

Pt. Oh, I don't know. The only one I do remember is one. It's not worth mentioning, but I'll tell you anyhow. It's one about a friend, a friend whom I've been thinking of going to see about a building in his neighborhood. I thought I'll ask him about it as well as about a girl. He knows her and I had it on my mind to ask him about her and her sister. Her sister is a little better than she is. Both sisters come down. We were all introduced to each other, see, and I like them both.

Dr. This is sort of a happy dream?

Pt. Yes.

Dr. How have things been going with you?

Pt. Well, last week I went out. My brother asked me to go with him dancing, first time in thirty years. At first I didn't want to go out. I was in my chair resting up, and I didn't want to go out, but he told me to go, see, and the urge to go out came.

Dr. Any fun?

Pt. Well, I had a little fun. I was thinking about my girl friend.

Dr. How are things coming with your girl friend?

Pt. She called me up once this last week and she said, "I've got to see you tonight." Kinda demanding; a demanding request, you see. I thought, "Well, I'll be a son of a gun." Immediately, somehow or other I got so many thoughts on my mind about what'll it be about. Boy did I get a headache, like that.

Dr. Did you see her?

Pt. Yes, I saw her.

Dr. What did she want?

Pt. She wanted to give me a present. She gave me a shirt and a tie. (*Laughs*)

Dr. What did you think?

Pt. Well, I thought, I thought maybe she could be pregnant. That was the main thing.

Dr. The fear that she might have gotten pregnant?

Pt. She might.

Dr. What would happen if she got pregnant?

Pt. Well, I don't know. Best to get rid of it.

Dr. And supposing you couldn't, would you marry her, if you couldn't?

Pt. No, because she's not what I really want.

Dr. How about your father this week?

Pt. It's been O.K. I have much to talk about. The symptoms come up before I know, but I calm myself down, and don't let it get the best of me.

Dr. You don't permit it to get the best of you. There will be setbacks because this little fellow inside of you isn't going to take it lying down. He doesn't want to leave, he wants to keep right where he is, because he's afraid of life, afraid of doing something wrong. He's going to try to hold you back all the time. You have to expect that. Don't be disappointed if you suddenly find yourself being held back. You'll know what it is if it comes. If you don't watch out for it, you are apt to slip back again and be discouraged. If you happen to slip back to a point where you don't want to go on at all, where you want to stay at home, where you want to work all the time, where you don't want to take any interest in outside things, you will know that it is the operation of this little fellow inside of you. The little fellow still wants to be small, wants to hold on to his mother's apron strings, wants to knuckle down to what his father tells him to do, and is afraid to go out and to do what he wants to do.

Pt. If there is this thing, if there is such a thing as being afraid, how will I know?

Dr. You, yourself, will be able to tell.

Pt. I think I can tell that.

Dr. How?

Pt. Whenever I get a headache that has something to do with this neurotic condition of mine, there's a funny feeling in here, you know. (*Points to head.*) Something gums up the works like, you know. Now I know when I have a headache from a cold, let's say, I don't have that feeling.

Dr. It's an entirely different feeling?

Pt. It's an entirely different feeling, and I know the difference.

Dr. All right, let us see what we've learned so far. Let's try to consolidate our gains. What have you learned so far? What have you learned so far about yourself and about your headaches?

Pt. Well, I learned that I should do what I want to do, and when I do it not to be afraid of what's going to happen later on. Get hold of the guy inside who's keeping you down; you just keep him back, that's all. Let him know that you know that he's behind all the trouble; then get him, knock him down somehow.

Dr. And what do you think has been causing your headaches?

Pt. What I think (*sigh*) is it's a lack of courage, not being quite a whole man, doctor. Fear of most any damn thing, like fear of eating because you won't be able to swallow, most any damn thing I can think of. How did I get this way?

Dr. Supposing I help you understand that. When a child is born into a family, he is helpless because he's little. He doesn't have any resources within himself, and he's got to be dependent upon his parents. He gets satisfactions from being dependent, from being given things by the parents. But there is another part of him that wants to grow up, that wants to be strong, that wants to be independent, that wants to break away from the ties of the parents and do things for himself. A child feels that is the masculine part that makes him aggressive, that makes it possible to stand on his own feet.

Now it happens that there are a lot of satisfactions in growing up, but there are also many satisfactions in being dependent upon the parents. When one is afraid to grow up, then the only way he can have security is by becoming more dependent upon the parents. Sometimes parents prevent the child from growing up. Sometimes they make it difficult for him to grow up, because they want him to be a child and are afraid for him to grow. The child may be frightened out of a desire to grow up, and he may be willing to accept prolonged dependency on the parents in order to feel safe. When this happens, he becomes afraid of counteracting

anything the parents want him to do. He becomes afraid
to do anything against what they say, because he doesn't
feel strong enough within himself to go out and fight his own
battles. He's afraid, for instance, that if he talks back to
his father, if he doesn't do what his mother says, if he does
what he wants to do when he wants to do it, his parents will
punish him, or they will abandon him and he'll starve. Well,
a little child will actually starve if nobody takes care of him.
But not an adult. However, the adult may still feel
emotionally that he will starve, feel panicky and anxious.
And that's where the headache and stomach symptoms are
tied together. They go back that far. The fear of starving
is associated with stomach tension and may create a symptom such as you have. This is not only happening to you,
but it has happened to countless thousands of people who
have grown up under circumstances in which they had to
develop a fear of becoming independent. This may cause
also feelings of inferiority about themselves and their sexual
functioning, their masculinity. You remember that first
dream you had here in which you were coasting up a hill
riding on your penis, a big penis?

Pt. Yes, I do.

Dr. Coasting up a hill, riding on the big penis is a symbol
that often represents being able to break out of this mess
you're in, by becoming a man, by becoming masculine. The
symbol of the big penis is the symbol of masculinity and of
growth from a little boy to a man. You were supposed to
have developed this feeling when you were in adolescence.
If you had done it then, you wouldn't have to do it now.
That's what that dream probably meant, and when you
were under hypnosis and you had that dream, you possibly
had the feeling that you would be able to make progress,
hence the dream. Do you follow me?

Pt. Yes, of course.

Dr. Very often a person with a problem of being tied

down to the family, particularly to the mother, feels as if he isn't big enough to grow.   He feels as if he's got a little penis. He actually feels inferior sexually.   In your case it isn't so much that.   I don't know to what extent you have had feelings about your own sexual organs?

Pt. No.

Dr. Deep down underneath there may have been a fear that somehow you weren't as much of a man as you could be.

Pt. As much of a man in general, but not sexually.

Dr. In some cases this kind of problem paralyzes a person completely.   He cannot even function sexually.   In your case it wasn't that bad.   It was bad enough, though, creating headaches.   And the headaches are a sign of a fear of some harm being done you.   What harm?   What the blazes can happen to you that hasn't happened already?

Pt. Did you read in the papers lately, two days ago, how there was a shooting and killing on a yacht?   A man was shot.

Dr. No.

Pt. Well, it was a headline, you couldn't miss it.   Well, that could happen to me.

Dr. Tell me about that.

Pt. You mean it can't happen to me?

Dr. How was he shot?

Pt. How was he shot?   Somehow he had an argument with her, with his girl, about another woman.   What the actual fight was I don't remember; I just looked at the headlines and saw somehow they got into an argument and she shot him.

Dr. Well, who's going to shoot you?

Pt. Who's going to shoot me?   Well, my girl friend maybe.

Dr. That girl friend of yours?

Pt. Why, isn't it possible?

Dr. It's possible, yes, it's possible, but it's not probable, unless she's a hatchet murderess. Why would she shoot you?

Pt. If she doesn't see me that one day a week, it means something terrible for her. I'd even bust with her now, but she isn't very well satisfied.

Dr. Do you see her because you feel that you're obligated to see her or because you want to?

Pt. Well, I want to see her and I feel sorry for her. I want to see her happy, because I know she doesn't have much money. I was being too good to her. Somehow or other she got to depend too much on me. She doesn't go out with other men that I know of.

Dr. Do you look upon your going out with other women as a threat to your relationship with her?

Pt. No, not exactly; the thing is that I know that when I find someone I'd like to tell her this is the end, something like that.

Dr. She'd be upset?

Pt. She probably will.

Dr. All right, but the question, is will she shoot you?

Pt. I don't know that. (*Laughs*)

Dr. This brings up the whole problem of your relations with women. Now supposing you go to sleep. Put your hands down, and watch one of your hands, particularly the right hand, keep gazing at the right hand. And as you do, the hand will become light and rise. You will go to sleep, go to sleep. The hand will keep rising and lifting straight up towards your face, straight up, and you'll be asleep, deeply asleep. Your legs feel heavy and tired, but the arm will continue to lift and rise, and you get sleepier and sleepier, and sleepier, from your head right down to your feet. Keep breathing steady and deep, very deep; get drowsy, drowsy, drowsy, from your head right down to your feet. You get so drowsy that you go into a deep, comfortable, relaxed sleep. Go deeply to sleep, and your hand will keep rising and lifting toward your face, and when it touches your face, your eyes get so heavy that it is difficult to keep them open. Your breathing gets automatic and deeper. You go into a restful comfortable sleep. Very tired, very sleepy, sleepy, very sleepy. Your hand moves up, and your breathing gets deeper and more automatic. Your arm moves toward the face, it's touching the face, and now you're asleep. In a moment I'll talk to you, and when I talk to you next you'll be still more deeply asleep. (*Pause*)

As you know, you have been progressing in your own development. You have become more assertive, more self confident, more capable of expressing yourself, more capable of living your own life. You have begun to see that many of the ideas you have about your parents right now are those imparted to you when you were very little. You see that there is absolutely no reason in the world why you cannot lead your own life, why you cannot be assertive and self confident, and do what you want to do.

I suggested that perhaps you might even test your parents sometimes and see how they adjust to you as an assertive person. Sure they regard you in the same light as they regarded you when you were a little boy. But that may be because you never let them regard you in any other light. The big problem is that for some reason you have been victimized by fear. The fear, according to your own estimate of the problem is that you will be injured if you do something that is wrong.

Just to give you a crude example let us take the case of your girl friend. Deep down underneath you feel you have a good relationship with your girl friend, but part of you is still the little boy in relationship to the grown woman. That part of you read the newspaper and noticed in it that someone had gotten shot by a woman he had crossed, when he did something that he wanted to do that was against the desire of the woman. Now what we have to watch out for is that

you aren't victimized by the same fear.   You probably will
not be shot if you stand up to this girl.   Nor will you be
hurt or killed or injured in any way if you stand up to your
mother or your father.   Nothing will happen to you in
reality.

Now in order for you to cure this headache, in order for
you to become a real person in your own right like anybody
else, it is necessary to take a more aggressive stand with
your parents, and to feel that you can do what you want to do
when you want to do it.   That holds good for your girl
friend, too.   She's been a good companion to you, but you
do not owe her your life.   You need not tie yourself down
to her the way you've tied yourself down to your parents.
If you want to, you can find other women, attractive ones,
women to whom you can relate yourself in the right way.
You really have a lot of good solid fight in you.   You've
got to liberate yourself and break this neurosis.   Your headache is, as you say, a sign of fear.   The fear must be conquered, you must conquer the fear.

Now I'm going to ask you to have a dream now.   I'm
going to ask you to have a dream, or a vision like a dream.
Go into a deep sleep, have a dream and as soon as you've
had the dream, indicate it to me by your left hand rising.
Go ahead, now, have the dream. (*Pause*) The hand comes
up, and down, straight down, straight down. I want you to
tell me that dream without you waking up. What was the
dream?

Pt.   It was as though I was walking on a cloud.   I
couldn't see with who.

Dr.   Was that the entire dream?

Pt.   Yep.

Dr.   All right, I am going to wake you up.   When you
wake up, you will have a sensation that you have been so
deeply asleep that you cannot remember a thing, until I tap
on the side of this chair four times.   At the fourth tap,

suddenly the dream will pop into your mind. I am going to count now from one to five. At the count of five, open your eyes and wake up. One, start waking up slowly; two, slowly, just as if you're coming out of a deep sleep; three; four; five. (*Patient opens his eyes.*) How do you feel?

Pt. Good.

Dr. What are you thinking of?

Pt. Nothing.

Dr. Any dreams?

Pt. I think so. I have a vision in my mind.

Dr. What do you see?

Pt. A figure.

Dr. What figure?

Pt. I can't make it out.

Dr. Now, watch. (*Rap, rap, rap, rap.*)

Pt. Now that figure is walking. (*Laughs*)

Dr. Yes.

Pt. Am I crazy or what? (*Laughs*)

Dr. Why do you say that?

Pt. (*Laughs*) The way things happen. How do I shake that guy off of me?

Dr. Which guy?

Pt. He's still there.

Dr. You mean that figure?

Pt. Yeah.

Dr. Who is that guy?

Pt. I think it's me. It's right here. (*Points to forehead.*)

Dr. Right on your forehead?

Pt. Yes.

Dr. Tell me the whole dream, do you remember it now?

Pt. Yes, that I was walking on a cloud, pretty spry, with a girl next to me, very close to me, very close.

Dr. Possibly the meaning is that you really want to be close to a girl, very close. You want to get the girl. Walking on a cloud is probably reaching out for her. You never felt you could ever get that far before. That's why it looked like walking on a cloud. You can have that. You have a right to it. You are a grown adult, you have a right to find a girl and to have happiness with her in an adult kind of relationship.

TENTH SESSION (April 23)

The patient expresses the conviction that he has his symptoms conquered. The need to develop assertiveness and self confidence is pointed out to him, and he evinces the interest to go further in therapy. The matter of his relationship with his girl friend is taken up and he evidences less fear of her. The patient mentions the inability to concentrate as a symptom that remains. Tests reveal no retentive or recall difficulty. Under hypnosis he relates this symptom to frustration.

Dr. How go things?

Pt. Well I'll tell you the truth, I've felt better. Things are getting along fine, at least it seems all right, all right with me.

Dr. No tensions, no anxieties, no headaches?

Pt. No.

Dr. You feel you know the core, the basis of your problem?

Pt. I think I do.

Dr. You know what your enemies are?

Pt. Sure, I know.

Dr. What are your enemies?

Pt. Myself, my own conscience.

Dr. Your own conscience, you feel, has prevented you from getting places, from being able to do the things you wanted to do.

Pt. It's true. I think from here on in, it's just a matter of time, and it'll go away. I know it's possible for it all to go away.

Dr. We have been able to see what caused your trouble, how it began, what's keeping it up now. The important thing is being able to develop. We can't be content with merely having your headache disappear. That's pretty much solved. We've got to go beyond relief of symptoms to a point where you can be much more self sufficient and able to do the things you want to do.

Pt. That's so.

Dr. All right. The next step is being able to go beyond losing your symptoms to a better kind of life. Now you've made very good progress. Many people at this point feel that they can go ahead on their own. I shall leave that up to you. You can stop now, but if you desire to go further, I shall be glad to go on with you.

Pt. I do, I mean I want to.

Dr. There still may be resistances against moving forward and making a proper kind of life for yourself.

Pt. You know what I'd like?

Dr. What?

Pt. I'd like to get in a state where if something happens, I don't have to fight it off. It would just come natural, by itself.

Dr. For instance?

Pt. For instance, say something happens in the family where, say I had an argument on account of a new item, well the headache may come. Now I know very well that if I fight the headache off, like while I'm arguing I tell myself, "It's not you he's arguing with, he's arguing with that kid, there," I fight it off that way and my headache won't appear, see? But I have to fight it off.

Dr. You fight it off and you can see that your headache disappears?

Pt. Precisely.

Dr. You want to get to a point where you won't have to fight so hard?

Pt. That's what I want.

Dr. It will come, but it takes time. Remember you

must be patient because this thing just didn't happen to you last Tuesday or last month. You know how far back it goes, back as far as you can remember. It will take time, but the important thing is that knowledge and insight are your best friends. If you really have insight, if you know what is happening to you, then never again will you be in the position that you've been. Insight is like having a map. You just don't wander around in the woods. With insight you can still get lost, but at least you can find your way out of the woods.

Pt.   That's right.

Dr.   Now what have you done about the other business?

Pt.   What do you mean about the other business?

Dr.   Your girl friend?

Pt.   Well, I just can't see any (*laughs*) solution.

Dr.   Is there a feeling maybe you better not break that off?

Pt.   Well, there is that feeling.

Dr.   You're afraid she'll shoot you?

Pt.   No. I'm not sure that she'll shoot me. (*Laughs*) Here's what I'm thinking. I could just say, "Hey, I don't want to continue any more." But I can't hurt her.

Dr.   If you don't watch out, that relationship is going to be exactly the same thing as your mother holding on to you. And that will cause headaches. If you don't see your way clear out of this thing, you'll be in the same boat that you've been in with your parents. Very insidiously, it repeats the same pattern. It's incredible how these things happen. But you don't have to give her up, if you really get something out of the relationship.

Pt.   I, I, I (*cough*), there is a desire to get away from her. Now I see it now, but if I had someone else.

Dr.   Are you letting your feeling about that relationship block you in finding someone else?

Pt.   Here's the thing. How can you just tell a woman,

"Look, I've found another woman, I want to get married, and I can't go with you?" Just how could the matter be handled?

Dr. You know how to handle a situation like that?

Pt. No, I'm asking.

Dr. I won't tell you how to handle it. You've got to handle it yourself.

Pt. All right, then.

Dr. You could stop seeing her if you really feel you don't want to.

Pt. So that's what a brush off is like?

Dr. That's a brush off.

Pt. Is there a better way?

Dr. I don't know, that's up to you to figure out.

Pt. You don't know?

Dr. Do you know any better way?

Pt. Frankly, it's something I would like to discuss out in the open with her.

Dr. Is she the kind of person that you can do that with?

Pt. She is. I'm not afraid to talk to her. Now it would hurt me more than it would hurt her if I gave her that brush off in that way.

Dr. You want to be very frank with her then, and when the time comes, you want to tell her that you've met somebody you'd like to start a relationship with.

Pt. Doc, actually I feel sorry for her, and I get to a point and say, "Yes, I know I've hurt her," I say to myself. That's how I feel about it.

Dr. Don't you think you were tied down to your mother too? You didn't want to hurt your mother either.

Pt. Well I wasn't sorry for my mother. I know she can take care of herself.

Dr. Yes, but you are afraid of hurting her, too. You don't want to hurt her.

Pt. You can't go around hurting people.

Dr. You've got to be a little tough, sometimes. It's better for you to hurt her a little bit by being frank than for you to go on seeing her when you don't want to, because in the long run that will hurt her more. Sincerity on your part and the desire to see her is an important thing in your relationship, and if you see her when you really don't want to, it would be bad for her and for you. The bad thing for you would be that your headaches would become extreme, if you felt forced to do something you really didn't want to do. You've got to look after yourself. You can't be good to anybody else unless you're good to yourself, too.

Pt. Yes, but where am I going to get that third party?

Dr. You know what also may occur? Resistance. You'll get tired at nighttime; you'll want to go to sleep earlier; you'll have no interest in going out. This resistance is a means of avoiding a showdown with your girl. There may be resistance about getting out of the house, mixing with people, finding new friends and so on. And that resistance has a purpose, a meaning. It is a way of blocking you from getting into a situation that will cause you pain. Why don't you talk it over with your girl if you want to?

Pt. I'd talk her out of it, I suppose.

Dr. You have been working pretty well all week? No headaches or anxiety? Any other troubles?

Pt. I'm getting on better with my father. He always has a tendency to boss me around. I can understand he's perfectly justified, sometimes, and when I do, I don't seem to find any objections to it.

Dr. You feel it's justified sometimes?

Pt. Yes. You know what? One thing is that sometimes it's difficult to concentrate yet. Is that a natural condition for me or what?

Dr. You find it difficult to concentrate? What do you mean by that?

Pt. I can't remember very much, like when it comes to figures, I can't remember them.

Dr. Supposing we test your retentive powers. I'll repeat consecutively certain figures, and ask you to repeat them. Four, zero, five, two, seven, nine, five.

Pt. Four, zero, five, two, seven, nine, five.

Dr. Now repeat them backwards.

Pt. Well, five, nine, seven . . . two . . . five, zero, four.

Dr. There seem to be no gross retentive errors. Supposing you go to sleep now. Gaze at your hand until the hand touches your face, when you'll be asleep, deeply asleep. The sleep will get deeper and deeper and deeper. It will get very much deeper. The hand will rise and lift, just like that, lift straight up in the air, higher, and higher, and higher. You're getting tired, very tired. You're getting sleepy. The hand will lift and you'll be asleep, deeply asleep.

I want you to go into a sufficiently deep sleep now so that you start dreaming. As soon as you dream, your left hand, this hand, will rise up about an inch to tell me that you dreamed. So have a dream and then your hand will rise up about an inch. (*Pause*) Your hand rises and comes down again, right down to your thigh, just like that.

Now listen, imagine yourself walking with me into a schoolroom. We walk over to a blackboard. I go over to the blackboard and I start writing down a series of numbers. Can you visualize yourself with me in a schoolroom?

Pt. Yes.

Dr. Good, now I'm going to write certain numbers on the blackboard. After I put the numbers down, look at them on the blackboard, and then repeat them back to me, just exactly the way you see them: Three, seven, two, four, five, eight, zero. Repeat those to me just exactly the way you see them.

Pt. Three, seven, two, four, five, eight, zero.

Dr. Listen to me. I'm going to put down numbers. As I write them down, look at them on the blackboard. Two, five, two, one, zero, one, three, five. Repeat that.

Pt. Two, five, two, one, zero, one, three, five.

Dr. Good. Now your ability to repeat these indicates that there probably is no organic reason for your not being able to concentrate. I want you to look at that blackboard, can you see those numbers still there?

Pt. Not very well.

Dr. Now I'm going to repeat them again. Two, five, two, one, zero, one, three, five. Can you see them now?

Pt. Not clear.

Dr. Repeat them.

Pt. Two, five, two, one, zero, one, three, five.

Dr. Good, when you wake up, I'm going to ask you to repeat those numbers to me. Remember them, remember them no matter what else comes up. Now, as you sit there, I want you to have another dream, and this dream will involve a situation at home where you want to concentrate on something and you can't concentrate. It is impossible for you to concentrate. I want you to go into a deep sleep, and as soon as you've had that dream, indicate it by your hand rising up about an inch. (*Pause*) Your hand has come up. I want you to tell me that dream without waking up. What did you dream?

Pt. Well, something that happened at the time when I was going to come here and I saw my father's ceiling dripping with water. I was more or less upset; I didn't know what I was going to do first.

Dr. Does that give you a feeling of frustration?

Pt. Yes.

Dr. So that it is a feeling of frustration that sometimes makes it difficult for you to concentrate.

Pt. That's it, that's it.

Dr. Now, you will be able to handle better and better your relationship with your folks. You are going to be able to liberate yourself and break away from the hold they have had on you. It is necessary for you to be more independent.

And I'm going to give you a strong suggestion that you be more independent. Furthermore it will be possible for you, if you desire, to tackle in this next week your relations with your girl friend. It would be helpful to you to be able to solve this thing and get it out of the way.

Also next week see about the matter of your concentration. See if you can, on the basis of your ability to handle frustration better, concentrate better on what you do. This will make you feel better and cause your self confidence to increase.

I am now going to count from one to five. At the count of five, open your eyes and wake up. Remember the numbers on the blackboard. I am going to count from one to five. At the count of five, open your eyes, and wake up. One, two, three, four, five. (*Patient awakens.*)

Pt. Want me to repeat a number? Two, five, two, one zero, one, three, five.

Dr. Good.

Pt. Guess I made sure there were eight. (*Laughs*)

Dr. Do you remember that first dream you had?

Pt. Yes.

Dr. What was it?

Pt. I was walking down the aisle, on a cloud as usual, with a girl. Then she walked away. I tried to call her back but she wouldn't come.

Dr. You tried to call her back, but she wouldn't come?

Pt. What I mean, well, I'm looking high enough, maybe not hard enough, I don't know. (*Laughs*)

Dr. You remember what I told you about resistance. Resistance is always there. You're not looking hard enough, may be that there is resistance, a desire to stay a little boy. There are values, there are virtues in being a little boy.

Pt. At this age? (*Laughs*)

Dr. It's too much of a strain to be a little boy. It takes too much out of you.

Pt.   I hope it does.   I find it easier to be the other way.

Dr.   Well you've just got to get him out of your system, but part of the little boy will be there for a while.   He doesn't want to give up so easily.

Pt.   Got to educate him a little bit more.   (*Laughs*)

Dr.   And it will be a good thing to get settled and straighten out your life.   That holds for your relationship with your girl friend.   How would you feel if she happened to find another man she would fall in love with?

Pt.   I wouldn't say anything.

Dr.   Probably be relieved?

Pt.   (*Laughs*)   Probably (*laughs*).   I think I would.   I mean, I see now that, ah, we should break off, and yet we can't do it.

Dr.   There's guilt, fear of hurting her, fear of being hurt.

Eleventh Session (April 28)

During the past week the patient mustered the courage to break off his relationship with his girl friend.   He experienced a great deal of emotional relief as a result of this action.   He remains free from headaches, but mentions the symptom of a dull feeling in his head which is different from a headache.   This has been with him since a blow to his head in childhood.   Psychological probing suggests that the symptom of dullness is the product of a fear of being imposed upon in a dependency relationship that he himself nurtures.   Under hypnosis the meaning of this symptom is demonstrated to him.

Pt.   Last week I went out three nights in succession, Friday, Saturday, and Sunday.   I didn't work.   I went to another dance and had a swell time, got home late, about two.   Saturday night I went out and I came home about one-fifteen.   And, ah, it was all right, no fear, nothing.   I suppose you're anxious to know about the good news, if any?

Dr.   If any?

Pt.   Well, doc, you know, I didn't think it would be so easy.   We actually broke off.   Actually it was easy, I

thought. I had tried to break off three other times. I
never could do it. It was rough, pretty rough going. This
time one good lift and everything, and the first thing you
know I was telling her that I wasn't going to see her any more,
see. Well, so far as she was concerned, here's what she
said, she said, for the past three or four months, ever since
she knew I was coming here, she could actually see me improving, see. She knew that I was getting better all along.
She knew the crisis was going to come between her and
myself, but she stuck it all along, see. She knew that one
day I'd tell her, and naturally she was more or less
prepared for it. She said there was relief, now that she
knew that we're through. "I want you to grow up, I want
you to get well, because your staying as you are isn't good.
I was on the border line not knowing when you were going
to throw me over. I just couldn't take it. I want you
to go."

Dr. So you've got a clean slate, now?

Pt. Yeah, and my leaving her so far hasn't bothered me.
The last time I left her, I just stood two days, then I couldn't
take it. I had to go call her up again; left her on Sunday,
and Tuesday I called her up. So far I haven't had any
bad effects.

Dr. If you can see that there's no need to feel guilty.

Pt. Well look, I did feel guilty, will you believe it, after
I told her, while she was crying. I think I can tell you,
you're my doctor, anyhow.

Dr. Sure.

Pt. While she was crying, I wasn't hurt at all. As a
matter of fact while she was crying, I had a feeling in me as
though I was doing something good, and I knew that her
tears weren't tears, of, shall I say, of regret. They weren't
tears that she was ashamed of what we had done. You see
they were tears because we were parting, because we really
loved, I am sure. And I felt good in that respect, because

I knew she was going away with a clean slate. I know I won't see her any more . . . .

Dr.   There actually was no real urgency about breaking off, but you wanted to keep a clean slate, didn't you?

Pt.   That's right.

Dr.   You weren't getting as much out of the relationship as you wanted.

Pt.   No, I'm a guy who, well, so far as our both enjoying ourselves, we both did, you see. The thing that I didn't like most of all was that I couldn't introduce her to anybody. I didn't want to, you see.   Anything we did we were always alone.

Dr.   Yes.

Pt.   We made as little friends as possible. That's what I hated most of all.

Dr.   Yes.

Pt.   That hiding business.

Dr.   Have you found anybody else? You're not hiding yourself, are you?

Pt.   No, I don't think I am.

Dr.   You want to give yourself the opportunity of going ahead with your own life, doing what you want to do?

Pt.   Certainly.

Dr.   You feel that you've liberated yourself from your family now?

Pt.   I believe that.

Dr.   You can do what you want to do and they will accept it?

Pt.   That's right.

Dr.   As you look back what were you so fearful about?

Pt.   Well I can't see why, I can't see why I was fearful.

Dr.   Could it have been just a childish misconception?

Pt.   Well I hope it was that. Last week I did things I'd done before and in a certain respect I've had some fear, but not like what it was. I was going to the garage door, the wind must have shut the door, see, and as I was going in, the door closes just to the point where it bent the fender. As I was going in I got an attack of fear that I shook off, it didn't bother me. No headache. Before I met you, things like that would start me worrying and give me headaches. It did not bother me. I told my dad about that Friday morning, and he said, "I don't believe a word of it. Either you must have gone in very, very fast, or the door was shutting and you didn't watch it, or you must have bumped up against the wall of the garage." Now, my version of it, he wouldn't accept. He had to put it into his own words which was totally wrong. I told him that it happened and that's all, I told him. I could actually feel a headache coming on, you see. As soon as I felt that coming on, I said don't be silly and it went away.

Dr. You could feel the headache coming on?

Pt. I could feel the headache, but it went right away.

Dr. The headache came as soon as you felt that he did not understand?

Pt. He didn't want to believe what I said.

Dr. What about the dull feeling in your head?

Pt. You know, I had a dull feeling in my head all the time, see. But now it comes occasionally.

Dr. Do you ever get any dizzy spells or flashes of light?

Pt. No.

Dr. Does the dullness come when you are in bed and you get up suddenly?

Pt. Not particularly.

Dr. It's just the dullness, no real headache?

Pt. There's no pain, no.

Dr. Did you ever have a hangover?

Pt. That's how I feel sometimes.

Dr. I see, we will have to understand that dull feeling to see if it is organic, if it's related to the blow to your head you got as a child.

Pt. Sometimes I can actually work it up. When I bend down or do something strenuous, something like that, I get little white spots, little spots the shape of small tears.

Dr. That may or may not be significant.

Pt. Well that's the only thing I ever get.

Dr. I may want to get an electro-encephalogram.

Pt. What's that?

Dr. That's a machine that measures brain waves. It will tell if there's any damage in the brain, as a result of the injury that you had, that causes spells of dullness. As far as the headaches are concerned, they are due to psychological causes. You, yourself, can see them related to your relations with your parents, with authority, with life, with the feeling that you were a licked person and have to go along with your tail between your legs. (*An electro-encephalogram obtained later showed no abnormal brain waves.*)

Pt. Yes, I can see that. What about the intelligence tests I took? Is there a sign I'm dull mentally?

Dr. Your tests, as a matter of fact, indicate a superior intelligence. Why did you ask me that?

Pt. Well I'll answer that. We talked about parting, see. As a matter of fact we had come to the conclusion that we were going to part, see, that is my girl and me.

Dr. Yes.

Pt. So immediately after we had decided we were going to part, she kissed me and after that I had a hint, shall I say? So I kissed her. Well then I had to make the fierce lover to her, see. And I came to a climax but she didn't. I know she didn't. When I stopped, I noticed that she was crying. I said, "What are you crying for?" And she said, "What I can't understand is, how could two people who could really make love to each other as we do here, actually part? How could they part?" So I said to myself, "Something wrong somewhere, should I have wanted her?"

Dr. Did you feel passionate?

Pt. Well, when I'm with her I always feel that way.

Dr. Why did you break this relationship up?

Pt. The truth of the matter is that I want to get married. Too, I don't know very much if I'm being hypocritical about it, but at least I thought or I think I had a fear that maybe some harm would come to me in that someone who may be a member of her family, or maybe her ex-husband, would not like the idea of my going out with her. That and actually I did not want to hurt her, that I'm positive about.

Dr. You had mentioned to me that you would feel much freer and much more sincere and honest if you acquainted her with the fact that you wanted to go out with somebody else. You aren't a hypocrite and you therefore decided to break the thing up. But if you are aroused by her sexually, if you have a feeling for her, there's nothing to be particularly ashamed of there. That doesn't indicate any lack of intelligence at all. You must see for yourself whether you want to be with her or not.

Pt. Want to know what, I do want to leave her because I am desiring to get married.

Dr. You feel then that the way you are built, you will feel freer to go out and find a relationship and get married if you weren't tied down to her?

Pt. I felt as though I'd never get well if I continued with her.

Dr. What do you think has to be accomplished now? Do you feel you are going in the right direction?

Pt. I feel, Doc, that before I came here, I didn't matter. I feel now though as I should matter and be alive. I feel as though I had a new life this morning. I'm very confident of that.

Dr. So the next step since you have freed yourself, and taken all the shackles off your arms and legs is to lead your own life.

Pt. That's right.

Dr. If you want to get married, that's your business.

Pt. That's right.

Dr. As far as the girl friend is concerned?

Pt. You cleared that up for me and I'm very happy about it.

Dr. What still has to be done, it seems to me, is complete liberation from your family, in addition to wanting to have a normal sex life and normal married life.

Pt. Well, I met a very pretty girl, see, at the dance. I went over to dance with her and she accepted. So we struck up a conversation and my brother and I, see, we're both at the tables there. He had asked one of the other girls to dance. It just happened that he danced with another girl on the floor, and he danced with her too, see. After I came back to the table, I found that he wasn't there with her. He was away. So I saw him come back with her, see. So I imagined that he must have asked her to go out. They were outside. So when we take the girls home that night, when they get into the ladies' room, see, I asked my brother what night he had asked this girl out, because if he hadn't asked her, I would. So he said, "Yes, I did ask her." I'm glad one of us did, because she's good, very nice. She's going to be nineteen, he said. Well immediately I felt as though she's too young for me, and whatever feeling I had for her, automatically disappeared. The desire to have her disappeared entirely.

Dr. You like a more mature kind of person?

Pt. I don't like them too young.

Dr. All right now, supposing you go to sleep. Just relax, watch your hand, and this time very rapidly begin to feel yourself dozing off, going into a deep sleep. Your arm slowly lifts and rises straight up in the air, and as it rises, you'll get drowsier and drowsier, until the hand touches your face, and then you go into a deep sleep. The hand is slowly beginning to lift, slowly lifting, like that. When it touches your face, your eyes will close and you'll be in a deep, restful, relaxed, comforable sleep. (*Patient's eyes close.*)

Listen to me. You have, up to this time, shown signal important gains that are significant to you—gains that reflect themselves in your whole attitude toward life. You've become a stronger person, a more mature person. You have grown and been able to liberate yourself from the shackles of your family and from the frustrating hold of the relationship with your girl friend.

You must go forward a little bit more, now. You must take another step toward further liberation, further self sufficiency.   In addition to that, it is necessary for you to see that your symptoms are the product of difficulties that you've gotten into, and frustrations that you've experienced. Now there is another thing we must understand, and that is the dull feeling in your head.   It may be that the dull feeling resulted from the blow you had when you fell down.   It may be an associated symptom that came as a result of psychological forces.   It is necessary to find out the nature of this dullness.   If it is an organic thing, and if it came from the blow on your head, then working in a psychological sense may not be the complete answer.   It will make it better, but it will not completely annihilate it.   If, on the other hand, there are psychological reasons for the dullness, as there were reasons for those pounding headaches, then we will, in understanding reasons, remove the symptom.

Dreams as you know are extremely significant. They often give us clues that we cannot find out from ordinary talk. Now I am going to give you the suggestion to dream about what it is that makes you feel completely well.   Imagine, for instance, that you have just gotten out of bed and that there's no dullness in your head. And you ask yourself, "What happened to me yesterday that accounts for the fact that I have no dullness in my head?" Now I want you to have a dream. Don't direct it, let it come. If the dream does not come spontaneously, then imagine yourself in a theater looking up at a stage. The curtain opens and you see a play. The play will be what might have happened to you that made you feel so well. As soon as you've either dreamed or seen that play, indicate it by your left hand rising up about an inch. (*Pause*) Now your hand rises up, and I want you to talk to me without waking up.

Pt. I felt as though I got up without a dull head and no one was home.

Dr. You got up without the dullness and no one was home. Now whatever the meaning and significance of that, if it's true that the dullness can disappear because nobody is home, then it must indicate that the dullness is related to a feeling that there's somebody in some relationship with you. The work that we have been doing together is to liberate you; to bring out from within strength and capacity to function that make for independent action. Even though you are in your home right now, the knowledge that such things are possible will in turn influence your ability to liberate yourself from your symptoms almost as if there is nobody at home to bother you. Your headaches will get better and better, and they will gradually disappear. The dullness will become less and less noticeable. As you sit there, imagine that you are alone at home, as if the people in your home do not impose themselves upon you. When you wake up, see if this has any effect whatsoever on your head, on the dullness, and feelings of pressure in your head. I'm going to count now from one to five. At the count of five, open your eyes and wake up. One, two, slowly wake up—three, four, five. (*Patient opens his eyes.*) How do you feel?

Pt. Feel awful lonely, but the dullness is gone.

Dr. You do? So that even though the dullness is gone, the feeling is of great loneliness? That may be very helpful, because those two things need not be associated. A person cannot live in a vacuum. You need people around, but because you may feel you need them so much, you may resent them.

Pt. I felt as though I had no reason to work or live.

Dr. Very interesting, isn't it? Remember when we talked about a mother, needing a mother?

Pt. Yes.

Dr. You must have felt just like a little boy feels when his mother goes away.

Pt. Exactly. Nothing to do, nothing to wait for. Just sit down and waste your life away, sort of.

Dr. Did you ever realize that you were dependent, very dependent?

Pt. You mean needing a mother around?

Dr. Or a motherly person.

Pt. Of course I know that.

Dr. So long as you need a mother around, you may get yourself into a position where you are a little boy and not a man. That's the danger.

Pt. But if I can substitute something else for her, it's all right, though?

Dr. Most men do.

Pt. When I come home, I usually find my meals ready. I'd like to be independent, I know, see, I know I can probably substitute something else.

Twelfth Session (May 5)

In the past week the patient was symptom free. He recounts an experience at work of being frightened by peculiar questions of a woman and her daughter who implied they knew him. He was disturbed by his reaction of fear. To build up a sense of inner strength, a nondirective technic is attempted with the patient. He is taught the technic of self hypnosis in line with developing his own resources. By a self-induced dream he learns that his fear reaction to the above experience is a projection of his own guilt feelings.

Pt. The thing you tackled is all right.

Dr. The what?

Pt. The thing you tackled before is all right. I mean, I see more and more what goes on in me.

Dr. Well let's see what that is.

Pt. O. K. I have to convince myself. Well this friend of mine in the store and I, we were talking. A woman and her daughter came into the store and were asking my father, they wanted to know who of the two sons, which one went to Missouri to open a store. He said none of them, both are here. And they asked me, too. They looked like the right type of people; I gave him all kinds of answers. The woman said, she said she was of the family and knew us well and yet she didn't know where we lived and all that stuff. Well, somehow it gave me the impression that these people were searching for something. So that night when I went home I couldn't rest. I was actually worried about it. I was wondering, what have they got on me, what is it? I know there isn't anything, because I've never been in Missouri, but nevertheless these people looked funny. Son of a gun I was afraid to go out of the house.

Dr. You were afraid they might hurt you.

Pt. I was afraid to go out of the house, and couldn't understand why I was afraid. It come to the point where I was afraid to stay home for fear they would come over, so I went out. I just roamed the streets, went to a show. Now what is so intelligent about that, if you think I am intelligent?

Dr. There's a difference between intelligence and emotions. An intelligent person can still succumb to fears. You were afraid that perhaps they might have misidentified you and might therefore hurt you in some way, weren't you? What hurt could they do? What is the worst thing you can think of?

Pt. I haven't the slightest idea. Somehow I was afraid of something.

Dr. Why were you afraid? What were you afraid of?

Pt. You answer that.

Dr. I don't know what you were afraid of. Perhaps you were afraid of accusations of some kind.

Pt. I guess I must have been.

Dr. What accusations?

Pt. I don't know.

Dr. Well how about other things this week?

Pt. Why dismiss it so easily?

Dr. Are we?

Pt. I can't understand if there's nothing to it, why do I react this way?

Dr. You mean succumbing to fears?

Pt. Yes.

Dr. Let us work the thing out and find out what it is that actually made you act the way you did. Let us work the thing out and see what it was you were afraid of. Perhaps the most significant thing was your own reaction, your own fear that you had acted like a sissy.

Pt. Exactly, that's what bothered me most of all.

Dr. There must be some terror so strong that it overwhelms your reason. Maybe we can find out what that terror is. What else happened during the week?

Pt. Nothing, I felt very well, no headaches, no dullness.

Dr. All right, supposing you go to sleep now. Take your time this time, and make sure you go into a deep sleep. Watch your hand, just keep gazing at your hand, and as you gaze at it, you'll notice that it will begin to feel light, will slowly rise, slowly lift and get light, will slowly rise, and move towards your face until you go into a deep, restful, relaxed sleep. Now the hand begins to sweep up, up, and as it goes up, your eyes will get tired, your whole body will get heavy and tired. You'll get sleepier, sleepier, sleepier, and go into a deep, restful, relaxed, comfortable sleep. Your hand moves up, straight up, up toward your face, higher,

higher, and higher, straight up, straight up towards your face. When it touches your face, you'll be asleep, deeply asleep. Your breathing gets deep now and automatic. You get drowsy, very tired and very sleepy. Your sleep is getting deeper and deeper. Your eyes are getting tired, the lids are just like lead. They're getting heavier and heavier and heavier. When your hand touches your face, you'll be asleep. Your hand moves up, up, up, towards your face. You are getting very, very sleepy. Your head feels like lead, your body feels heavy. Deeper and deeper asleep, very sleepy, very tired. Your body will get heavy, and relaxed. Go into a comfortable sleep, into a very deep sleep in which you'll experience a feeling of deep sleep. (*Patient's eyes close.*)

Now I'm going to take your right arm down, and I'm going to stretch your left arm out in front of you. You'll notice that your arm gets stiff and rigid. I stretch it out in front of you like this. It becomes fixed and rigid in that position. I'm going to stroke it, and you'll see how fixed and rigid it becomes, so that when I reach the count of five, it will have become so fixed and rigid that it will be impossible for you to raise it up, no matter how hard you try. One, two, three, stiff and rigid, four, five. Even though you try to raise it up in the air, it remains exactly as it is, until I stroke it. Then it will come down, as I stroke it, it will slowly come down, just this way. Now go to sleep deeply, and when I talk to you next, you will be very deeply asleep. (*Pause*)

Now listen very carefully to me. It is essential to go into an area of your life that may be painful to you. From time to time you have brought me information to the effect that you feel certain terrors and fears that are so powerful that you cannot control them. I am going to give you a suggestion to work out what is behind these terrors. Visualize the same event that happened to you, of these people inquiring about you, and falsely making assumptions about you. Then you will have a dream which will indicate the significance of why you ran away, of what the terror is. Have a dream, and as soon as you've had the dream, indicate it by your hand rising up about two inches. (*Pause*) Now your hand is rising in the air. Even though you are asleep, I want you to tell me exactly what it was that you dreamed, without waking up.

Pt. Two people, mother and daughter, just made all kinds of accusations. First my mother and father were there, then suddenly people in general came in.

Dr. Yes.

Pt. They listened to all these accusations at me.

Dr. What sort of accusations were they?

Pt. All kinds, my going out with my girl and that stuff. I felt very guilty as if I had done something very wrong.

Dr. All right, now listen to me. We have come to a period in our work together here when it is essential for you to begin to work out your own destiny through your own resources. You came to me because you came to an impasse where you needed professional help. We removed your symptoms, but the bigger thing is that we must build up your self esteem, your own feeling of bigness inside of yourself, so you won't be like a little boy, so you won't run away, so you won't be afraid. And that's the big thing we're attempting to achieve, isn't it? You don't want to be a little boy, do you?

Pt. No.

Dr. You want to be a grown man. You want to be able to feel the security and the capacity of acting that comes from being grown up.

Pt. Yes.

Dr. That is the thing we are striving for. One way we can approach this is by a modification of the hypnotic technic. When a person is sick emotionally, he wants and expects the doctor to direct him, to tell him what is wrong and how he can change. The doctor becomes the authority who knows the answers. We have gone through this stage. But if we are going to achieve the goal of your being really strong and grown up, you have to think things out for yourself. You must change your relationship to the doctor where you work things out for yourself, with the doctor cooperating with you on an equal basis. Right here and now we can start this, so you can see that you are able to figure things out for yourself, and make your own choices and decisions.

I shall teach you the technic of self hypnosis, so that when you have a problem to work out you can put yourself to sleep the same way I suggested it for you. You can also give yourself suggestions to dream, to find out what things mean to you. Then when you have accomplished what you set out to do, you can give yourself a suggestion to wake up, and wake up with the understanding what is going on to help you overcome the particular problem that confronts you at the time.

Now, I'm going to count from one to five. At the count of five, your eyes will open and you'll bring your hand back to your thigh. Then I want you to give yourself the suggestion that your are going to be able to go to sleep. Just say it to yourself that you will watch your hand, will keep your eyes riveted on it so that your hand automatically, perhaps without any effort at all, will rise straight up in the air, and you'll get drowsy, your eyelids will get heavy and you'll go to sleep. And as soon as your hand touches your face, you'll go into a deep, deep sleep, during which you'll give yourself a suggestion to dream about a particular problem. I'm going to give the suggestion now that you put yourself to sleep first, in the way that I described, then give yourself the suggestion that you work out an understanding of yourself even further through the medium of dreams. As soon as you've worked that out, you will suddenly lose your tiredness, your eyes will open and you'll wake up. Do you understand me?

Pt. Yes.

Dr. Good. I am going to count from one to five, and at the count of five, open your eyes, bring your hand down to your thigh, watch it and then give yourself the suggestion that you're sleepy, that you're going to sleep. One, two, three, four, five. (*Patient brings his hand down, gazes at his hand as it rises and touches his face, closes his eyes, and after a long pause opens them.*)

Pt. Um hum.

Dr. Tell me all about your experience.

Pt. Well I think I know what made me react the way I did to people inquiring about me. I got it by dreaming about it.

Dr. All right. Tell me what your conclusions are now.

Pt. The conclusions are that I was more or less afraid of what people might think of my actions. I am afraid what they think about me all the time. I just came to the conclusion that I'm always guilty even when I do no wrong. I can see that I look around for things to be guilty about. But really what have I got to worry about?

Dr. So it's your conscience that causes your trouble. There isn't any reason for your worry?

Pt. No.

Dr. Perhaps you had the problem of being concerned about what other people think of you and you reacted in an irrational way, not a reasonable way.

Pt. Exactly, a very irrational way.

Dr. But the irrationality was produced by your emotions. Isn't there a possibility that deep down underneath you think you're a pretty dumb guy?

Pt. Yes, yes.

Dr. Do you think you're dumb?

Pt. I don't think I'm dumb, but I'm not as smart as I might be.

Dr. Well, you've had an intelligence test, and it shows that you're an intelligent person. You can't deny that, but inwardly you may have certain fears and feelings that you're not at all intelligent. That is part of your emotional problem. How long has it been that you've felt there is something wrong with your intelligence?

Pt. I've always felt that.

Dr. You've always felt that.

Pt. Yes, I know I'm intelligent to a certain extent in that I could cope with the people. I don't find it too difficult. But sometimes when I concentrate I find it difficult. When I try to follow conversations and someone's talking, I can't follow the conversation. There's something definitely wrong somewheres.

Dr. A particular conversation that is in line with what you know, or is it any conversation in general?

Pt. Well (*coughs*), I'd almost go as far as any conversation is concerned.

Dr. You feel that you just can't keep up with a lot of people. How much education have you had?

Pt. High school.

Dr. You graduated high school? How old were you?

Pt. Seventeen and a half, eighteen.

Dr. Have you ever wanted to better yourself educationally, go to night school?

Pt. Yes.

Dr. What happened there?

Pt. Well, I, you see, somehow or other I feel as though, well, I'd be ridiculed, too old.

Dr. You'd like to go to night school, but you feel that you're too old? Do other adult people go to night school?

Pt. Sure.

Dr. Are they older than you are?

Pt. All the more intelligent I suppose.

Dr. Older and more intelligent. So that perhaps it isn't only the oldness, but it's the fear that you would be lacking in intelligence. You won't be able to make the grade.

Pt. That could be too.

Dr. You have a problem then, in your own self evaluation, the sort of person you think you are.

Pt. Well, I know I was going with a girl once—matter of fact I went out with her for a few months and somehow or other I always knocked myself down to her. As a matter of fact even today I never, I never give the appearance that I'm conceited or that I know too much. I'd more or less rather knock myself down than to build myself up.

Dr. Do you have any desire at all to build yourself up?

Pt. Yes.

Dr. All right supposing you figure that out. Put yourself to sleep, and give yourself the suggestion that you're going to dream about what you would really like to be inside without any camouflage, without any kidding of yourself, what you would like to be, if you could have your wish. Imagine the kind of a person you would be, what your expectations are. Let's see if you can work that out. Put yourself to sleep and give yourself the suggestion to dream of yourself as the kind of person you'd really like to be. (*Patient puts himself to sleep, then awakens.*)

Pt. I had a dream of how I'd like to be. I have gaiety, have two or three children. My wife, she's very happy, always laughing. Saw people coming in and out of our house, me going to theirs and playing with their children. Go out to the country, have a good time, come back and enjoy myself.

Dr. You feel then that you are not making exorbitant demands of life, that you are asking as much as any human being has the right to ask. Perhaps you felt you had no right to this, that you were not as good as others.

Pt. Well, only when my headache occurred.

Dr. Only where your headaches occurred.

Pt. I think I am just as good as the next fellow.

Dr. Perhaps the headache concealed a lot of things. Perhaps it was a mask behind which you hid, a symbol. Perhaps because you sometimes can't follow the drift of conversation you may think you are not as smart as others.

Pt. Some people start a conversation where they mention about two or three different people, see. They mention one person to the other, what the other did to this one. I can't follow that routine.

Dr. In other words you get confused.

Pt. Exactly. I don't know who said what and why they said it.

Dr. That makes you feel stupid.

Pt. Yup.

Dr. Do you really feel dumb?

Pt. I, I'd like to open another store. And it seems as though my mother and father, they're for it. They're for it when they talk about it, but when they come to actually doing something about it, we don't go ahead. My brother, he's got exactly the same thing. He'd like to open a store. He's always talking about it, but he never gives a suggestion, never, never does anything about it. One day I made a suggestion to let's go see if we can do something about it. Right away my mother says, "Oh, what good is it? The boys will rob you, the men will rob you, and I don't like the idea. You can't control the men." Things like that, I mean; it just knocks the, just knocks it out of you, and right there I said I'd go on my own. But I haven't had the courage to go on my own.

Dr. We have spent this session on your seeing that you can through your own effort do those things that can be of value for you. This week, if you so desire, put yourself to sleep and give yourself suggestions to work out a problem. Do you think you can do it?

Pt. Sure thing, I think I can.

THIRTEENTH SESSION (May 13)

*The sensation of dullness in the head has been markedly relieved
in the past week. The patient, however, is still concerned with a
fear he is not as intelligent as the average person. He recognizes
the fact that his headaches have constituted for him a smoke screen
behind which he hid his feelings of self devaluation and of low
intelligence. Through self hypnosis he learns more about the
reasons for his fear of low intelligence. He expresses a desire for
self improvement and for development of his abilities. Believing
he is capable of handling his problems, he requests an appointment in three weeks to see whether he can manage by himself.*

Pt. Last week I didn't go out much, but I did go dancing
the other day. I came to a bar here in New York, and, well,
I went in, paid my money, sat around, looked at the women,
didn't like 'em and walked out. I came home and went to
sleep. Everything has been going well with my family.
I've had no headaches or dullness.

Dr. Any dreams?

Pt. No.

Dr. What would you like to work on today?

Pt. Well, I think I'd like to discuss my intelligence.

Dr. What aspect?

Pt. That I feel I'm not average.

Dr. That feeling is an emotional feeling. The intelligence test that you got here, what we call the Bellevue-
Wechsler test, shows an intelligence quotient of one hundred
and twelve which is above average. This test considers
your concentrative ability, your ability to remember things,
as well as your reasoning powers. Your evaluation of yourself is not in line with the facts. You feel for some reason
that you can't think well, that you can't concentrate. There
may be times during the day when perhaps this is true, but
it doesn't show up on your intelligence test. How do you
figure that out?

Pt. All right, every question there I had to reread at least,
at least twice, and as many as four times.

Dr. This test considers the time element. In other words if you had read through it once and had made more errors, your inaccuracies would have brought your score down to the same thing.

Pt. Do you think so?

Dr. We can't account for a normal or above normal I. Q. on any other basis.

Pt. About how many did I get wrong out of all of them?

Dr. I don't know, I just have the score here. Maybe you'd really like an I. Q. of 199.

Pt. No, about 150.

Dr. You'd like an I. Q. of 150? Do you know how many people in this country have an I. Q. of 150?

Pt. I'd say about a fourth.

Dr. Well it's probably closer to a fourth of one per cent. Do you know what an I. Q. of 150 means? It approaches genius mentality.

Pt. (*Laughs*)

Dr. Perhaps you'd like to be a genius.

Pt. No, just average.

Dr. With your I. Q. you have the capacity for development.

Pt. And develop into something?

Dr. And develop into something. Why haven't you taken any more education? Perhaps it was because you felt you couldn't absorb learning.

Pt. That was one reason. Now (*cough*), you said that if I read the thing and immediately answered probably I'd made more mistakes doing them all, and my score would go back to what it originally was.

Dr. Perhaps it does take you longer to size up a problem or situation than the average person; but the fact is that you are more accurate when you deliberate longer about a thing. This may be a personal way of thinking and reasoning for you.   It is not abnormal.   However, the big problem is an emotional one.   Your emphasis on intelligence may be one way of saying you are convinced there is something seriously wrong with you.   You may be convinced that there is something wrong with your brain.

Pt.   It's the inability to remember certain things.   I can't remember very much.   As I was telling you before I try to remember prices of particular items, wholesale prices, and the salesman comes along, and starts quoting me prices, and I can't know one price from another, see?   And that's where that confusion sets in.

Dr.   You get very confused then?

Pt.   Well, I'm lost, I mean that's when I would get a headache most of the time.   I mean everything else is gone except that particular thing.

Dr.   You get a headache now when you get confused like when a salesman baffles you with prices?

Pt.   If it's about something that I don't know. Something I know what I'm talking about, you understand, or I try to make believe that I do, does not bother me.

Dr.   Let us look into this thing and see what may be behind it.   Can other people, when a wholesale price is mentioned to them, remember the previous prices?

Pt.   A major portion of the items that move very fast they should remember it, see.   I remember some, but not all.   It is as if I have no interest.

Dr.   If you have no interest, and if you don't particularly care to remember, it is natural that you may not remember.

Pt.   When you know that your own welfare depends on remembering something, why don't you?   Well, I know that's my welfare, that I've got to remember in order to exist.   It's the truth, price means everything today.   If you haven't got the right price, well, we'll just close up.

Dr. Do you have the desire to be in the hardware business?

Pt. I don't know, but I don't know what else I would do.

Dr. Do you feel your parents force you to be in the business?

Pt. They depend on me, and I suppose I do want to be in it.

Dr. If you really desire to be in the business, if you want to concentrate, if you are convinced you are not really unintelligent, there is no reason why you cannot do a good job in remembering those items you desire. Perhaps the problem is that you really feel you are stupid and not as good as other people.

Pt. The funny part of it was I didn't get panicky for one simple reason. I blamed all my maladies on my headache. I said to myself, "I know very well if my headache goes away, I'll be perfectly normal." So I'm not afraid. Now I don't have this headache and I can't make excuses and I I think maybe I blame my intelligence.

Dr. So you see that deep down underneath you seem to feel that you're not as good as other people.

Pt. It would seem so, but I have to tell you I don't really believe that, especially now.

Dr. Perhaps you'd like to be better than other people.

Pt. I'd like to be as good.

Dr. Then we come to this. We've been working with your headache. The headache's disappeared completely or to a large extent. Now you believe you are as good as others as far as not having headaches is concerned. How about in a physical sense? Do you feel that you are physically as good as any other person?

Pt. Yes, I do.

Dr. You're convinced of that.

Pt. Yes, that I'm convinced of.

Dr. So it now comes to the area of your mental functioning, your intellectual functioning. If you could be convinced that you were able to function as good as other people, that you had just as much sense, that you were just as smart, you would be satisfied?

Pt. (*Laughs*) I guess you are convincing me.

Dr. Now, last time you were able to put yourself to sleep, weren't you?

Pt. Yes.

Dr. This time I'd like to have you do exactly the same thing. I'd like to have you do exactly the same thing. I'd like to have you give yourself the same suggestions you did last week. Watch your hand and go to sleep. (*Patient brings his hands to his thighs, the right hand rises, touches his face and his eyes close.*) The reason you are now doing the work is that we must function like two equals. I am not going to tell you what to do. I shall not make decisions for you. I am not going to outline the goals you are to follow. I expect you to take over and to think things out for yourself. As you know, you have been able to achieve certain gains from coming to therapy. So far you've been able to get rid of your headaches; you've been able to liberate yourself from your parents; you're more assertive, self confident and capable of taking a stand with people. You are able to do what you want to do when you want to do it. Things are much better for you all around. You have been able to handle the situation with your girl, and you even see the possibility of making a life for yourself.

However, a block remains. You still feel that you can't make the grade, that you can't concentrate. Previously you said when your headaches disappear then everything would be all right. We learned your headaches were associated with a fear that you were not functioning intellectually. You have overcome your headaches and are better. We still want to know more about what goes on in you inside. Supposing you ask yourself that, and if you want to solve it, give yourself the suggestion to dream.   As soon as you dream, tell me about it without waking up.   (*Pause*)

Pt.   A man with a briefcase in his hand goes around like a merry go round.   He goes around in a circle.

Dr.   Do you know who he is?

Pt.   No.

Dr.   If you want to find out, tell yourself you are going to count from one to five.   As you count from one to five, you'll see the man's name in letters that scramble around and fall into place.   You'll be able to recognize the letters.   At the count of five, you'll suddenly see in front of you the letters scrambling around, and you'll be able to see the man's name, the one with the briefcase going around in a circle.   You'll see what his name is.   (*Pause*)

Pt.   His name is Jimmy Meyers.

Dr.   How do you spell the last name?

Pt.   M-e-y-e-r-s.

Dr.   Do you know him?

Pt.   Yes.

Dr.   Who is he?

Pt.   A salesman.

Dr.   Does he go around in circles?

Pt.   Yeah.

Dr.   What sort of person is he?

Pt.   Well he's a salesman, the kind that sells merchandise.

Dr.   Now what do you believe is going on in you?

Pt.   (*Long pause.*)   I had a dream.   I was in the center at a table surrounded by men, high, outstanding men.

Dr.   You saw yourself at a round table with high outstanding men.

Pt.   I'm in the center.

Dr.   You are in the center.   What does that do to you, to be in the center?

Pt.   It doesn't affect me at all.

Dr. Do you think you come up to them at all? Do you think that you stand up to any high, outstanding men?

Pt. I think I could. I am not afraid of salesmen. They go around in circles, most of the time anyways.

Dr. Perhaps there is a feeling in you now that you can stand up to high, outstanding men, but the fear may be still there that you won't be able to. Perhaps if you desire, you yourself can give yourself a suggestion to explore how far back this feeling goes that you cannot stand up to high out-standing men. (*Long pause.*)

Pt. I was twelve years old.

Dr. You were twelve years old. Tell me about it.

Pt. So I had to go and see what the salesman was selling, and I was afraid to go. My mother asked me to go out, she couldn't.

Dr. And what happened?

Pt. Well I went and I didn't know what I was doing. That is exactly what I feel now, I see it, see it.

Dr. You thought that you couldn't do it.

Pt. I wasn't prepared to, see?

Dr. Do you wish to get to a point where you could feel just as good as anybody that ever lived?

Pt. Yes, yes.

Dr. You will be able to, but you must do it by tackling life actively. You must go ahead and do those things that give you a better estimate of yourself. You must be the one to decide what to do. If you have a desire to be an out-standing person or a successful person, then you will prepare yourself and do everything that is essential. Perhaps you will want to do such things as taking a course, even though there may be a fear that you cannot get through the course. Perhaps you will want to go to school, or perhaps simply want to go ahead on your own and take a chance with your own business. Whatever it is, if you have a real desire to go forward, you will then want to prepare yourself and work at

it.   It will not come by magic, you've got to work at it.
You will have a stronger and stronger desire to feel that you
are functioning well, to feel as smart as other people, as
intelligent.

In a moment I will wake you up.   If you have a desire to
go forward, you will have the determination to do what is
necessary.   You may want to do it by going to school,
taking a course, opening a store, getting a job, by studying
for yourself, or other ways.   It is necessary that you make
the decision, and you will want to, if you are not satisfied with
the way things have been.

Pt.   I want to.

Dr.   I am going to count from one to five, at the count of
five, open your eyes, and wake up.   One, two, three, four,
five.   (*Patient opens his eyes.*)   Don't you think it is important to go forward?

Pt.   That's right.

Dr.   Now what plans can you make concretely to better
yourself?

Pt.   Well I was just thinking of devising a system.   What
it really is when you come down to think of it, is just a matter
of efficiency and nothing else.   Devise a system where if
there's anything I want, a certain item I want, well, I can
write down the item, my last price that I paid for it, and
when the salesman comes to quote a price, I'll have it there
in front of me.

Dr.   Why don't you do that?

Pt.   That's what I will do.   I know the price, and I know
when that particular salesman comes in, well, if I can refer
to the paper, he can't put nothing over on me at all.   I feel
as though I'm up to him now. I can face him.   I can know
what I'm talking about, see? I'll solve that sort of trouble.
I think this is the last barrier, and I know I will get over it. I
want to try things on my own for a while.   If I can't manage,
I will call you.   Say I see you in three weeks, see, or before
then if things don't go well.

Dr. You feel you understand yourself enough now so you can tackle things on your own. You want to try to manage your own affairs to see if you can stay free of headaches and other symptoms, and see if you can act in a more assertive, self confident way?

Pt. Exactly, doctor, I feel that I can do it now.

FOURTEENTH SESSION (June 3)

The patient reports a sustained consistent improvement to a point where he has no complaints of any kind. He believes he has mastered his problems and that he can face the future without trepidation. He realizes that he can develop in his personality growth still further, and he is certain that his growth will proceed through his own spontaneous efforts. A check-up Rorschach test shows that structural changes in the personality have occurred.

Dr. Well, what's happened?

Pt. Well, nothing, nothing else has happened to me, I mean I felt I was doing what I wanted to do. That's reason to feel nice. And I think I can get rid of most everything that's bothered me.

Dr. You've got rid of most everything that used to bother you?

Pt. Well those fears, for instance, you know. Coming home late and wondering what the folks would say, and doing what I want to do, and you know.

Dr. And you feel a great deal better?

Pt. Sure.

Dr. Can you tell me in which way you feel better?

Pt. Well I feel better in that I'm more free to do those things I actually want, that way. I don't see myself restricted or tied down. Naturally I am learning to fight that last problem we had. The headache and dullness is all gone.

Dr. The last problem we had is what?

Pt. Well, I'm licking it in time. I find that I'm actually learning what I'm doing. That's what is most important.

Dr. In general you are quite satisfied and happy about this?

Pt.   Sure.

Dr.   I see. How long since you have been here now?

Pt.   I haven't seen you for three weeks now.

Dr.   And in that time you are satisfied with the way things have been going?

Pt.   More than satisfied.   I know I've got it licked.

Dr.   All right, what remains to be done now, what do you feel remains to be done?   Do you feel that maybe there is a problem in your relations to women?

Pt.   Well, frankly I don't think that's there.   Some don't appeal to me because they aren't good looking enough, or they don't carry themselves well or have poise or know how to talk.   I mean things like that. When I find the right woman, I know I will get married. It's coming.

Dr.   Have you met any of them that were good looking enough?

Pt.   I met one this Sunday, for instance, a very good looking girl at a dance.   I stood around more than an hour with the manager and then I spotted her, I enjoyed her company very much.   Somehow I enjoy myself with a good looking woman, and I can't do it otherwise when they are not good looking.   Now I haven't had my mind on that headache for a long time.   Just take it for granted it's going to go away, see?   And it doesn't bother me more that way.   And I was to a show.   About six, seven years ago, I saw. . . I don't know if you saw the picture or not, with Edward G. Robinson?

Dr.   I don't seem to recall it.

Pt.   And he was, there was something wrong with him, insane sort of, you know, and he used to have headaches, and he'd go like this, his eyes would come out of his head.   I remember when I first saw it about six, seven years ago. That picture had me worried, I mean actually worried.   Was it possible I might lose my eyesight?   Then I'd get a headache and by the time I got out I was sick, you know.   Well

I saw that picture again last week, and I looked at the picture, and I enjoyed it this time. It didn't even bother me. And inside of me I was telling myself I must be better. Wolberg I betcha he (*laughs*) fixed the "Sea Wolf" too.

Dr. You felt that I had fixed the "Sea Wolf"? (*Laugh*)

Pt. It didn't upset me at all.

Dr. Have you had any dreams since I saw you last?

Pt. Well none that I can remember, but, ah, those that I did have, they were mostly pleasant dreams, or dreams that I could understand, see, things that would happen to me the same day, pleasant things like talking to a person. I'd dream that I'm talking to him again. But nothing to scare me, nothing that really presents itself as a problem.

Dr. You feel then you have made progress. After all your progress has continued even though you haven't seen me for three weeks now. You can see yourself really opening up and not being afraid.

Pt. Well yesterday I went to see the Show in Madison Square Garden. That's the first time I saw a Show in my life, and I've been in business all my years, all these years. I rather enjoyed it, too. Met quite a number of people, and I wasn't afraid to go up and talk to them, you know. I feel good about that.

Dr. What would complete the picture?

Pt. Getting married.

Dr. You'd like to get married?

Pt. But I think it's very bad just wanting to get married, because say I go some place to a function where there are women. Well I know if I let myself loose, and if I wasn't too particular with whom I was going, I could have better times. Somehow or other when I go up there with the sole purpose of finding a good looking girl, I often am disappointed.

Dr. So that you sometimes actually cross yourself up, don't you?

Pt. In a way, yes. It's a very simple thing to get myself another woman. It's the simplest thing, and start fooling around again, but I don't want that. I want to be serious about someone.

Dr. You'd like to exercise discriminatory tastes and wait until the right person came along.

Pt. That's right.

Dr. And you feel that until that time comes, you're just as satisfied to have things go along this way.

Pt. They're so improved, as a matter of fact, I think it's a normal life I'm leading as far as my parents are concerned.

Dr. You think you lead a normal life now as far as your parents are concerned. And you find that they have been able to adjust themselves to your new found health. What about your father? You used to be quite afraid of your father.

Pt. Well, not that I'm afraid of him but, it's just that as before. You know he keeps on reminding you that you did wrong, you know, and, ah, well, I know it irks me, understand, but I don't feel so bad about it that I get a headache.

Dr. Not even though you get yourself into situations that irritate him, it doesn't create headaches and you are not afraid of him?

Pt. No.

Dr. Why do you think it doesn't create headaches?

Pt. Well I don't let it worry me anymore, don't you see?

Dr. You don't let it worry you. All right now, what more do we have to do?

Pt. I can't see anything to do.

Dr. Do you feel that you've got enough out of this now so that you can go ahead on your own?

Pt. I certainly do, thanks to you.

Dr. You do feel that?

Pt. Yes I do.

Dr. Supposing you put yourself to sleep now. Give

yourself the suggestion to go to sleep so that you feel that you sink into a very, very deep, restful, relaxed, comfortable sleep. As soon as you are asleep, I'll talk to you. (*Patient puts himself into a trance.*) As you sit there, I'm going to suggest to you that you go back, back, back in your life. Just turn back the pages, turn back the clock, to the point where you first came to see me. You will have forgotten everything else that happened. It will be exactly as it was then, and as you enter the room and talk to me, I'm going to give you the suggestion that you imagine you sit in the front row of a theater and notice that overhead, in front of you is a stage. The curtains open up and you notice a scene. You notice a small boy and his mother. The boy wants to do something, and the mother says, "No." Now I want you to notice that scene, and see what goes on. As soon as you have visualized what is happening, tell me about it without waking up.

Pt. The little boy that's on the stage there, and he wants to do something, but his mother is at the side of the curtains and he is naturally afraid.

Dr. He's afraid?

Pt. Yeah, moving back and forth, and don't know which way to go.

Dr. He runs back and forth and doesn't know which way to go. Does anything else happen to him that you can see?

Pt. He's almost trembling.

Dr. Is he capable of doing anything about it? Does he want to?

Pt. No.

Dr. He's not capable of doing anything about it. Now listen closely to me. I'm going to ask you at this point to look up at the stage, and again you are at the period when you first came here. As you look up at the stage, you're going to notice an image of yourself. You're going to see somebody up there who resembles yourself. I want you to describe him to me.

Pt.   Well it's a boy just standing there and being rocked by waves, sort of.

Dr.   A boy standing there being rocked by waves.

Pt.   Just standing there and don't know what to do.

Dr.   How old a boy is it?

Pt.   Looks young, about twelve.

Dr.   Now listen closely to me.   You are going to grow up now.   You are going to grow up to the present day.   You are back in Dr. Wolberg's office.   It is the present day.   And I'm going to give you the same suggestion.   I want you to feel yourself going back into that theater and noticing the same scenes.   First you will notice the curtains open up, and you'll notice again a scene of a boy who is being told what to do by his mother.   I want you to tell me what happens.

Pt.   The boy is still in the waves, the waves seem to come more fiercely.

Dr.   The waves seem to do what?

Pt.   Pound him more fiercely.

Dr.   Now listen carefully to me.   Watch that boy and notice that he feels the way you, yourself feel.   The boy looks exactly like you.   Soon certain things will happen.   I want you to notice the boy and see if anything happens to him now when his mother talks to him.   It will be as if the boy feels like you feel now.

Pt.   Do anything you want to do.

Dr.   What do you see as you notice that boy up on the stage?

Pt.   I repeat what I said, yes, I bounced two waves at my feet, just made them stop.

Dr.   You bounced the waves at your feet?

Pt.   And made 'em stop.

Dr.   And then what happened?

Pt.   And I walked on the stage, sort of.

Dr.   You walked on the stage.

Pt.   There's my mother.

Dr. Yes.

Pt. And I asked her whether she wants to go home or what she wanted to do; she didn't care one way or the other. I could do what I want.

Dr. So that you felt you were capable of doing something about the situation? Now, I want you to notice, as you look up at the stage, a person. It will come to you in a flash. Tell me just exactly what you see.

Pt. Well I'm full of life. There's so many things to do, and plenty of energy to do it, plenty of enthusiasm.

Dr. You feel yourself to be full of life, plenty of things to do.

Pt. That's right.

Dr. Have you changed any in the way you look to yourself?

Pt. I feel more confident in myself.

Dr. You feel more confident of yourself. You feel then that you have been able to achieve a real change in your personality?

Pt. There's been, there's so many things, I don't know which one to pick on first.

Dr. Now have a dream, and I want you in that dream to be able to feel what progress you actually have made. As soon as you've had that dream, I want you to wake yourself up. Then tell me the dream, and in telling me the dream, you will then decide whether you want to continue coming to see me, or whether you feel that you've made enough prog- ress so that you can stop. Do you understand me?

Pt. Yes.

Dr. As you have the dream, your eyes will open. You'll tell me the dream, and then in a flash, you, yourself, will make a decision as to whether you want to continue with these treatments for a while longer, or whether you want to stop now. Go ahead, have the dream and then wake up. (*Pause, following which the patient opens his eyes.*)

Pt.   Well, I had a dream.

Dr.   What about?

Pt.   Well, I made, I made pretty good progress.   As a matter of fact I don't think I could have made better progress, all the things that have happened.   I notice the fear of my mother disappeared, my fear of my father disappeared, and I know I can combat those salesmen.   I feel as though I'm on the right road.

Dr.   You're on the right road?

Pt.   I think I'll try it on my own doctor.

Dr.   Fine.   Before you go, I want to show you the cards the psychologist showed you before.   Tell me what they looked like.   This is the first card.

Pt.   Looks like a bat, wings on the side.   A woman's shape in the middle with arms outstretched.

Dr.   This is the second.

Pt.   Two dogs bumping their noses together.   A butterfly below.

Dr.   This is the third card.

Pt.   There are two men in formal clothes bowing to each other.   A bow-tie.   I remember saying a kidney.

Dr.   This is the fourth.

Pt.   This is a family shield.   It is like a rug, rough.   A spine in the center.   A head here, funny animal.

Dr.   This is the fifth.

Pt.   A bat flying.

Dr.   This is the sixth.

Pt.   A rug here.   An insect.   A male organ.

Dr.   The seventh.

Pt.   Two dolls with hair up.   Two dogs.

Dr.   This is the eighth.

Pt.   These are animals like a buffalo moving up.   A corset with the laces.   A flower, nice orchid.

Dr.   The ninth.

Pt.   Two people with witches' hats on.   The inside is like a violin.   I remember seeing the hearts here, but it doesn't look so much like it.   Two animals.

Dr.   This is the tenth card.

Pt.   Two caterpillars here.   Blue crabs on each side. Funny animals glaring at each other on top.   An egg with a yolk.   A deer.

(*It will be noted that there are material changes in the Rorschach record as compared to the original productions.   The patient has shown a marked clinical improvement.   He is functioning symptom free and with greater assertiveness and self confidence. Furthermore, he has been so prepared that should he in the future become aware of, and desire help for, deeper problems, he will be properly motivated to utilize this help constructively.   On the other hand, it is possible that with the impetus given him by therapy, his self development will proceed without need for further professional aid.*)

REFERENCES

[1]ERICKSON, M. H.: The investigation of a specific amnesia.   Brit. J. M. Psychol. *13:* 143–50, 1933.

[2]——: A study of experimental neurosis hypnotically induced in a case of ejaculatio praecox.   Brit. J. M. Psychol. *15:* 34–50, 1935.

[3]——: Development of apparent unconsciousness during hypnotic reliving of a traumatic experience.   Arch. Neurol. & Psychiat. *38:* 1282–88, 1937.

[4]——: Hypnotic investigation of psychosomatic phenomena: A controlled experimental use of hypnotic regression in the therapy of an acquired food intolerance. Psychosom. Med. *5:* 67–70, 1943.

[5]——, AND HILL, L. B.: Unconscious mental activity in hypnosis—psychoanalytic implications.   Psychoanalyt. Quart. *13:* 60–78, 1944.

[6]——, AND KUBIE, L. S.   The permanent relief of an obsessional phobia by means of communications with an unsuspected dual personality.   Psychoanalyt. Quart. *8:* 471–509, 1939.

[7]—— AND ——: The successful treatment of a case of acute hysterical depression by a return under hypnosis to a critical phase of childhood.   Psychoanalyt. Quart. *10:* 583–609, 1941.

[8]EISENBUD, J.: Psychology of headache.   Psychiatric. Quart. *11:* 592–619, 1937.

[9]KUBIE, L. S.: The use of hypnagogic reveries in the recovery of repressed amnesic data.   Bull. Menninger Clin. *7:* 172–82, 1943.

[10]LINDNER, R. M.: Rebel Without a Cause: The Hypnoanalysis of a Criminal Psychopath.   New York, Grune & Stratton, 1944.

[11]GILL, M. M., AND BRENMAN, M.: Treatment of a case of anxiety hysteria by a

hypnotic technique employing psychoanalytic principles.　Bull. Menninger Clin. *7:* 163–71, 1943.

[12]FISHER, C.: Hypnosis in treatment of neuroses due to war and to other causes. War Med. *4:* 565–76, 1943.

[13]WOLBERG, L. R.: Hypnoanalysis.　New York, Grune & Stratton, 1945.

[14]*Idem.*

[15]KUBIE, L. S.: *op. cit.,* reference 9.

[16]LINDNER, R. M.: *op. cit.,* reference 10.

[17]ERICKSON, M. H.: The method employed to formulate a complex story for the induction of an experimental neurosis in a hypnotic subject.　J. Gen. Psychol. *31:* 67–84, 1944.

[18]BREUER, J., AND FREUD, S.: Studies in Hysteria.　Washington, D. C., Nerv. & Ment. Dis. Pub. Co., 1936.

[19]BROWN, W.: Psychology and Psychotherapy.　London, Arnold, 1921.　Pp. 21–22.

[20]WINGFIELD, H. E.: An introduction to the Study of Hypnotism.　Ed. 2. London, Balliere, Tindall & Co., 1920.

[21]HADFIELD, J. A.: Functional Nerve Disease.　Ed. by Crichton-Miller, London, 1920.

[22]KARUP, F.: Ztschr. f. d. ges. Neurol. u. Psychiat. *90:* 638, 1924.

[23]TAYLOR, W. S.: Behavior under hypnoanalysis, and the mechanism of the neurosis. J. Abnorm. & Social Psychol. *18:* 107–24, 1923.

[24]SMITH, G. M.: A phobia originating before the age of three cured with the aid of hypnotic recall.　Charac. & Personal. *5:* 331–37, 1936–7.

[25]ERICKSON, M. H.: *op. cit.,* reference 3.

[26]——: *op. cit.,* reference 4.

[27]——, AND KUBIE, L. S.: *op. cit.,* reference 7.

[28]——, AND——: *op. cit.,* reference 6.

[29]LINDNER, R. M.: *op. cit.,* reference, 10.

[30]GRINKER, R. R.: Treatment of war neuroses.　J. A. M. A. *126:* 142–145, 1944.

[31]HORSLEY, J. S.: Narco-Analysis.　London, Oxford, 1943.

[32]LINDNER, R. M.: *op. cit.,* reference 10.

[33]LIVINGOOD, F. G.: Hypnosis as an aid to adjustment.　J. Gen. Psychol. *12:* 203–7, 1941.

[34]HORSLEY, J. S.: *op. cit.,* reference 31.

THE FUTURE OF HYPNOSIS

THE FUTURE of hypnosis as a form of medical therapy is linked to a recognition of its utilities and limitations. These volumes have attempted to define areas in which hypnosis may be successfully applied. Hypnosis has been described as an important medical procedure, but only in its use as an adjunct to those other psychotherapeutic approaches which have been proven to be founded on solid clinical ground. Only by employing the trance as an augmentation and a reinforcement for psychotherapy is its inclusion in the psychotherapeutic armamentarium fully justified.

These volumes have, furthermore, emphasized the dangers of applying hypnosis indiscriminately without regard for the dynamics of the patient's emotional problem. While hypnosis is a catalyst to psychotherapy, it is no substitute for psychotherapy. It will not cover up deficiencies in the personality, knowledge and technical skill of the physician. Nor will it eliminate the need for a careful analysis of the patient's neurotic difficulty and a precise application of therapeutic methods which only adequate training and experience make possible.

Used conservatively in its rightful context, hypnotherapy can play an important role, and it is this value which is endangered by the exaggerated claims made for it by irresponsible persons. Fantastic publicity in lay magazines and books have tended to take hypnosis, in the minds of the lay public, out of the class of a practical scientific phenomenon and to place it into the category of metaphysical magic. This gives it both a false danger and a false value for those individuals who, possibly not trained to discount unscientific data, hope to benefit by nonexistent mystic virtues.

It is this unfortunate source of misinformation which has been partly responsible for the discrimination against medical hypnosis in the past and for its depreciation as a medical procedure.

Further, because of the nature of hypnosis, and the possibility of utilizing it in a dramatic and spectacular manner on public platforms, as well as in private parlors, it is constantly in danger of falling into the disrepute which has frequently halted its progress in the past. Quacks, charlatans and showmen, who see in hypnosis no more than a profitable evening's entertainment, or a means of self glorification, as well as editors and publishers who conceive of the subject as a spell-binding circulation-builder, help to undermine its reputation as a serious medical practice.

What are needed at this time are protective laws which would safeguard both the public and the medical profession, in the same manner as they are protected by the Federal Food, Drug and Cosmetics Act, the Harrison Anti-narcotic Act and the State Medical Practice Laws. Such laws would restrict the use of hypnotherapy to members of the medical profession in the same way that drugs and narcotics are restricted to medical prescription administered under medical supervision.

Furthermore, as in the Federal Food, Drug and Cosmetic Act, there should also be a legal curb against extravagant claims. The public should not be misled into believing that it is the state of hypnosis itself which is therapeutic; they should learn that it is only the therapeutic steps taken while the patient is in hypnosis in which there may lie the possibility of a cure. False claims, such as have mitigated against the usefulness of hypnotherapy in the past, are of real danger to the public, since they cause either overoptimism or over-reluctance on the part of the patient who might be considerably benefited by hypnotherapy if he approached it without distorted motivation.

The understanding of the limitations as well as the virtues of hypnosis by the medical profession as well as by the law makers will help safeguard present-day advances made in hypnotherapy as a medical science. In this way hypnosis will avoid becoming an antiquated and useless therapy which seems to have been its historical destiny.

INDEX

Italic numbers are references to volume II